Treatment-Related Stroke

Including Iatrogenic and In-hospital Strokes

Treatment-Related Stroke

Including Iatrogenic and In-Hospital Strokes

Edited by

Alexander Tsiskaridze
Professor, Department of Neurology, Ivane Javakhishvili Tbilisi State University, Tbilisi, Georgia
Arne Lindgren
Professor of Neurology, Department of Clinical Sciences, Lund University, Sweden; Senior Consultant,
Department of Neurology and Rehabilitation Medicine, Skåne University Hospital, Lund, Sweden
Adnan I. Qureshi
Executive Director, Zeenat Qureshi Stroke Institute, St Cloud, MN; Professor of Neurology, Neurosurgery, and Radiology,
University of Minnesota, Minneapolis, MN, USA

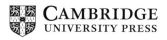

CAMBRIDGE
UNIVERSITY PRESS

CAMBRIDGE
UNIVERSITY PRESS

University Printing House, Cambridge CB2 8BS, United Kingdom

Cambridge University Press is part of the University of Cambridge.

It furthers the University's mission by disseminating knowledge in the pursuit of education, learning and research at the highest international levels of excellence.

www.cambridge.org
Information on this title: www.cambridge.org/9781107037434

© Cambridge University Press 2016

First published 2016

Printed in the United Kingdom by TJ International Ltd. Padstow Cornwall

A catalog record for this publication is available from the British Library

Library of Congress Cataloging in Publication data
Tsiskaridze, Alexander, editor. | Lindgren, Arne (Neurologist), editor. | Qureshi, Adnan I., editor.
Treatment-related stroke : including iatrogenic and in-hospital strokes / edited by Alexander Tsiskaridze, Arne Lindgren, Adnan Qureshi.
Cambridge ; New York : Cambridge University Press, 2016. |
Includes bibliographical references and index.
LCCN 2016002558 | ISBN 9781107037434 (hardback)
| MESH: Stroke | Perioperative Period – adverse effects | Iatrogenic Disease | Intraoperative Complications
LCC RC388.5 | NLM WL 356 | DDC 616.8/1–dc23
LC record available at http://lccn.loc.gov/2016002558

ISBN 978-1-107-03743-4 Hardback

....

To our families and mentors.

Contents

Contents

Contributors

Pablo Ajler, MD, PhD
Assistant Professor and Neurosurgeon,
Hospital Italiano de Buenos Aires, Buenos Aires,
Argentina

Andrei V. Alexandrov, MD
Semmes-Murphey Professor and Chairman,
Department of Neurology, The University of
Tennessee Health Science Center, Memphis,
TN, USA

Rushna Ali, MD
Resident, Department of Neurosurgery, Henry Ford
Hospital, Detroit, MI, USA

Tommy Andersson, MD, PhD
Neurosurgeon and Neuroradiologist. Senior
Consultant, Karolinska University Hospital,
Stockholm, Sweden

Kristian Barlinn, MD, MSc
Department of Neurology, Carl Gustav Carus
University Hospital, Dresden, Germany

David Bergqvist, MD, PhD, FEBVS
Professor Emeritus in Vascular Surgery, University
Hospital, Uppsala, Sweden

David J. Blacker, MBBS, FRACP
Neurologist and Stroke Physician, Sir Charles
Gairdner Hospital; Clinical Professor of Neurology,
University of Western Australia; Medical Director,
Western Australian Neuroscience Research Institute,
Nedlands, Australia

J. Alfredo Caceres, MD
Zeenat Qureshi Stroke Institute and CentraCare
Health System, St Cloud, MN, USA

Patrícia Canhão, MD, PhD
Associate Professor of Neurology, Department of
Neurosciences and Mental Health, Service of
Neurology, Hospital de Santa Maria, University of
Lisbon, Lisbon, Portugal

Fernando de M. Cardoso, MD, PhD
Hospital Quinta D'Or, Rio de Janeiro, Brazil

Gabriel R. de Freitas, MD, PhD
Hospital Quinta D'Or/D'Or Institute for Research
and Education (IDOR), Rio de Janeiro, Brazil

Elisabetta Del Zotto, MD, PhD
Neurorehabilitation Unit, Rehabilitation Center
"E. Spalenza", Don Gnocchi Foundation, Rovato,
Brescia, Italy

Jelle Demeestere
Department of Neurology, University Hospitals
Leuven, Leuven, Belgium

José M. Ferro, MD, PhD
Chairman and Full Professor of Neurology,
Department of Neurosciences and Mental Health,
Service of Neurology, Hospital de Santa Maria,
University of Lisbon, Lisbon, Portugal

Fernando D. Goldenberg, MD
Co-Director, Neuroscience ICU, The University of
Chicago Medicine, Chicago, IL, USA;
Director of Neurocritical Care, Hospital Italiano de
Buenos Aires, Buenos Aires, Argentina

Morten L. Hansen, MD, PhD
Department of Cardiology, Gentofte Hospital,
Cogenhagen, Denmark

Nabeel A. Herial, MD
Department of Neurology, UC San Diego Health
System, San Diego, CA, USA

Steen Husted, MD, DMSci
Department of Medicine, Hospital Unit West,
Herning, Denmark

Muhib Alam Khan, MD
Clinical Assistant Professor, Neuroscience Institute,
Spectrum Health Michigan State University,
Providence, RI, USA

Björn Kragsterman, MD, PhD
Department of Surgical Sciences, Section of Vascular
Surgery, University Hospital, Uppsala, Sweden

Stephan C. Knipp, MD
Consultant in Cardiothoracic Surgery,
Department of Thoracic and Cardiovascular Surgery,
West German Heart and Vascular Center,
University of Duisburg-Essen, Essen, Germany

Federico Landriel, MD
Neurosurgeon, Hospital Italiano de Buenos Aires,
Buenos Aires, Argentina

Arne Lindgren, MD, PhD
Professor of Neurology, Department of Clinical
Sciences, Lund University, Lund, Sweden
Senior Consultant in Neurology, Department of
Neurology and Rehabilitation Medicine, Skåne
University Hospital, Lund, Sweden

Shraddha Mainali, MD
Division of Vascular Neurology, Weil-Cornell
Medical College, New York, NY, USA

Robert Mikulik, MD, PhD
Director of Stroke Program, Department of Neurology,
St. Anne's University Hospital, Brno, Czech Republic

Anastasios Mpotsaris, MD, PhD
Radiologist and Neuroradiologist, Acting Head,
Department of Neuroradiology, University Hospital
of Cologne, Cologne, Germany

Lars Neeb, MD
Department of Neurology, Charité
Universitätsmedizin Berlin, Berlin, Germany

Norbert Nighoghossian, MD, PhD
Professor, Neurovascular Unit, Hopital Neurologique,
Pierre Wertheimer University, Lyon, France

Alessandro Pezzini, MD
Associate Professor of Neurology, Department of
Clinical and Experimental Sciences, Neurology Clinic,
University of Brescia, Brescia, Italy

Adnan I. Qureshi, MD
Professor of Neurology, Department of Neurology,
University of Minnesota, MN, USA

Mushtaq H. Qureshi, MD
Zeenat Qureshi Stroke Research Center, University of
Minnesota, Minneapolis, MN, USA

Uwe Reuter, MD, PhD, MBA
Department of Neurology, Charité
Universitätsmedizin Berlin, Berlin, Germany

Magdy Selim, MD, PhD
Professor of Neurology, Harvard Medical School,
Boston, MA, USA;
Chief, Stroke Division, Department of Neurology, Beth
Israel Deaconess Medical Center, Boston, MA, USA

Fazeel M. Siddiqui, MD
Department of Neurology, UT Southwestern Medical
Center, Dallas, TX, USA

Mario D. Terán, MD
Neurocritical Care Staff Physician, Hospital Italiano
de Buenos Aires, Buenos Aires, Argentina

Vincent Thijs, MD
Department of Neurology, Austin Health,
Heidelberg, Victoria, Australia
Florey Institute of Neuroscience and Mental
Health, University of Melbourne, Heidelberg,
Australia

Alexander Tsiskaridze, MD, PhD, DSc, FESO
Professor of Neurology, Department of Neurology,
Ivane Javakhishvili Tbilisi State University, Tbilisi,
Georgia

Christian Weimar, MD
Department of Neurology, University Hospital Essen,
Essen, Germany

Claudio Yampolsky, MD
Chief of Neurosurgical Department, Hospital
Italiano de Buenos Aires, Buenos Aires,
Argentina

Preface

Iatrogenic stroke is considered to be uncommon but can occur in many different settings and may have unexpected and disastrous consequences. However, until now there has been no major comprehensive book dedicated to this topic. We are therefore very grateful for the opportunity to for the first time be able to present a book with special focus on iatrogenic stroke.

Iatrogenic derives from the ancient Greek word *iatros* (physician). It means an effect induced inadvertently by a physician or surgeon or by medical treatment or diagnostic procedures in a patient.

During the last decades, there have been impressive advances in medicine, leading to better outcomes for patients afflicted with what were earlier perceived as incurable diseases. Many new drugs, surgical techniques, and medical devices have been introduced in the diagnostic and therapeutic armamentarium. Also, diagnosis and treatment are now accessible to a much larger proportion of patients worldwide. Challenging and complex interventions are increasingly performed in elderly patients and in subjects with multiple comorbidities. This is particularly true in the fields of acute stroke care, secondary stroke prevention, surgery, intensive care, and oncology.

As all medical interventions have an inherent risk, and also known as well as sometimes unexpected adverse effects, the risk of iatrogenic stroke has increased in parallel with the availability of advanced treatments and general improvement in medical care. Iatrogenesis can be reduced by improving patients' safety and by risk reduction programs, but there is sometimes an inevitable pay-off of the diagnostic and therapeutic escalade in complex and critical patients.

Many very experienced and well known authors have contributed to the different chapters of this book. Without their help and the support from Cambridge University Press this project would not have been possible to accomplish. We hope that this book will provide a comprehensive overview of the topic and be of use for many stroke neurologists and other physicians working with stroke patients and patients with risk of stroke and thereby help reduce the risk of iatrogenic stroke.

Arne Lindgren, Adnan I. Qureshi, Alexander Tsikaridze, José M. Ferro, and Patrícia Canhão
Lund, Minneapolis, Tbilisi, and Lisbon

Stroke after general surgery

Magdy Selim and Arne Lindgren

Introduction

Stroke during the perioperative period is a devastating complication of surgery. It offsets the potential benefits of surgery and results in dramatic increases in mortality and healthcare costs. There is a paucity of information about stroke in patients undergoing general surgery such as abdominal, thoracic, orthopedic, dental, and gynecological procedures. In this chapter, we review the incidence, predisposing risk factors, etiological mechanisms, and preventive and management strategies of stroke in patients undergoing general, non-cardiovascular, non-neurosurgical procedures.

The prevalence and burden of stroke in general surgery patients

The true incidence rate of stroke in patients undergoing general surgery is uncertain. The reported incidence rates vary from <1% up to 4.8% [1–10], depending on the nature of the study – retrospective vs. prospective, whether a detailed neurological examination or diagnostic brain imaging was performed, and whether advanced imaging using diffusion-weighted magnetic resonance imaging (DWI-MRI) was obtained. The vast majority of published studies have been retrospective and lacked detailed neurological and radiological assessments, in particular DWI-MRI. It is therefore likely that the actual rates of stroke after general surgical procedures are higher than reported as many patients with minor or rapidly resolving deficits due to stroke might be misdiagnosed with "post-operative confusion" or "residual effects of anesthesia." In our own experience, approximately 13% of surgical patients seen by the neurology service for postoperative confusion were found to have a stroke.

Stroke in surgical patients is associated with high morbidity and mortality – about 26% up to 60% in patients with history of prior stroke [3,7]. It increases the cost of care as these patients tend to have longer length of hospitalization, often require an intensive level of care, and frequently require transfer to rehabilitation or long-term care facilities upon discharge.

Risk factors for stroke in general surgery patients

Although surgery and anesthesia themselves contribute to stroke risk, the patient's baseline comorbidities play a dominant role. Table 1.1 summarizes the patient-related risk factors for stroke after general surgical procedures. Overall, they do not significantly differ from the risk factors predisposing to stroke in the general population. However, a case-control study of 61 patients with ischemic strokes after urogenital, gastrointestinal, orthopedic, and pulmonary surgical procedures and 122 age-, sex-, and procedure-matched controls showed that surgery substantially increases the risk of stroke (odds ratio = 2.9) [4], indicating that the risk of stroke after surgery does not simply represent the random chance of stroke occurrence in the general population.

Advanced age (usually >70 years), preoperative history of stroke or transient ischemic attack (TIA), and atrial fibrillation emerge as the most important risk factors for stroke in patients undergoing general surgery [1–5,8].

The type of surgery also influences the risk of perioperative stroke. The stroke risk is higher in head and neck resection and orthopedic procedures, in particular hip replacement, than in other general surgical procedures.

Treatment-Related Stroke, ed. Alexander Tsiskaridze, Arne Lindgren and Adnan Qureshi. Published by Cambridge University Press. © Cambridge University Press 2016.

Table 1.1 Patient-related risk factors for stroke in general surgery patients.

Risk factor	Comments
Age	Older age is a marker of increased comorbidities, and is often associated with restricted cerebral autoregulation and subclinical vascular disease, which makes older patients more susceptible and vulnerable to cerebral ischemic insult
Sex	Women appear to be at greater risk for perioperative stroke. This may be attributed to a prothrombotic state due to estrogen or use of hormone replacement therapy
Previous history of stroke or TIA	Previous stroke or TIA suggests existing pathological cerebrovascular condition(s), which may predispose to stroke recurrence during the perioperative period
Diabetes mellitus	Diabetics have macro- and microvascular disease, and impaired autoregulation, which increase their risk for stroke after surgery
Smoking and chronic obstructive pulmonary disease	Smoking and COPD are associated with increased risk of perioperative complications including stroke
Hypertension	Chronic hypertension is often associated with heart failure and impaired cerebral autoregulation. Significantly elevated blood pressure can also cause a hemorrhagic stroke
Peripheral vascular disease	This is a marker of generalized atherosclerosis, which could involve the cerebral vasculature
Renal insufficiency – preoperative serum creatinine >2 mg/dL (176 μmol/L)	Patients with renal failure are at greater risk of electrolyte derangements, perioperative atrial arrhythmias, and fluctuations in blood pressure
Atrial fibrillation (AF)	Patients with chronic AF on oral anticoagulation are at significant risk if anticoagulation is withheld before surgery. Perioperative electrolyte derangements, in particular high magnesium levels, and preoperative withdrawal of some medications, such as beta-blockers, can lead to the development of postoperative AF de novo
Heart failure	Heart failure and low cardiac output can lead to hemodynamic instability, impaired cerebral perfusion, and intracardiac clot formation in the setting of perioperative dehydration, hypovolemia, and blood loss
Carotid stenosis	Carotid stenosis is associated with increased risk for perioperative stroke in patients with preoperative symptoms of stroke or TIA, i.e., symptomatic carotid stenosis. The relationship between asymptomatic carotid stenosis and stroke risk after surgery is less certain
Perioperative discontinuation of antithrombotic therapy	Abrupt discontinuation of antithrombotic therapy has been associated with increased risk of ischemic stroke, particularly in patients with cardiovascular risk factors

Lengthy procedures may also carry a higher risk for perioperative stroke. The variables that affect cerebral blood flow and oxygen consumption during surgery, such as changes in intraoperative blood pressure, ventilation, oxygenation, fluid status, and depth of anesthesia, are more likely to occur during longer surgeries. A retrospective review of the outcome of various major elective non-cardiac surgeries in 797 patients found a strong association between operation time and the POSSUM score (a quantitative score of preoperative risk of morbidity and mortality due to premorbid medical conditions) regarding negative outcome, defined as hospital stay >10 days with a morbid condition including stroke or death. The incidence of negative surgical outcome was 10.3% in operations lasting <220 minutes vs. 38.2% in those with a duration of >220 minutes [9].

Individual risk factors should not be viewed in isolation during preoperative assessment of stroke risk. Unlike cardiac surgeries, predictive models for preoperative estimation of stroke risk in patients undergoing general surgical procedures have not been fully studied. Press *et al.* [11] compared various models that are widely used to assess the cardiac risk of patients undergoing non-cardiac surgical procedures, and reported that a revised cardiac risk index [12] (Table 1.2) can predict non-cardiac, medical, surgical, and neurological complications including stroke. However, the use of this revised cardiac risk index in predicting stroke in general surgery patients requires validation. It has been suggested that $CHADS_2$ or CHA_2DS_2-VASc scores can better predict major perioperative events including mortality in patients with atrial fibrillation [13].

Table 1.2 The revised cardiac risk index.

Six independent predictors of perioperative complications:

1. High-risk type of surgery

2. History of ischemic heart disease

3. History of congestive heart failure

4. History of cerebrovascular disease

5. Preoperative treatment with insulin

6. Preoperative serum creatinine >2.0 mg/dL (176 μmol/L)

The presence of two or more of these factors can aid with preoperative evaluation of patients undergoing non-urgent major non-cardiac surgery. Perioperative complication rates were reported as moderate (7%) in patients with two factors; and high (11%) in patients with more than two factors [12].

Pathophysiology and etiological mechanisms of stroke in general surgery patients

Most strokes after general surgery are ischemic – only a few are hemorrhagic [1–3]. The mechanisms of stroke in patients undergoing general surgery are variable, and depend on the nature of the surgical procedure, patient's risk factors, and intra- and postoperative course. Figure 1.1 summarizes the potential mechanisms of perioperative stroke in general surgery patients.

Hypotension can result in low flow and subsequent borderzone infarcts. Intraoperative hypotension (IOH) is frequently misconceived as a cause for perioperative stroke. While IOH might contribute to stroke risk in cardiac surgery patients, studies in general surgery

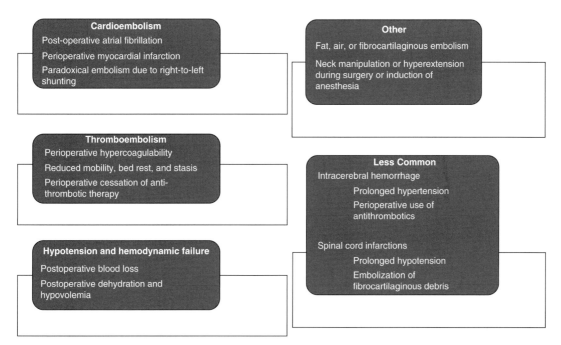

Figure 1.1 Potential mechanisms of stroke in general surgery patients

patients showed little or no association between IOH and perioperative stroke risk [1,4].

Hypotension during the postoperative period might be more important than hypotension induced by anesthesia or hypotension during the highly monitored and controlled intraoperative period. A case-control study in 24,241 patients who underwent non-cardiac, non-neurological surgeries found that the duration that the mean blood pressure was decreased more than 30% from baseline was associated with the occurrence of postoperative stroke [14].

The timing and topography of stroke in general surgery patients provide clues to its pathophysiology and etiology. Several studies reported that the majority of perioperative strokes occur during the postoperative period [1–4]. In one study, only 10 out of 61 strokes in patients who had general surgery occurred during the procedure [4]. The median time interval between the procedure and stroke onset/detection was 2 days; maximum 16 days. Brain imaging (CT or MRI) was negative in 5 patients, and showed infarcts in a single arterial territory in 48 patients, infarcts in multiple territories in 6 patients, and borderzone (watershed) infarcts in only 7 patients. A review of 10 published studies found that only 5.8% of patients (14 out of 242) awoke with a stroke from a general surgical procedure [15]. These findings indicate that intraoperative mechanisms are rarely the immediate cause of perioperative stroke; that postoperative events are more important; and that most strokes after general surgery are related to thromboembolism.

The major cause of thromboembolism appears to be cardiac embolism. In one study, cardiac embolism was the cause of perioperative stroke in 42% of cases, and most were related to postoperative atrial fibrillation [1]. Another cause is perioperative myocardial infarction as a result of supply–demand mismatch due to hypertension, hypotension, or tachycardia during the perioperative period.

However, thromboembolism may be multifactorial. The perioperative period is characterized by adrenergic stimulation, increased prothrombotic activity, platelet activation, and reduced fibrinolytic activity resulting in transient hypercoagulability [16]. This is further exacerbated by reduced mobility, bed rest, stasis, dehydration, and withholding of antiplatelets or anticoagulants perioperatively. A population-based study showed that among 2,197 patients with ischemic stroke, 5.2% had withdrawal of antiplatelet or antithrombotic medications (in nearly half of these cases stopped for procedures) during the 60 days preceding their acute stroke onset, presumably due to rebound hypercoagulability [17]. A surgery-related hypercoagulability increases the risk of thrombogenesis and perioperative vascular events including paradoxical cerebral embolism via a patent foramen ovale in patients who develop lower extremity or pelvic venous embolism during the postoperative period.

Blood loss, hypovolemia, dehydration, and prolonged hypotension can contribute to hemodynamic failure during the perioperative period. This can reduce cerebral perfusion and cause subsequent stroke especially if cerebral collateral perfusion is inadequate or autoregulation fails, or in the presence of pre-existing cerebrovascular arterial occlusive lesions. Hemodynamic failure and subsequent hypoperfusion may also increase the risk for thromboembolism by reducing the wash out of microemboli [18]. Neck manipulations and hyperextension during surgery and induction of anesthesia may also play a role, either by kinking or aggravating rupture of a pre-existing plaque in the presence of carotid or vertebral artery stenosis, or causing arterial dissection. Fat, air, or fibrocartilaginous embolism during orthopedic and spine procedures are other sources of embolization.

It is important to point out that stroke following general surgical procedures may not always be localized to the brain. Occasionally, spinal cord infarction might complicate general surgical non-aortic procedures, such as orthopedic and spinal surgery [19–20]. This is often attributed to significant and prolonged hypotension or embolization of fibrocartilaginous debris.

Prevention of stroke in general surgery patients

Preoperative assessment

Prevention of perioperative stroke in patients undergoing general surgery should include closer evaluation of the patient's risk profile, and a detailed neurological history for signs or symptoms of prior stroke/TIA before posing an indication to surgery. A history suggestive of prior stroke/TIA should prompt neurological consultation and detailed neurological assessment with brain and vascular imaging, particularly if these neurological events were not previously investigated or prior workup was incomplete. Patients with previously undiagnosed symptomatic hemodynamically significant carotid stenosis might benefit from preoperative carotid revascularization, if the general surgery is elective and can be delayed.

The timing of surgery in a patient who had a recent stroke should be carefully considered based on the urgency of surgery and its risks, the cause and size of the infarct, stability of stroke symptoms, and whether anticoagulation is required. Cerebrovascular reserve can be tenuous during the days to weeks following a stroke, and may increase the risk of stroke recurrence during the perioperative period. Although there are no systematic studies or outcome data to guide this decision, it is advisable to delay elective surgery in patients who had a recent stroke/TIA for six to eight weeks after stroke symptom onset to allow the cerebral autoregulation to recover before encountering the hemodynamic stresses of surgery. A recent study indicated that the risk of adverse outcomes following surgery may be increased up to nine months after a previous acute stroke [21].

Risk factor management

Close monitoring and optimal management of the identified risk factors in the perioperative period is essential to minimize the risk for stroke, and the stroke's sequelae if it occurs. Measures should be taken to prevent arrhythmias, thromboembolic complications, and sharp fluctuations in blood pressure, fluid volume status, and electrolytes during the perioperative period. Special considerations include the following:

Glycemic control Close attention should be paid to glycemic control in the perioperative period. Preoperative hyperglycemia and impaired fasting glucose levels, independent of diabetes and other comorbidities, are associated with increased risk for perioperative stroke, myocardial infarction, and death [22]. Hyperglycemia is also associated with worse outcome after stroke [23].

Perioperative management of atrial fibrillation Patients with chronic atrial fibrillation undergoing surgery require close monitoring during the perioperative period. Anti-arrhythmia and rate-controlling medications, such as β-blockers, should often be continued without interruption, and electrolytes and fluid status should be carefully monitored and corrected on an ongoing basis. Most patients with chronic atrial fibrillation on oral anticoagulation should continue to receive anticoagulation during the perioperative period. Bridging therapy with heparin or heparinoids (as detailed below), and promptly restarting oral anticoagulation after surgery, as soon as the risk of bleeding from the surgical site is minimal and hematocrit is stable, are recommended especially in patients at intermediate or high risk for thromboembolism (Table 1.3). Clinical prediction rules, such as $CHADS_2$ or CHA_2DS_2-VASc scores could help to estimate stroke risk in the perioperative setting [13] and those with low scores may not necessarily need bridging therapy [24]. In some situations for patients with AF, bridging may even increase the risk of adverse events [25].

Patients who develop atrial fibrillation de novo postoperatively may have increased risk of subsequent stroke both after non-cardiac and cardiac surgery [26]. Initiation of anticoagulation may be warranted, especially in high-risk patients such as those with a history of stroke/TIA. Anticoagulation therapy should continue for 30 days after the return of normal sinus rhythm based on the recommendations of the American College of Chest Physicians [27] and the American Association for Thoracic Surgery guidelines [28].

Perioperative management of antithrombotic agents The perioperative management of patients taking an antithrombotic agent before undergoing an elective surgery is often challenging. The decision of whether to discontinue antithrombotic therapy before a surgical procedure should be based on careful assessment of the risk of bleeding complications vs. the benefit of preventing thromboembolic events during the perioperative period. Temporary cessation of antithrombotics in anticipation of a surgical procedure is associated with increased risk of thromboembolic events either due to the indication for treatment itself, rebound hypercoagulability due to discontinuation of the antithrombotic agent, or surgery-induced hypercoagulable state [16,17,29,30]. Given that bleeding is a treatable perioperative complication, the decision-making should place a high value on preventing thromboembolism in patients at high or moderate risk for thromboembolism, and preventing bleeding in patients at low risk for thromboembolism (Table 1.3) [31]. The time off antithrombotic therapy should be minimized in patients on antiplatelets or anticoagulants to decrease the risk of systemic thromboembolism and stroke during the perioperative period.

Table 1.3 Thromboembolic risk categories for patients taking antithrombotic therapy.

Thromboembolism risk category	Indication for antithrombotic therapy			
	Prosthetic heart valve	Atrial fibrillation	Venous embolism	Perioperative bridging therapy
High	• History of stroke/TIA • Any mitral valve • Caged ball or single leaflet aortic valve	• History of stroke/TIA • Rheumatic valvular heart disease • CHADS$_2$ score >4	• Recent venous embolism (within 3 months) • Thrombophilia	Strongly recommended
Moderate	• Bi-leaflet aortic valve and ≥1 stroke risk factor	• ≥2 stroke risk factors • CHADS$_2$ score 3–4	• Venous embolism within 3–12 months • Active cancer • Recurrent venous thromboembolism	Strongly recommended
Low	• Bi-leaflet aortic valve and no stroke risk factors	• No history of stroke/TIA • CHADS$_2$ score <3	• Single venous embolic event >12 months ago • None of the above	Optional – may sometimes be recommended, if feasible

Adapted from the American College of Chest Physicians Clinical Practice Guidelines [31].

There are no large randomized controlled trials to guide the optimal strategy for management of antithrombotic therapy, in particular anticoagulants, during the perioperative period. The decision of when to stop or continue antithrombotics during the perioperative period should be individualized, and should always involve a discussion involving the patient and the physicians involved in his/her care weighing the risks of thromboembolic events in that particular patient vs. the risks of major perioperative bleeding complications.

Perioperative management of antiplatelet agents

There is accumulating evidence to suggest that continuation of aspirin perioperatively outweighs the risks of its discontinuation. Interruption of aspirin preoperatively is associated with increased risk of ischemic stroke within the following days, particularly in patients with multiple cardiovascular risk factors [17,29]. In a retrospective, cross-sectional, case-control study of 648 patients, aspirin interruption yielded an odds ratio of 3.4 for ischemic stroke/TIA within a mean of 9±7 days of its interruption [29]. On the other hand, continuation of aspirin therapy during the perioperative period does not seem to increase the risk of intraoperative bleeding during cataract surgery [32], and only prolonged the duration of self-limiting hematuria and rectal bleeding in patients undergoing transrectal prostate biopsy [33]. Kovich and Otley [34] reported increased risk of thromboembolic complications, including stroke/TIA, among patients in whom use of aspirin and warfarin was discontinued for dermatological procedures, and no increase in hemorrhagic complications when these agents were continued perioperatively. A prospective study in 213 patients undergoing tooth extractions concluded that the procedure can be performed safely in patients taking aspirin alone, warfarin alone, or aspirin and warfarin in combination. All cases of postoperative bleeding were controlled easily by using local hemostatic measures [35]. In addition, preoperative use of aspirin did not result in increased perioperative blood loss in patients who underwent unexpected urgent gynecological procedures [36]. Bridging with use of low molecular weight heparin (LMWH) for patients with coronary stents undergoing non-cardiac surgery seems to increase the risk for perioperative complications [37]. Therefore continuation of aspirin therapy seems to be acceptable in many procedures, in particular dental, dermatological, ophthalmologic, and endoscopic procedures with or without biopsy [38].

There are insufficient data to make specific recommendations regarding the use of other antiplatelet agents, such as clopidogrel and dipyridamole. In the Clopidogrel in Unstable Angina to Prevent Recurrent Events (CURE) trial, the risk of major bleeding complications following coronary revascularization procedures was increased among patients treated with clopidogrel vs. aspirin, when the drug was discontinued less than five days before the procedure [39]. It is unclear how to manage this drug preoperatively in patients undergoing general surgery, and whether withholding it for at least five days prior to major general surgery is required as is the case with cardiac procedures. However, continuing clopidogrel and aspirin during the perioperative period has been advised in patients with a bare metal coronary stent who require surgery within six weeks of stent placement and in patients with a drug-eluting coronary stent who require surgery within 12 months of stent placement to prevent stent-related coronary thrombosis [31].

Perioperative management of oral anticoagulation Is surgery feasible on anticoagulation? Larson *et al.* [40] studied 100 consecutive patients at high risk for thromboembolic events who continued warfarin therapy, targeting a goal for the INR of 1.5 to 2.0, perioperatively while undergoing invasive procedures including hip replacement, gastrointestinal, vascular, and even cardiothoracic surgery. This moderate intensity of anticoagulation was considered safe and feasible. Only six patients had bleeding complications (two major; four minor) and two patients had thromboembolic events. These findings suggest that some patients can be maintained on oral anticoagulation during the perioperative period, if necessary. However, the clinical question is often whether or not to use anticoagulation bridging therapy during the preoperative period. A systematic review reported a 1.6% rate of thromboembolic events among 1,868 surgical patients receiving warfarin (0.4% for continuation of oral anticoagulation, 0.6% for discontinuation of warfarin, 0% for discontinuation of warfarin and bridging therapy with intravenous heparin, and 0.6% for discontinuation of warfarin and bridging therapy with LMWH).

The overall rate of stroke was 0.4%, and major bleeding rate while receiving therapeutic doses of warfarin was 0.2% for dental procedures and 0% for cataract extraction surgery [41].

The American College of Chest Physicians Evidence-Based Clinical Practice Guidelines [31] has made the following recommendations regarding perioperative management of anticoagulation:

1. In patients who require temporary interruption of oral anticoagulation and preoperative bridging therapy, the use of subcutaneous (SC) low molecular weight heparin (LMWH), which can be administered in an outpatient setting, is preferable to intravenous (IV) unfractionated heparin (UFH) from a cost-containment perspective.

2. Bridging warfarin with therapeutic-dose SC LMWH (for example, dalteparin 200 IU/kg qd or enoxaparin 1.5 to 2.0 mg/kg qd) or IV UFH is recommended preoperatively in patients with a mechanical heart valve, or atrial fibrillation, or venous thromboembolism, or clotting disorder at high risk for thromboembolism.

   - The last preoperative dose of SC LMWH should approximate half the total daily dose instead of 100% and should be administered 24 hours before the procedure.
   - If IV UFH is used as a bridging anticoagulation, it should be stopped approximately 4 hours before surgery.

3. In patients with a mechanical heart valve, or atrial fibrillation, or venous thromboembolism at low risk for thromboembolism, no bridging over bridging with therapeutic-dose SC LMWH or IV UFH is recommended.

4. Continuation of warfarin during the perioperative period in patients undergoing minor dental or dermatological procedures, or cataract removal.

There is also evidence to suggest that patients can be maintained on oral anticoagulation for other procedures, such as lithotripsy and low-risk endoscopic procedures such as diagnostic colonoscopy and sigmoidoscopy [38–42].

Little is known about the management of newer anticoagulants, such as direct thrombin or factor Xa inhibitors, during the perioperative period and their impact on perioperative bleeding risks. The duration for which these drugs need to be withheld prior to a procedure depends on baseline renal function and creatinine clearance.

Perioperative management of blood pressure
Patients with poorly controlled hypertension preoperatively have an exaggerated hypertensive response to the induction of anesthesia and pain. Hypertensive patients are also more likely to experience more fluctuations in blood pressure, including hypotension, intraoperatively. During the postoperative period, blood pressure and heart rate tend to increase as patients recover from anesthesia and as a result of excessive release of catecholamines due to surgical stress response and pain. In an observational study of 797 patients undergoing non-cardiac surgeries, intraoperative systolic hypertension and tachycardia were independently associated with increased risk for perioperative morbidity, including stroke [43]. In another study, the duration that the intraoperative mean blood pressure was decreased more than 30% from baseline was associated with the occurrence of postoperative stroke [9]. The optimal intraoperative target range for blood pressure is uncertain. Some recommend maintaining mean or systolic blood pressure within 20% of the preoperative baseline blood pressure [15].

Optimal control of blood pressure preoperatively, coupled with careful monitoring of blood pressure intra- and postoperatively is of critical importance to prevent hypertension or hypotensive episodes and to maintain adequate cerebral perfusion. Therefore antihypertensive agents should be continued up to the time of surgery to maintain a near-normal blood pressure. Special caution should be considered with: (1) abrupt preoperative discontinuation of some antihypertensive medications, such as clonidine, that may result in rebound hypertension; and (2) initiation of acute therapy with extended-release metoprolol (de novo) shortly before surgery, as this might be associated with increased risk of postoperative stroke [44].

Intraoperative interventions

Intraoperative factors can lead to perioperative arrhythmias, respiratory compromise, hypotension or hypertension, reduced cerebral perfusion, and thromboembolism, all of which can be associated with increased stroke risk. Taking additional precautionary measures to avoid these complications can help to reduce the risk for perioperative stroke.

These include: (1) considering local instead of general anesthesia when possible; (2) taking measures to maintain near-normal BP, heart rate, and respiratory and fluid status during surgery; and (3) attempting to minimize the duration of surgery when feasible.

The use of local anesthesia is associated with less postoperative morbidity and a shorter hospital stay, thereby decreasing postoperative thromboembolic complications and arrhythmias. Regional anesthesia also allows clinical monitoring of neurologic function by assessing level of consciousness, speech, and strength of hand grip during surgical procedures, thus allowing timely detection and the taking of necessary measures to correct inadequate cerebral perfusion. A population-based, case-control, retrospective study of 1,455 stroke patients and 1,455 age- and gender-matched controls identified risk factors associated with ischemic stroke in patients undergoing surgery involving general or local anesthesia, using a conditional logistic regression model to estimate the odds ratio of surgery and anesthesia for perioperative stroke, while adjusting for other known risk factors. After adjusting for classical stroke risk factors, the odds ratio for stroke during the perioperative period was 3.9 in an analysis that excluded matched pairs, where the case and control underwent "high risk" surgery (cardiac, vascular, or neurologic procedures), also "low-risk" surgical procedures were found to be a significant independent risk factor for stroke (odds ratio = 2.9) [45].

Postoperative management

Continued and close monitoring of patients for postoperative arrhythmia, development of heart failure, neurologic status, vital signs and fluid volume status, electrolytes, hemostatics, and blood sugar in the days after major surgery is essential to implement immediate corrective actions. It should be emphasized for personnel performing the monitoring that there is a risk that stroke symptoms in the postoperative phase can be undiagnosed because these symptoms are misinterpreted as "general deterioration" due to, for example, anesthesia or metabolic imbalance. Rapid identification of postoperative neurological complications including focal neurological deficits is essential and allows timely management to optimize the patient's recovery. It is also important to identify and treat remedial causes of postoperative hypertension such as pain, agitation, bladder distension, hypoxia, etc.

Early postoperative use of prophylactic strategies to minimize the risk of systemic thromboembolism is recommended to prevent potential paradoxical embolism and stroke. A prospective study of patients undergoing gynecologic surgery showed that the incidence of thromboembolic complications, especially deep vein thrombosis (DVT), can be reduced by using elastic stockings, early postoperative mobilization, hematocrit and volume control, and heparin [46]. A randomized trial in patients undergoing major abdominal surgery has shown that combined treatment drug strategies (compression stockings and LMWH) for preventing thromboembolic complications after surgery are more effective than either strategy alone [47]. Similarly, a Cochrane database systematic review showed that the use of compression stockings is effective in diminishing the risk of thromboembolic events in hospitalized patients after various surgeries, and that using stockings with another method of DVT prophylaxis is more effective than using stockings alone [48].

Management of acute stroke in general surgery patients

The general supportive management principles of acute stroke – *timely* resuscitation of salvageable brain tissue and prevention and management of complications to improve recovery – are the same during the perioperative period. Improved and early recognition of stroke by the surgical staff and immediate consultation of the stroke team (or a neurologist familiar with acute stroke treatment) for suspected stroke are crucial to facilitate early treatment. Brain imaging should be performed as soon as possible to rule out intracranial hemorrhage or an undiagnosed brain lesion.

Many patients with ischemic stroke following general surgery may not be candidates for intravenous thrombolysis, which is often contraindicated during the first two weeks after a major procedure. However, the use of endovascular revascularization strategies, especially thrombectomy, appears to be a reasonable and safe alternative for the management of hyperacute ischemic stroke in the perioperative setting [43].

Summary

Stroke after general surgical procedures is not as uncommon as once thought. It usually occurs postoperatively, largely due to thromboembolism, and intraoperative events are rarely the direct immediate cause. Increased awareness of the etiology and pathophysiology of the predisposing risk factors and mechanisms of perioperative stroke and rapid recognition of its onset are vital to prevent it and to improve outcomes.

References

1. Hart R, Hindman B. Mechanisms of perioperative cerebral infarction. *Stroke.* 1982; **13**:766–73.

2. Larsen S F, Zaric D, Bosen G. Postoperative cerebrovascular accidents in general surgery. Stroke. *Acta Anaesthesiol Scand.* 1988; **32**:698–701.

3. Parikh S, Cohen J R. Postoperative stroke after general surgical procedures. *NY State J Med.* 1993; **93**:162–5.

4. Limburg M, Wijdicks E F, Li H. Ischemic stroke after surgical procedures: Clinical features, neuroimaging, and stroke factors. *Neurology.* 1998; **50**:895–901.

5. Kikura M, Oikawa F, Yamamoto K, *et al.* Myocardial infarction and cerebrovascular accident following non-cardiac surgery: Differences in postoperative temporal distribution and risk factors. *J Thromb Haemost.* 2008; **6**:742–8.

6. Nosan D K, Gomez C R, Maves M D. Perioperative stroke in patients undergoing head and neck surgery. *Ann Otol Rhonol Laryngol.* 1993; **102**:717–23.

7. Bateman B T, Schumacher H C, Wang S, Shaefi S, Berman M F. Perioperative acute ischemic stroke in non-cardiac and non-vascular surgery: Incidence, risk factors, and outcomes. *Anesthesiology.* 2009; **110**:231–8.

8. Polanczyk C A, Marcantonio E, Goldman L, *et al.* Impact of age on perioperative complications and length of stay in patients undergoing noncardiac surgery. *Ann Intern Med.* 2001; **134**(8):637–43.

9. Reich D L, Bennett-Guerrero E, Bodian C A, *et al.* Intraoperative tachycardia and hypertension are independently associated with adverse outcome in noncardiac surgery of long duration. *Anesth Analg.* 2002; **95**(2):273–7.

10. Brooks D C, Schindler J L. Perioperative stroke: Risk assessment, prevention and treatment. *Current Treatment Options in Cardiovascular Medicine.* 2014; **16**:282.

11. Press M J, Chassin M R, Wang J, Tuhrim S, Halm E A. Predicting medical and surgical complications of carotid endarterectomy: comparing the risk indexes. *Arch Intern Med.* 2006; **166**(8):914–20.

12. Lee T H, Marcantonio E R, Mangione C M, *et al.* Derivation and prospective validation of a simple index for prediction of cardiac risk of major noncardiac surgery. *Circulation.* 1999; **100**(10):1043–9.

13. van Diepen S, Youngson E, Ezekowitz J A, McAlister F A. Which risk score best predicts

perioperative outcomes in nonvalvular atrial fibrillation patients undergoing noncardiac surgery? *Am Heart J.* 2014; **168**(1):60–7.

14. Bijker J B, Persoon S, Peelen L M, et al. *Anesthesiology.* 2012; **116**(3):658–64.

15. Ng J L, Chan M T, Gelb A W. Perioperative stroke in noncardiac, nonneurosurgical surgery. *Anesthesiology.* 2011; **115**(4):879–90.

16. Hinterhuber G, Böhler K, Kittler H, Quehenberger P. *Dermatol Surg.* 2006; **32**(5):632–9.

17. Broderick J P, Bonomo J B, Kissela B M, et al. Withdrawal of antithrombotic agents and its impact on ischemic stroke occurrence. *Stroke.* 2011; **42**(9): 2509–14.

18. Sedlaczek O, Caplan L, Hennerici M. Impaired washout-embolism and ischemic stroke: further examples and proof of concept. *Cerebrovasc Dis.* 2005; **19**(6):396–401.

19. Kim J S, Ko S B, Shin H E, Han S R, Lee K S. Perioperative stroke in the brain and spinal cord following an induced hypotension. *Yonsei Med J.* 2003; **44**(1):143–5.

20. Langmayr J J, Ortler M, Obwegeser A, Felber S. Quadriplegia after lumbar disc surgery. A case report. *Spine.* 1996; **21**(16):1932–5.

21. Jorgensen M E, Torp-Pedersen C, Gislason G H, et al. Time elapsed after ischemic stroke and risk of adverse cardiovascular events and mortality following elective noncardiac surgery. *JAMA.* 2014; **312**(3):269–277.

22. Biteker M, Dayan A, Can M M, et al. Impaired fasting glucose is associated with increased perioperative cardiovascular event rates in patients undergoing major non-cardiothoracic surgery. *Cardiovasc Diabetol.* 2011; **10**:63.

23. Gentile N T, Seftchick M W, Huynh T, Kruus L K, Gaughan J. Decreased mortality by normalizing blood glucose after acute ischemic stroke. *Acad Emerg Med.* 2006; **13**(2):174–80.

24. Douketis J D, Spyropoulos A C, Kaatz S, et al. Perioperative bridging anticoagulation in patients with atrial fibrillation. *New England Journal of Medicine.* 2015; **373**(9):823–33.

25. Steinberg B A, Peterson E D, Kim S, et al. Use and outcomes associated with bridging during anticoagulation interruptions in patients with atrial fibrillation: Findings from the outcomes registry for better informed treatment of atrial fibrillation (ORBIT-AF). *Circulation.* 2015; **131**(5):488–94.

26. Gialdini G, Nearing K, Bhave P D, et al. Perioperative atrial fibrillation and the long-term risk of ischemic stroke. *JAMA.* 2014; **312**(6):616–22.

27. Epstein A E, Alexander J C, Gutterman D D, Maisel W, Wharton J M, American College of Chest Physicians.

Anticoagulation: American College of Chest Physicians guidelines for the prevention and management of postoperative atrial fibrillation after cardiac surgery. *Chest.* 2005; **128**(2 Suppl):24S-27S.

28. Frendl G, Sodickson A C, Chung M K, et al. AATS guidelines for the prevention and management of perioperative atrial fibrillation and flutter for thoracic surgical procedures. *J Thorac Cardiovasc Surg.* 2014; **148**(3):e153–93.

29. Maulaz A B, Bezerra D C, Michel P, Bogousslavsky J. Effect of discontinuing aspirin therapy on the risk of brain ischemic stroke. *Arch Neurol.* 2005; **62**(8): 1217–20.

30. Genewein U, Haeberli A, Straub P W, Beer J H. Rebound after cessation of oral anticoagulant therapy: the biochemical evidence. *Br J Haematol.* 1996; **92**(2):479–85.

31. Douketis J D, Spyropoulos A C, Spencer F A, et al.; American College of Chest Physicians. Perioperative management of antithrombotic therapy: Antithrombotic Therapy and Prevention of Thrombosis, 9th ed: American College of Chest Physicians Evidence-Based Clinical Practice Guidelines. *Chest.* 2012; Feb;**141**(2 Suppl):e326S–50S. Erratum in: *Chest.* 2012; **141**(4):1129.

32. Assia E I, Raskin T, Kaiserman I, Rotenstreich Y, Segev F. Effect of aspirin intake on bleeding during cataract surgery. *J Cataract Refract Surg.* 1998; **24**(9): 1243–6.

33. Giannarini G, Mogorovich A, Valent F, et al. Continuing or discontinuing low-dose aspirin before transrectal prostate biopsy: results of a prospective randomized trial. *Urology.* 2007; **70**(3):501–5.

34. Kovich O, Otley C C. Thrombotic complications related to discontinuation of warfarin and aspirin therapy perioperatively for cutaneous operation. *J Am Acad Dermatol.* 2003; **48**(2):233–7.

35. Bajkin B V, Bajkin I A, Petrovic B B. The effects of combined oral anticoagulant-aspirin therapy in patients undergoing tooth extractions: a prospective study. *J Am Dent Assoc.* 2012; **143**(7):771–6.

36. Ferraris V A, Swanson E. Aspirin usage and perioperative blood loss in patients undergoing unexpected operations. *Surg Gynecol Obstet.* 1983; **156**(4):439–42.

37. Capodanno D, Musumeci G, Lettieri C, et al. Impact of bridging with perioperative low-molecular-weight heparin on cardiac and bleeding outcomes of stented patients undergoing non-cardiac surgery. *Thromb Haemost.* 2015; **114**(2):423–31.

38. Armstrong M J, Schneck M J, Biller J. Discontinuation of perioperative antiplatelet and anticoagulant therapy in stroke patients. *Neurol Clin.* 2006; **24**(4):607–30.

39. Yusuf S, Zhao F, Mehta S R, *et al.* Clopidogrel in Unstable Angina to Prevent Recurrent Events Trial Investigators. Effects of clopidogrel in addition to aspirin in patients with acute coronary syndromes without ST-segment elevation. *N Engl J Med.* 2001; **345**(7):494–502. Erratum in: *N Engl J Med* 2001; **345**(23):1716.

40. Larson B J, Zumberg M S, Kitchens C S. A feasibility study of continuing dose-reduced warfarin for invasive procedures in patients with high thromboembolic risk. *Chest.* 2005; **127**(3):922–7.

41. Dunn A S, Turpie A G. Perioperative management of patients receiving oral anticoagulants: a systematic review. *Arch Intern Med.* 2003; **163**: 901–8.

42. The American Society for Gastrointestinal Endoscopy. Guideline: Management of antithrombotic agents for endoscopic procedures. 2009; doi:10.1016/j. gie.2009.09.040. www.asge.org/uploadedFiles/Publicat ions_and_Products/Practice_Guidelines/PII S0016510709025498.pdf.

43. POISE Study Group, Devereaux P J, Yang H, Yusuf S, *et al.* Effects of extended-release metoprolol succinate in patients undergoing non-cardiac surgery (POISE trial): a randomised controlled trial. *Lancet.* 2008; **371**(9627):1839–47.

44. Wong G Y, Warner D O, Schroeder D R, *et al.* Risk of surgery and anesthesia for ischemic stroke. *Anesthesiology.* 2000; **92**:425–32.

45. Stentella P, Frega A, Cipriano L, *et al.* Prevention of thromboembolic complications in women undergoing gynecologic surgery. *Clin Exp Obstet Gynecol.* 1997; **24**:58–60.

46. Celebi F, Balik A A, Yildirgan M I, *et al.* Thromboembolic prophylaxis after major abdominal surgery. *Ulus Travma Derg.* 2001; **7**:44–8.

47. Amarigiri S V, Lees T A. Elastic compression stockings for prevention of deep vein thrombosis. *Cochrane Database Syst Rev.* 2000; CD001484.

48. Chalela J A, Katzan I, Liebeskind D S, *et al.* Safety of intra-arterial thrombolysis in the postoperative period. *Stroke.* 2001; **32**(6):1365–9.

Stroke after open arterial surgery

David Bergqvist and Björn Kragsterman

The majority of vascular surgical patients are elderly, and most of them undergo reconstructions because of atherosclerotic vascular disease. Although the indication for the surgical procedure is symptoms from one vascular area, atherosclerosis is a generalized disease often with involvements of other vascular beds that are only occasionally symptomatic [1–5].

Perioperative care and pharmacological prophylaxis have improved, but serious complications still do occur after vascular surgery. Patients with cerebrovascular involvement of their disease may suffer perioperative stroke, but atrial fibrillation is another possible source of cerebral embolism in vascular patients. A special problem is stroke after carotid endarterectomy (CEA), where the aim of the operation actually is to prevent stroke.

Stroke is devastating with disability to patients and families and with an increased mortality. A stroke further generates high health economic costs, being a financial burden both for the patients and society. There has been a discussion whether patients with asymptomatic carotid artery stenosis should undergo prophylactic CEA in relation to major cardiovascular surgery. However, there is no evidence supporting the use of prophylactic CEA in coronary artery bypass surgery as recently shown in a meta-analysis [6]. A small randomized trial on prophylactic CEA in patients undergoing major vascular surgery arrived at the same conclusion [7].

The aim of this chapter is to analyze the occurrence of stroke after open peripheral arterial surgery, with the exception of cardiac and intracranial vascular surgery. This will be made using two sources of information: a systematic review of published postoperative complications and an analysis of stroke as a postoperative complication reported to the Swedish vascular surgical registry (Swedvasc). The focus will be on stroke during the first 30 postoperative days or in hospital.

Methods

Definitions In the literature review we have accepted stroke as defined by the authors. Very rarely there is an attempt to differ between alternative stroke diagnoses or etiologies.

Whenever possible, intraoperative and postoperative stroke have been separated. Stroke is described as a new neurological deficit lasting for more than 24 hours occurring within 30 days of surgery. An intraoperative stroke is apparent already when the patient recovers from anesthesia, a postoperative stroke occurs after an initial free interval after awakening from anesthesia.

A literature search was performed as recommended in health technology assessment [8]. PubMed and Medline and reference lists of identified articles were used. The search terms regarding vascular surgery and various types of complications such as stroke did not, however, reveal many useful references. Therefore incidences of perioperative stroke have been collected from large trials and reports of series on reconstructions for lower limb ischemia, aortic aneurysm, thoracic aortic surgery, and carotid artery disease.

As a general comment it is remarkable that many published series are focused on the function of the reconstruction (which is understandable as it reflects the technical aim of the surgical procedure) but do not report on general complications (which are important regarding the total existence and quality of life of patients).

We also performed an analysis of the Swedvasc registry. In Swedvasc perioperative cerebrovascular

Treatment-Related Stroke, ed. Alexander Tsiskaridze, Arne Lindgren and Adnan Qureshi. Published by Cambridge University Press. © Cambridge University Press 2016.

events include intra- and postoperative deficits, which are registered at 30 days. They are defined as: TIA (hemispheric deficits resolved <24 hours), amaurosis fugax (sudden loss of ipsilateral vision resolved <24 hours), crescendo-TIA (daily TIAs or stroke in evolution/progressive stroke), minor stroke (hemispheric deficit resolved >24 hours or minor focal remaining symptoms), and major stroke (hemispheric permanent symptoms). Posterior circulation (vertebro-basilary) events are only registered as "yes/no," and not further specified. Similarly, the complication of perioperative cerebral bleeding is a separate variable, but often registered in combination with appropriate hemispheric symptoms. The perioperative events are registered differently according to the location of surgery:

I) Infrainguinal surgery includes one variable with major stroke "yes/no"
II) Surgery for abdominal aortic aneurysm (AAA) has two variables with cerebrovascular event "yes/no," and when "yes" followed by a classification (defined as above)
III) Carotid artery surgery has variables of ispi- and contralateral event (defined as above), vertebro-basilar event and cerebral bleeding.

Swedvasc covers all centers performing vascular surgery in Sweden since 1994. The registry has been validated on several occasions, both externally and internally, and has very good quality for carotid and aortic surgery, whereas infrainguinal surgery is somewhat less well registered. For this chapter, data from Swedvasc have been analyzed from the period May 2008 to March 2012.

Results of literature search

Non-cerebrovascular arterial surgery

Table 2.1 demonstrates the data from the studies on arterial reconstructive surgery, carotid artery revascularization excluded (see below). Because of variations in time for follow-up, the results are not directly comparable, but when looking at studies reporting in-hospital and 30-day stroke rates, the range is between 0% and 2%, the highest proportion, however, coming from a very small study. Longer duration of follow-up after surgery leads to increased stroke rates, which also has to do with the natural course of the disease, and from a surgical complication point of view 30 days is traditionally used as the time for reporting postoperative complications.

Surgery of the thoracic aorta

From a stroke complication point of view the thoracic aorta can be divided into two parts: the aortic arch and the descending aorta. The arch surgery directly or indirectly involves the extracerebral vessels and is often performed in extracorporeal circulation with its specific problems, which will not be covered in this chapter, while the descending thoracic aorta in this respect is more comparable to the abdominal aorta. As can be seen in Table 2.2 the risk of postoperative stroke seems to be somewhat higher after arch surgery than after surgery of the descending thoracic aorta, the latter showing a similar frequency as surgery of the abdominal aorta (Table 2.1). Independent risk factors for stroke after aortic arch surgery are chronic obstructive pulmonary disease (COPD), prolonged hypothermic circulatory arrest time, resection into the proximal descending aorta, and permanent postoperative dialysis [9]. Based on results from a non-randomized study there seems to be a lower stroke rate at open arch replacement if retro- or antegrade cerebral perfusion is used compared to hypothermia and circulatory arrest [10]. In a large series (37 states in the US) of aneurysmal surgery of the descending aorta [11], there was no differences in stroke rate, whether the aneurysm was ruptured or intact, but the mortality was significantly higher after rupture (45% vs. 10%). Nor did the frequency depend on hospital case load. It should also be noted that patients with rupture were five years older (median 72 years vs. 67 years), but there are no data on the number of fatal strokes. A pre-existing old cerebral infarction enhances the vulnerability of the brain when total arch replacement is performed [12]. Cheng *et al.* [13] performed a recent systematic review and meta-analysis of endovascular vs. open repair of descending thoracic aortic disease, but unfortunately there were no randomized trials, and they moreover included several diagnoses including trauma. The overall stroke proportion after open surgery was 6.2% in the 1,012 patients who could be included in the analysis.

Open carotid artery surgery (CEA, carotid endarterectomy)

In Table 2.3 stroke after open carotid revascularization is listed and here all data are on 30-day or peri-procedural results, but again there are differences in definitions and whether or not death is included. The overall stroke incidence varies from 1.4% to

Table 2.1 Stroke after non-carotid arterial surgery.

Author	Year	No of patients	Type of surgery	No of strokes	%	FU
Plate [46]	1988	1,066	Surviving AAA repair	14	1.3	1 year
Harris [47]	1992	1,390	Non-carotid	11	0.8	Within 2 weeks
Parikh [28]	1993	6,407	Various non-carotid vasc	5	0.07	Perioperative
Pomposelli [48]	2003	1,032	Bypass to dorsal pedal artery	3	0.3	30 days
Liapis [49]	2003	208	Open AAA repair	0	0	30 days
Liapis [49]	2003	208	Open AAA repair	6	2.8	Median 50 months
Durazzo [36]	2004	44	Various	1	2	30 days
Blankensteijn [50]	2005	174	Open AAA repair	0	0	In hospital
EVAR [51]	2005	539	Open AAA repair	6 (fatal)	1.1	Mean 3.3 years
Jensen [52]	2007	413	Femoral popliteal bypass	0	0	30 days
Biancari[a] [53]	2007	5,709	Op CLI	66	1.7	30 days
Cherr [54]	2008	257	Lower limb revasc	9	3.5	Mean 28.3 months
Lederle [55]	2009	437	Open AAA repair	4	0.9	1 year
Lange [56]	2009	296	Femoral distal bypass	0	0	In hospital
Gisbertz [57]	2009	55	Femoral popliteal bypass	0	0	30 days
Brown [58]	2011	626	Open AAA	51	8.1	Mean 5.1 years
Becquemin [59]	2011	149	Open AAA	0	0	In hospital

[a] Report from the Finnish vascular registry.

FU: follow-up; AAA: abdominal aortic aneurysm; CLI: critical limb ischemia

4.9%, the latter figure being 2.8% if only permanent stroke is included.

The American College of Surgeons' National Surgical Quality Improvement Program (NSQIP) reported data from 2007 and 2008 in 13,316 patients, with a combined stroke and/or death rate within 30 days of 2.8%, and a postoperative stroke rate of 1.4% [14]. Preoperative renal failure, chronic corticoid steroid medication, history of COPD, and impaired sensorium were independent risk factors for postoperative stroke.

In another study by Parlani et al. [15] from an Italian database there were no significant differences in stroke or death between diabetic and non-diabetic patients, disabling stroke being seen in 0.7% and 0.5% respectively.

Looking at the indication for surgery, a meta-analysis by Rothwell et al. [16] found the risk of fatal postoperative stroke to be significantly higher after surgery for symptomatic than asymptomatic carotid artery disease (0.9% vs. 0.47%).

Naylor et al. [17] performed an overview of the results from the ECST and NASCET trials and found no relation between degree of carotid artery stenosis and 30-day risk of death/stroke. The temporal distribution of postoperative stroke/death in the NASCET trial was as follows: one third upon recovery from anesthesia, one third the first postoperative day, and one third within the next 29 days (86% occurred during the first week). A similar temporal pattern was seen in the ECST trial.

In a recent meta-analysis on surgical technique in 16,200 procedures in 15,000 patients, eversion vs. conventional CEA were compared in both randomized studies (n = 6) and cohort studies (n = 13). There was a significant benefit in risk of perioperative

Table 2.2 Stroke after surgery on the thoracic aorta.

Author	Year	Number	Type	No of strokes	%	FU
Svensson [60]	1993	832	DTA	29	3.0	30+ days
Borst [61]	1994	132	DTA	0	0	Perioperative
Kouchoukas [62][a]	2001	161	DTA/TAAA	3	1.9	30 days
Brandt [63]	2004	22	DTA pathology	2	9	30 days
Coselli [64]	2004	387	DTA	7	1.8	Perioperative
Estrera [65]	2005	300	DTA	7	2.3	Perioperative
Stone [66]	2006	93	Most aneurysms	7	7.5	30 days
Schermerhorn [11]	2008	2,549	DTA, aneurysm		2.9	In hospital
Sundt [10]	2008	347	Arch replacement	29	8	Early 30 days
Khaladi [67]	2008	501	Arch surgery	48	9.6	30 days
Kulik [68]	2011	218	TAAA	8	3.7	Perioperative
Patel [9]	2011	721[b]	Arch reconstruction	34	4.7	Early
Nakamura [12]	2011	143	Total arch replacement	9	6.3	In hospital
Thomas [69]	2011	209[c]	Total arch replacement	13[d]	6.2	Perioperative

DTA: descending thoracic aorta; TAAA: thoracoabdominal aneurysm; FU: follow-up
[a] hypothermic circulatory arrest
[b] 284 dissection, 416 aneurysm
[c] 159 elective
[d] 12 ischemic, 1 hemorrhagic

Table 2.3 Stroke after open carotid surgery.

Author	Year	No of patients	No of strokes	%	FU
Naylor [17]	2003	3,216 (ECST, NASCET)	102 (disabling ± death)	3.1	Perioperative
Kragsterman [70]	2004	1,518	75	4.9[a]	30 days
ACST [71]	2004	1,560	40 (any stroke ± death)	2.8	30 days
Brott [72]	2010	1,240	21 (ipsilateral)	1.6	Periprocedural
Halliday [73]	2010	1,532	38	2.5	Perioperative
Gupta [14]	2011	13,316	186	1.4	30 days
Parlani [15]	2012	1,116	29	2.6	Perioperative
Sharpe [40]	2012	1,600	22	1.4	30 days

[a] permanent stroke 2.8% (n = 43)
ECST: European Carotid Surgery Trial; NASCET: North American Symptomatic Carotid Endarterectomy trial; FU: follow-up

Table 2.4 Perioperative major stroke after infrainguinal procedures in relation to operative technique. Data from Swedvasc from the period May 2008 to March 2012.

Procedure	No	Major stroke
Open	6,508	0.8%
Embolectomy	1,667	1.6%
TEA	2,756	0.7%
Patch	4,106	0.8%
Bypass	2,925	1.1%
Prosthetic	925	0.6%
Vein in-situ	1139	0.2%
Vein reversed	772	0.8%
Other	652	1.4%
Exploration	409	0.5%

TEA: thromboendarterectomy

Table 2.5 Perioperative major stroke after infrainguinal procedures in relation to indication. Data from Swedvasc from the period May 2008 to March 2012.

Indication	No	Major stroke
Acute ischemia	1,623	1.3%
TASC I	182	0.0%
TASC IIa	414	1.7%
TASC IIb	1,060	1.5%
TASC III	31	0.0%
Chronic ischemia	4,904	0.6%
Claudication	1,618	0.7%
Rest pain	1,054	0.9%
Ulcer/gangrene	2,232	0.4%
Popliteal aneurysm	483	0.4%
Acute	118	0.0%
Elective	360	0.6%

TASC: Trans-Atlantic Inter-Society Consensus trial document on management of peripheral arterial diseases

Table 2.6 Perioperative outcome of stroke and TIA after procedures for AAA in relation to surgical technique. Data from Swedvasc from the period May 2008 to March 2012.

Procedure	No	Major	All stroke	Stroke/TIA
Open	2,615	0.3%	0.5%	1.1%
Tube	1,546	0.2%	0.5%	1.0%
Aortobiiliacal	757	0.3%	0.4%	1.5%
Aortobifemoral	215	0.5%	0.5%	0.5%
Renal artery implantation	78	0.0%	0.0%	2.6%
Converted to open	17	0.0%	0.0%	0.0%

Tube: aortoaortic graft

stroke for eversion endarterectomy, the Peto odds ratio being 0.46 (95% CI 0.35–0.62) [18]. Death and stroke-related deaths as well as late mortality and late carotid artery occlusion were also diminished for the eversion group. The randomized and non-randomized studies were consistent in their findings.

In another meta-analysis comparing carotid artery stenting (n = 3754) with CEA (n = 3723) the absolute incidence of stroke is not given but the overall analysis favors CEA (OR 1.53, 95% CI 1.23–1.91). In online supplementary tables the short-term stroke incidence seems to be 3.9% [19]. This finding is true also for octogenarians [20].

Swedvasc results

Infrainguinal procedures in Swedvasc comprised 17,255 cases, of which 6,508 were open procedures included in this analysis. The overall rate of major stroke was 0.8%, depending on the type of surgery, ranging from 0.2% for in-situ vein bypass to 1.6% for embolectomy (Table 2.4). Analyzing stroke in relation to the indication for surgery, those with acute indication had the highest stroke rate of 1.3%, and among these individuals, the Trans-Atlantic Inter-Society Consensus (TASC) group II patients had a stroke rate of 1.7% (Table 2.5).

Operations for abdominal aortic aneurysm (AAA) comprised 5,230 registered cases, of which 2,615 open procedures are included in this analysis. In Table 2.6 the overall 30-day complication rates are listed, which for major stroke was 0.3% (range 0.0% to 0.5% depending on type of reconstruction), all stroke 0.5% (0.0% to 0.5%), and for all stroke/TIA 1.1% (0.0% to 2.6%). When analysing stroke complications according to indication, the ruptured cases had the highest rate with major stroke in 0.2%, all stroke in 0.5% and all stroke/TIA in 1.5% (Table 2.7).

Procedures for carotid artery stenosis were registered in 4,363 cases, of which 4,098 were open operations and included in the analysis.

The overall complication rates were 2.7% for ipsilateral stroke, 1.3% for major stroke, 3.2% for all stroke, and 4.5% for all stroke/TIA, with little differences concerning type of surgery (Table 2.8). Outcome vs. indication for the surgery is listed in Table 2.9, with the lowest stroke rates occurring in patients with amaurosis fugax and the highest in patients undergoing reoperation for bleeding with major stroke 8.0%, all stroke 10.2%, and all stroke/TIA 11.7%.

The timing of carotid surgery in relation to the symptom onset is of importance. In a recent analysis of Swedvasc data from 2008 to 2011, it was shown that surgery for carotid artery stenosis within 0 to 2 days after a qualifying event had a significantly increased risk of mortality and stroke: 11.5% vs. 4.4% [21].

Table 2.7 Perioperative outcome of stroke and TIA after procedures for AAA in relation to indication. Data from Swedvasc from the period May 2008 to March 2012.

	No	Major stroke	All stroke	Stroke/TIA
Non-ruptured	1,736	0.3%	0.5%	0.9%
Symptomatic	295	0.0%	0.0%	0.7%
Ruptured	875	0.2%	0.5%	1.5%

AAA: abdominal aortic aneurysm

Table 2.8 Perioperative outcome of (ipsi- and contralateral) stroke and TIA after procedures for carotid artery stenosis in relation to open or endovascular technique. Data from Swedvasc from the period May 2008 to March 2012.

Procedure	No	Ipsilateral stroke	Major stroke	All stroke	Stroke/TIA
Open	4,098	2.7%	1.3%	3.2%	4.5%
CEA	2,954	2.5%	1.3%	3.2%	4.3%
Eversion EA	1,087	2.9%	1.5%	3.3%	4.9%

CEA: carotid endarterectomy; EA: endarterectomy

Table 2.9 Perioperative outcome of (ipsi- and contralateral) stroke and TIA after procedures for carotid artery stenosis in relation to indication. Data from Swedvasc from the period May 2008 to March 2012.

Indication	No	Ipsilateral stroke	Major stroke	All stroke	Stroke/TIA
Asymptomatic	574	1.9%	1.0%	2.3%	3.8%
Asymptomatic (>6 months)[a]	129	2.3%	1.6%	3.9%	4.7%
Symptomatic	3,401	2.8%	1.4%	3.4%	4.6%
Amaurosis fugax	667	1.0%	0.4%	1.2%	2.1%
TIA	1,390	3.2%	1.6%	3.8%	5.3%
Crescendo-TIA	72	2.8%	2.8%	4.1%	6.9%
Minor stroke	1,173	3.5%	1.6%	4.1%	5.1%
Major stroke	100	1.0%	1.0%	1.0%	3.0%
Re-operation for bleeding	137	10.2%	8.0%	10.2%	11.7%

[a] Patients with previous stroke/TIA >6 months prior to decision for CEA/CAS.

Other cerebrovascular complications registered during the time period were cerebral bleeding in 0.6%, most included in the perioperative strokes, but in 0.1% (5/4363) without coupled stroke/TIA registration. Events in the posterior circulation (vertebro-basilary distribution area) were not specified of type (i.e., yes/no) but registered in 0.3%, of which 0.2% (9/4363) did not have another stroke/TIA registration.

Discussion

The etiology of stroke after vascular surgery is multifactorial, and often involves hemodynamic/rheological mechanisms, such as a sudden blood pressure drop, which may trigger an ischemic insult, or prothrombotic alterations in the coagulation/fibrinolysis systems as a response to the surgical trauma. Other causes are embolism from the heart or atherosclerotic ulcerations/thrombosis in the carotid artery bifurcation or aortic arch. In the literature, only rarely have there been attempts to differentiate between various mechanisms of postoperative stroke. In carotid endarterectomy there are potential local/technical issues with embolism from the endarterectomised area with platelet aggregation or from technical problems such as intimal flaps or a stenosis in closure of the arteriotomy without a patch.

Other problems when scrutinizing the literature are the variations in definition of peri/postoperative stroke and the time chosen for the follow-up period during which stroke is registered. Differences in these two fundamental criteria may explain some of the dissimilarities between publications. In a systematic review of short-term results after abdominal aortic aneurysm surgery [22], neurological complications are seen in 0% to 14% but this figure included cerebrovascular accidents, encephalopathy, neurological complications, organic brain dysfunction, paraplegia, seizure, stroke, and TIA, thus making a meaningful analysis impossible. This disagreement in reported mortality and morbidities is also pointed out by Blankensteijn [23], stressing the importance of the relation between frequency and study design/level of evidence. For instance, it is remarkable that in a large Medicare population of 22,830 open abdominal aneurysm repairs with a preoperative cerebrovascular disease rate of 16.8%, there is no reported postoperative stroke [24]. Another problem is that only rarely do reports on mortality include figures on fatal stroke.

As clearly demonstrated by the Swedvasc data for CEA, although all within the 30-day period, differently defined outcomes on perioperative cerebrovascular events result in complication rates ranging from 0.4% (major stroke rate in patients with amaurosis fugax as indication for surgery) to 6.9% (all stroke/TIA rate in patients with crescendo TIA as indication). Most publications from recent years on stroke rates in registries include the widely recommended complication rates of stroke (independent of ipsi- or contralateral) but the different types of surgery (aortic/infrainguinal/carotid) have still not the same outcome variables. A consensus on definitions and study designs would be most welcome and a joint aim for neurologists, vascular surgeons, as well as journal editors.

Although not included in this chapter, other studies show that stroke may also occur as a complication after non-vascular surgery in elderly patients (for further details on stroke after general surgery, please see Chapter 1). The true incidence does not seem much lower than after vascular surgery, indicating that the surgical trauma in itself is a risk situation, and this must be considered when discussing stroke as a complication to arterial surgery. In a study of 21,903 different surgical procedures, of which only a minority was cardiovascular, the risk for postoperative ischemic stroke was 0.44% and increased with age, history of ischemic stroke, and hyperuricemia [25]. However, as this study was performed in Japan the results may not be immediately representative for Western countries. In a recent review the incidence of stroke after non-vascular surgery varied between 0.05% and 4.0% [26]. The problem with the included studies is the great variation in several factors such as the period of analysis (the oldest is from 1959), the heterogenic patient population and types of surgery, the length of follow-up, diagnostic criteria and whether the study design is retro- or prospective. Many of these differences may explain at least parts of the variations in stroke rates, but the review is included to illustrate that stroke may complicate any type of surgery, and not just vascular. Predisposing factors were age, previous stroke, atrial fibrillation, vascular disease, and neck surgery. In the study by Bijker et al. [27] general and carotid artery surgery together with resection of head and neck tumors were included. Although a detailed analysis is impossible due to the summarized results, in a multivariate analysis the only significant independent risk factor for postoperative stroke (42 cases of 48,241 patients) was blood pressure drop of more than 30% from baseline, which in itself is important information.

When recalculating data from the study by Parikh [28] it was possible to compare perioperative stroke among 6,407 non-carotid arterial operations with 18,234 non-vascular operations; perioperative stroke rates were 0.07% in both groups. Larsen *et al.* [29], in a prospective analysis, found six strokes (four major) in 2,453 patients (0.2%) undergoing various types of general surgery. They also made a comparison with other studies, the oldest from 1962, and stated that the frequency of stroke had been consistent over the years. In a case-control study with 61 cases of ischemic stroke after non-vascular general surgery, previous cerebrovascular disease, chronic obstructive pulmonary disease, and peripheral vascular disease were significant risk factors [30]. For further details on stroke after general surgery, please see Chapter 1.

In the Swedvasc data, the stroke rate was lowest for AAA surgery with 0.4% for elective and 0.5% for acute (including ruptured). The highest rates were after carotid artery surgery with an overall stroke rate of 3.2%, and among these the indication of crescendo-TIA and minor stroke had a rate of 4.1%.

Patients undergoing arterial surgery should generally be on antiplatelet prophylaxis, basically to prevent coronary artery complications, but also as prophylaxis against occlusion of the reconstruction [31] and preventing neurological complications after carotid surgery [32]. After the latter type of surgery clopidogrel added to aspirin significantly reduces cerebral embolism as measured with transcranial Doppler [33,34]. Clopidogrel plus aspirin increases time to skin closure because of impaired local hemostasis but does not increase the postoperative bleeding risk [34].

Statins have emerged as an important part of best medical treatment for the atherosclerotic patient, and there is increased evidence that they can also reduce perioperative complications after vascular surgery [35–37]. Two retrospective studies have come to the same conclusion where statins use had a protective effect on perioperative stroke with an OR 0.35 to 0.55 [38,39].

During carotid artery surgery it is especially important to be technically perfect, paying attention to details. One way of reaching perfection of the repair is to use some method for completion control, i.e., how well the carotid artery stenosis has been removed. Techniques most often used are duplex ultrasonography, transit time ultrasound flow measurement, angiography, and angioscopy. The true utility of these methods remains a matter for debate with proponents demonstrating excellent results [40], whereas others suggest that they might worsen the outcome [41,42]. However, in clinical practice it seems to be center routines or surgeons' preferences that influence the pattern of completion control. In the Vascular Study Group of New England, 51% of the surgeons performed completion imaging rarely, 22% selectively, and 27% performed it routinely [42].

When analysing carotid artery studies it is important that indication and time for surgery are defined, which is not always the case [43]. Urgency CEA for evolving symptoms has a significantly higher risk than CEA for stable symptomatology (stroke and/or death 19.2% vs. 3.9%), but there is no difference between early (<3 to 6 weeks) and late (>3 to 6 weeks) CEA in stable patients. However, too early surgery (within 2 days after the qualifying event) may increase the risk for stroke and death considerably [21].

One question, which has been discussed, is whether screening for carotid artery stenosis should be recommended before major cardiac or vascular surgery. However, there is no evidence that preoperative prophylactic CEA reduces the risk of postoperative stroke [6,7]. Moreover, there is no relationship between the presence of a cervical bruit and the incidence of perioperative stroke [44]. A somewhat different approach is taken in the European Society for Vascular Surgery guidelines [45], which recommend that treatment of peripheral artery disease should not be delayed in case of asymptomatic carotid artery stenosis, but patients with symptomatic >70% stenosis should undergo CEA before surgery for peripheral artery disease (or possibly as a simultaneous procedure).

Concluding remarks

Stroke after arterial surgery unfortunately does occur, one reason being that the patients are at high risk as the majority have advanced and often generalized arteriosclerotic disease. Although there are no randomized trials – and probably never will be – on how to minimize the stroke risk after arterial surgery, it seems important to have a treatment strategy that involves pharmacological optimization with antiplatelet prophylaxis and possibly statins to reduce not only the stroke risk but also other cardiovascular events and mortality. When performing aortic arch and carotid artery surgery the surgical procedures should be as atraumatic as possible to prevent embolism provoked by the surgical manipulation of the artery.

References

1. CAPRIE Steering Committee. A randomised, blinded, trial of clopidogrel versus aspirin in patients at risk of ischaemic events (CAPRIE). *Lancet*. 1996; **348**(9038): 1329–39.

2. Sigvant B, Wiberg-Hedman K, Bergqvist D, *et al.* A population-based study of peripheral arterial disease prevalence with special focus on critical limb ischemia and sex differences. *J Vasc Surg*. 2007; **45**(6): 1185–91.

3. Steg P G, Bhatt D L, Wilson P W, *et al.* One-year cardiovascular event rates in outpatients with atherothrombosis. *JAMA*. 2007; **297**(11):1197–206.

4. Diehm C, Allenberg J R, Pittrow D, *et al.* Mortality and vascular morbidity in older adults with asymptomatic versus symptomatic peripheral artery disease. *Circulation*. 2009; **120**(21):2053–61.

5. Clark C E, Taylor R S, Shore A C, Ukoumunne O C, Campbell J L. Association of a difference in systolic blood pressure between arms with vascular disease and mortality: a systematic review and meta-analysis. *Lancet*. 2012; **379**(9819):905–14.

6. Naylor A R, Bown M J. Stroke after cardiac surgery and its association with asymptomatic carotid disease: an updated systematic review and meta-analysis. *Eur J Vasc Endovasc Surg*. 2011; **41**(5):607–24.

7. Ballotta E, Renon L, Da Giau G, *et al.* Prospective randomized study on asymptomatic severe carotid stenosis and perioperative stroke risk in patients undergoing major vascular surgery: prophylactic or deferred carotid endarterectomy? *Ann Vasc Surg*. 2005; **19**(6):876–81.

8. Bergqvist D, Rosén M. Health technology assessment in surgery. *Scand J Surg*. 2012; **101**(2):132–7.

9. Patel H J, Nguyen C, Diener A C, *et al.* Open arch reconstruction in the endovascular era: analysis of 721 patients over 17 years. *J Thorac Cardiovasc Surg*. 2011; **141**(6):1417–23.

10. Sundt T M 3rd, Orszulak T A, Cook D J, Schaff H V. Improving results of open arch replacement. *Ann Thorac Surg*. 2008; **86**(3):787–96.

11. Schermerhorn M L, Giles K A, Hamdan A D, *et al.* Population-based outcomes of open descending thoracic aortic aneurysm repair. *J Vasc Surg*. 2008; **48**(4):821–7.

12. Nakamura K, Nakamura E, Yano M, *et al.* Factors influencing permanent neurologic dysfunction and mortality after total arch replacement with separate arch vessel grafting using selective cerebral perfusion. *Ann Thorac Cardiovasc Surg*. 2011; **17**(1):39–44.

13. Cheng G, Zhang L. [Adverse events related to bevacizumab and the management principles in non-small cell lung cancer]. *Zhongguo Fei Ai Za Zhi*. 2010; **13**(6):563–7.

14. Gupta P K, Pipinos I I, Miller W J, *et al.* A population-based study of risk factors for stroke after carotid endarterectomy using the ACS NSQIP database. *J Surg Res*. 2011; **167**(2):182–91.

15. Parlani G, De Rango P, Cieri E, *et al.* Diabetes is not a predictor of outcome for carotid revascularization with stenting as it may be for carotid endarterectomy. *J Vasc Surg*. 2012; **55**(1):79–89.

16. Rothwell P M, Slattery J, Warlow C P. A systematic comparison of the risks of stroke and death due to carotid endarterectomy for symptomatic and asymptomatic stenosis. *Stroke*. 1996; **27**(2):266–9.

17. Naylor A R, Rothwell P M, Bell P R. Overview of the principal results and secondary analyses from the European and North American randomised trials of endarterectomy for symptomatic carotid stenosis. *Eur J Vasc Endovasc Surg*. 2003; **26**(2):115–29.

18. Antonopoulos C N, Kakisis J D, Sergentanis T N, Liapis C D. Eversion versus conventional carotid endarterectomy: a meta-analysis of randomised and non-randomised studies. *Eur J Vasc Endovasc Surg*. 2011; **42**(6):751–65.

19. Economopoulos K P, Sergentanis T N, Tsivgoulis G, Mariolis A D, Stefanadis C. Carotid artery stenting versus carotid endarterectomy: a comprehensive meta-analysis of short-term and long-term outcomes. *Stroke*. 2011; **42**(3):687–92.

20. Usman A A, Tang G L, Eskandari M K. Metaanalysis of procedural stroke and death among octogenarians: carotid stenting versus carotid endarterectomy. *J Am Coll Surg*. 2009; **208**(6):1124–31.

21. Stromberg S, Gelin J, Osterberg T, *et al.* Very urgent carotid endarterectomy confers increased procedural risk. *Stroke*. 2012; **43**(5):1331–5.

22. Adriaensen M E, Bosch J L, Halpern E F, Myriam Hunink M G, Gazelle G S. Elective endovascular versus open surgical repair of abdominal aortic aneurysms: systematic review of short-term results. *Radiology*. 2002; **224**(3):739–47.

23. Blankensteijn J D. Mortality and morbidity rates after conventional abdominal aortic aneurysm repair. *Semin Interv Cardiol*. 2000; **5**(1):7–13.

24. Schermerhorn M L, O'Malley A J, Jhaveri A, *et al.* Endovascular vs. open repair of abdominal aortic aneurysms in the Medicare population. *N Engl J Med*. 2008; **358**(5):464–74.

25. Kikura M, Takada T, Sato S. Preexisting morbidity as an independent risk factor for perioperative acute

thromboembolism syndrome. *Arch Surg.* 2005; **140**(12):1210–7.

26. Ng J L, Chan M T, Gelb A W. Perioperative stroke in noncardiac, nonneurosurgical surgery. *Anesthesiology.* 2011; **115**(4):879–90.

27. Bijker J B, Persoon S, Peelen L M, *et al.* Intraoperative hypotension and perioperative ischemic stroke after general surgery: a nested case-control study. *Anesthesiology.* 2012; **116**(3):658–64.

28. Parikh S, Cohen J R. Perioperative stroke after general surgical procedures. *N Y State J Med.* 1993; **93**(3):162–5.

29. Larsen S F, Zaric D, Boysen G. Postoperative cerebrovascular accidents in general surgery. *Acta Anaesthesiol Scand.* 1988; **32**(8):698–701.

30. Limburg M, Wijdicks E F, Li H. Ischemic stroke after surgical procedures: clinical features, neuroimaging, and risk factors. *Neurology.* 1998; **50**(4):895–901.

31. Sobel M, Verhaeghe R. Antithrombotic therapy for peripheral artery occlusive disease: American College of Chest Physicians Evidence-Based Clinical Practice Guidelines (8th Edition). *Chest.* 2008; **133**(6 Suppl):815S-43S.

32. Lindblad B, Persson N H, Takolander R, Bergqvist D. Does low-dose acetylsalicylic acid prevent stroke after carotid surgery? A double-blind, placebo-controlled randomized trial. *Stroke.* 1993; **24**(8):1125–8.

33. Sharpe R Y, Dennis M J, Nasim A, *et al.* Dual antiplatelet therapy prior to carotid endarterectomy reduces post-operative embolisation and thromboembolic events: post-operative transcranial Doppler monitoring is now unnecessary. *Eur J Vasc Endovasc Surg.* 2010; **40**(2):162–7.

34. Payne D A, Jones C I, Hayes P D, *et al.* Beneficial effects of clopidogrel combined with aspirin in reducing cerebral emboli in patients undergoing carotid endarterectomy. *Circulation.* 2004; **109**(12):1476–81.

35. O'Neil-Callahan K, Katsimaglis G, Tepper M R, *et al.* Statins decrease perioperative cardiac complications in patients undergoing noncardiac vascular surgery: the Statins for Risk Reduction in Surgery (StaRRS) study. *J Am Coll Cardiol.* 2005; **45**(3):336–42.

36. Durazzo A E, Machado F S, Ikeoka D T, *et al.* Reduction in cardiovascular events after vascular surgery with atorvastatin: a randomized trial. *J Vasc Surg.* 2004; **39**(5):967–75.

37. Sillesen H, Amarenco P, Hennerici M G, *et al.* Atorvastatin reduces the risk of cardiovascular events in patients with carotid atherosclerosis: a secondary analysis of the Stroke Prevention by Aggressive Reduction in Cholesterol Levels (SPARCL) trial. *Stroke.* 2008; **39**(12):3297–302.

38. Kennedy J, Quan H, Buchan A M, Ghali W A, Feasby T E. Statins are associated with better outcomes after carotid endarterectomy in symptomatic patients. *Stroke.* 2005; **36**(10):2072–6.

39. McGirt M J, Perler B A, Brooke B S, *et al.* 3-hydroxy-3-methylglutaryl coenzyme A reductase inhibitors reduce the risk of perioperative stroke and mortality after carotid endarterectomy. *J Vasc Surg.* 2005; **42**(5): 829–36.

40. Sharpe R, Sayers R D, McCarthy M J, *et al.* The war against error: a 15 year experience of completion angioscopy following carotid endarterectomy. *Eur J Vasc Endovasc Surg.* 2012; **43**(2):139–45.

41. Rockman C B, Halm E A. Intraoperative imaging: does it really improve perioperative outcomes of carotid endarterectomy? *Semin Vasc Surg.* 2007; **20**(4): 236–43.

42. Wallaert J B, Goodney P P, Vignati J J, *et al.* Completion imaging after carotid endarterectomy in the Vascular Study Group of New England. *J Vasc Surg.* 2011; **54**(2):376–85, 85 e1–3.

43. Bond R, Rerkasem K, Rothwell P M. Systematic review of the risks of carotid endarterectomy in relation to the clinical indication for and timing of surgery. *Stroke.* 2003; **34**(9):2290–301.

44. Turnipseed W D, Berkoff H A, Belzer F O. Postoperative stroke in cardiac and peripheral vascular disease. *Ann Surg.* 1980; **192**(3):365–8.

45. Liapis C D, Bell P R, Mikhailidis D, Sivenius J, *et al.* ESVS guidelines. Invasive treatment for carotid stenosis: indications, techniques. *Eur J Vasc Endovasc Surg.* 2009; **37**(4 Suppl):1–19.

46. Plate G, Hollier L H, O'Brien P C, Pairolero P C, Cherry K J. Late cerebrovascular accidents after repair of abdominal aortic aneurysms. *Acta Chir Scand.* 1988; **154**(1):25–9.

47. Harris E J, Jr., Moneta G L, Yeager R A, Taylor L M, Jr., Porter J M. Neurologic deficits following noncarotid vascular surgery. *Am J Surg.* 1992; **163**(5):537–40.

48. Pomposelli F B, Kansal N, Hamdan A D, *et al.* A decade of experience with dorsalis pedis artery bypass: analysis of outcome in more than 1000 cases. *J Vasc Surg.* 2003; **37**(2):307–15.

49. Liapis C D, Kakisis J D, Dimitroulis D A, *et al.* Carotid ultrasound findings as a predictor of long-term survival after abdominal aortic aneurysm repair: a 14-year prospective study. *J Vasc Surg.* 2003; **38**(6): 1220–5.

50. Blankensteijn J D, de Jong S E, Prinssen M, *et al.* Two-year outcomes after conventional or endovascular repair of abdominal aortic aneurysms. *N Engl J Med.* 2005; **352**(23):2398–405.

51. Endovascular aneurysm repair versus open repair in patients with abdominal aortic aneurysm (EVAR trial 1): randomised controlled trial. *Lancet.* 2005; **365**(9478):2179–86.

52. Jensen L P, Lepantalo M, Fossdal J E, *et al.* Dacron or PTFE for above-knee femoropopliteal bypass. a multicenter randomised study. *Eur J Vasc Endovasc Surg.* 2007; **34**(1):44–9.

53. Biancari F, Salenius J P, Heikkinen M, *et al.* Risk-scoring method for prediction of 30-day postoperative outcome after infrainguinal surgical revascularization for critical lower-limb ischemia: a Finnvasc registry study. *World J Surg.* 2007; **31**(1):217–25.

54. Cherr G S, Wang J, Zimmerman P M, Dosluoglu H H. Depression is associated with worse patency and recurrent leg symptoms after lower extremity revascularization. *J Vasc Surg.* 2007; **45**(4):744–50.

55. Lederle F A, Freischlag J A, Kyriakides T C, *et al.* Outcomes following endovascular vs open repair of abdominal aortic aneurysm: a randomized trial. *JAMA.* 2009; **302**(14):1535–42.

56. Lange C P, Ploeg A J, Lardenoye J W, Breslau P J. Patient- and procedure-specific risk factors for postoperative complications in peripheral vascular surgery. *Qual Saf Health Care.* 2009; **18**(2):131–6.

57. Gisbertz S S, Ramzan M, Tutein Nolthenius R P, *et al.* Short-term results of a randomized trial comparing remote endarterectomy and supragenicular bypass surgery for long occlusions of the superficial femoral artery [the REVAS trial]. *Eur J Vasc Endovasc Surg.* 2009; **37**(1):68–76.

58. Brown L C, Thompson S G, Greenhalgh R M, Powell J T. Incidence of cardiovascular events and death after open or endovascular repair of abdominal aortic aneurysm in the randomized EVAR trial 1. *Br J Surg.* 2011; **98**(7):935–42.

59. Becquemin J P, Pillet J C, Lescalie F, *et al.* A randomized controlled trial of endovascular aneurysm repair versus open surgery for abdominal aortic aneurysms in low- to moderate-risk patients. *J Vasc Surg.* 2011; **53**(5):1167–73 e1.

60. Svensson L G, Crawford E S, Hess K R, Coselli J S, Safi H J. Variables predictive of outcome in 832 patients undergoing repairs of the descending thoracic aorta. *Chest.* 1993; **104**(4):1248–53.

61. Borst H G, Jurmann M, Buhner B, Laas J. Risk of replacement of descending aorta with a standardized left heart bypass technique. *J Thorac Cardiovasc Surg.* 1994; **107**(1):126–32.

62. Kouchoukos N T, Masetti P, Rokkas C K, Murphy S F, Blackstone E H. Safety and efficacy of hypothermic cardiopulmonary bypass and circulatory arrest for operations on the descending thoracic and thoracoabdominal aorta. *Ann Thorac Surg.* 2001; **72**(3):699–707.

63. Brandt M, Hussel K, Walluscheck K P, *et al.* Stent-graft repair versus open surgery for the descending aorta: a case-control study. *J Endovasc Ther.* 2004; **11**(5):535–8.

64. Coselli J S, LeMaire S A, Conklin L D, Adams G J. Left heart bypass during descending thoracic aortic aneurysm repair does not reduce the incidence of paraplegia. *Ann Thorac Surg.* 2004; **77**(4):1298–303.

65. Estrera A L, Miller C C, 3rd, Chen E P, *et al.* Descending thoracic aortic aneurysm repair: 12-year experience using distal aortic perfusion and cerebrospinal fluid drainage. *Ann Thorac Surg.* 2005; **80**(4):1290–6.

66. Stone D H, Brewster D C, Kwolek C J, *et al.* Stent-graft versus open-surgical repair of the thoracic aorta: mid-term results. *J Vasc Surg.* 2006; **44**(6):1188–97.

67. Khaladj N, Shrestha M, Meck S, *et al.* Hypothermic circulatory arrest with selective antegrade cerebral perfusion in ascending aortic and aortic arch surgery: a risk factor analysis for adverse outcome in 501 patients. *J Thorac Cardiovasc Surg.* 2008; **135**(4): 908–14.

68. Kulik A, Castner C F, Kouchoukos N T. Outcomes after thoracoabdominal aortic aneurysm repair with hypothermic circulatory arrest. *J Thorac Cardiovasc Surg.* 2011; **141**(4):953–60.

69. Thomas M, Li Z, Cook D J, Greason K L, Sundt T M. Contemporary results of open aortic arch surgery. *J Thorac Cardiovasc Surg.* 2012; **144**(4):838–44.

70. Kragsterman B, Logason K, Ahari A, *et al.* Risk factors for complications after carotid endarterectomy: a population-based study. *Eur J Vasc Endovasc Surg.* 2004; **28**(1):98–103.

71. Halliday A, Mansfield A, Marro J, *et al.* Prevention of disabling and fatal strokes by successful carotid endarterectomy in patients without recent neurological symptoms: randomised controlled trial. *Lancet.* 2004; **363**(9420):1491–502.

72. Brott T G, Hobson R W, 2nd, Howard G, *et al.* Stenting versus endarterectomy for treatment of carotid-artery stenosis. *N Engl J Med.* 2010; **363**(1):11–23.

73. Halliday A, Harrison M, Hayter E, *et al.* 10-year stroke prevention after successful carotid endarterectomy for asymptomatic stenosis (ACST-1): a multicentre randomised trial. *Lancet.* 2010; **376**(9746):1074–84.

Chapter 3

Postoperative stroke in neurosurgery

Federico Landriel, Pablo Ajler and Claudio Yampolsky

Introduction

A stroke can be defined as a sudden permanent irreversible neurological deficit triggered by the death of brain tissue cells as a consequence of sustained inadequate blood perfusion. The most common cause of stroke in general is an ischemic infarct, an event accounting for 85% of cases, followed by hemorrhagic cerebrovascular accidents as a less frequent (15% to 30%) but more lethal cause. It is estimated that 8.7% of all strokes occur when the patient has already been hospitalized for other causes [1]. Stroke as a neurosurgical postoperative complication is relatively common, with cerebrovascular disease frequently appearing as an underlying condition. Postoperative stroke manifests differently from the general pattern, with hemorrhage being the most frequent event, followed by ischemia, herniation, and brain tissue edema. General risk of postoperative hemorrhage ranges between 0.8% and 1.1%, with intracerebral hematoma (ICH) accounting for 43% to 60% of the cases, extradural hematoma (EDH) for 28% to 33%, subgaleal hematoma for 11%, mixed hematomas for 8%, subdural hematoma (SDH) for 5% to 7%, and intrasellar hematoma for 5%; general mortality stands at 32% [2,3]. The mechanism of these complications is often related to an alteration of the physiological regulation of brain vascular circulation, autoregulation, and vasomotricity, varying according to the nature of different tumoral, vascular, infectious, or traumatic conditions, their localization and the surgical technique used for their treatment.

Preoperative assessment

Risk factors for stroke are to be determined before any scheduled surgery is performed especially those that can be modified. Hypertension is the most common and significant risk factor to be taken into account as it relates independently to the occurrence of stroke [4]. Its diagnosis, control, and management are vital in the preoperative assessment to prevent and minimize the occurrence of stroke during intra- and postoperative care.

A patient's coagulation profile must be assessed preoperatively. Coagulopathies such as thrombocytopenia, von Willebrand disease, disseminated intravascular coagulation (DIC), hemophilia, lupus and other such conditions must be screened for and managed in conjunction with the hematologist specialist and hemotherapy department. A basic coagulation profile includes prothrombin time, partial thromboplastin time, bleeding time, platelet count or another more sophisticated method of platelet function assessment. Thrombocytopenia is defined as a platelet count $<150,000$ mm^3 potentially leading to spontaneous subarachnoid hemorrhage or ICH, although it this uncommon with counts $>30,000$ mm^3 [5]. Alcoholism may be associated with an increased risk of ischemic or hemorrhagic stroke as a result of an alteration in liver function and coagulation mechanisms [6]. Although antiplatelet treatment with aspirin and/or clopidogrel reduces the risk of ischemic stroke in patients at high risk [7], administration of this therapy should, if it is without risk for the patient, be discontinued within five to seven days prior to a scheduled surgery as these antiplatelet drugs inhibit platelet function permanently [8]. Patients receiving anticoagulants and/or thrombolytics should be evaluated individually to assess the risk vs. benefits of the treatment suspension prior to surgery. Platelet replacement is advisable for patients with a platelet count $<10,000$ mm^3 even in the absence of bleeding, for those with $<20,000$ mm^3 and spontaneous bleeding, and for those with $<30,000$ mm^3 and at risk of bleeding (presenting

Treatment-Related Stroke, ed. Alexander Tsiskaridze, Arne Lindgren and Adnan Qureshi. Published by Cambridge University Press. © Cambridge University Press 2016.

with petechiae, continuous bleeding of wounds, retinal hemorrhage, etc.). Subjects with thrombocytopenia <50,000 mm^3 should be transfused within 12 hours of surgery or in the event of lumbar puncture, or if low platelet counts occur within 48 hours of surgery postoperatively, or in the event of losing >1 blood volume (= blood loss >150 mL/minute or = 50% blood volume loss in three hours) in less than 24 hours postoperatively. In pediatric patients 1 unit of platelets transfusion/m^2 increases platelets by approximately 10,000 mm^3, whereas in adults values range from 5,000 mm^3 to 10,000 mm^3.

Intraoperative management

Several neurosurgical conditions present with loss of autoregulation and changes in vascular reactivity, which result in intra- and postoperative blood pressure modifications playing a decisive role in the development of complications. Skull fixation with pins, laryngoscopy, intubation, extubation, and emergence from anesthesia can cause hypertension, increased cerebral blood flow (CBF) and volume, and increased intracranial pressure (ICP). There are several parameters to be managed and modulated by anesthesiologists during surgery. Continuous monitoring of blood pressure and pCO$_2$ modification can prevent these critical variations in cerebral perfusion pressure (i.e., it can be reduced during aneurysm clipping or increased to improve the perfusion of collaterals during cross-clamping). CO$_2$ is one of the most powerful vasodilators and the response to pCO$_2$ variation is preserved even with impaired autoregulation. Hyperventilation reduces pCO$_2$, decreasing CBF and cerebral blood volume, which additionally modifies ICP, and thus should be used carefully during stereotactic procedures and neuronavigation as it can shift intracranial contents [9]. Different neuroprotecting agents as well as variations in a patient's body temperature may provide some protection against ischemic brain injury; mild hypothermia reduces the cerebral metabolic rate of oxygen by 7% per degree centigrade. Hyperglycemia can aggravate ischemic deficits, especially when it is acute [10]; hence it should be diagnosed and managed before, during, and after surgery. Hypovolemia can worsen vascularization in compromised but recoverable ischemic territories (ischemic penumbra); however, fluid overload in patients operated in the prone position can increase facial edema, with a subsequent risk of posterior ischemic optic neuropathy.

Postoperative follow-up

Postoperative nausea and vomiting increase ICP, thereby incrementing the risk of hematoma of the surgical lodge in recently operated patients (Figure 3.1). This can be avoided through nasogastric intubation and antiemetic agents. Brief hypertension events may be undetected postoperatively, mainly if they occur during patient emergence from anesthesia or within the first 12 hours of postoperative intensive care and constitute one of the most common causes of hemorrhagic stroke. Vital signs should be monitored thoroughly on a permanent basis.

Any postoperative change in a patient's neurological status, especially when it follows a period of initial good outcome, should be studied. Hemorrhagic causes such as ICH, EDH, or SDH, ischemic events such as an arterial or venous infarction (particularly after procedures performed around venous sinuses), edema, pneumocephalus, vasospasm, acute hydrocephalus, and seizures should be excluded.

A postoperative stroke in the posterior fossa can have a worse outcome than a supratentorial stroke because this cavity is smaller in size, and a reduced quantity of mass effect can be lethal, since it results in direct compression of the brainstem or indirectly produces acute hydrocephalus by obstructing CSF flow, causing tonsillar herniation. Symptoms and signs associated with increased pressure in the posterior fossa commonly include increased systemic blood pressure and changes in the breathing pattern, whereas anisocoria and neurological deficit may sometimes occur only in later stages. To approach this sudden complication, we recommend immediate intubation, external ventricular drainage, and reoperation, where applicable (Figure 3.2).

Approach-related complications

Skull fixation with pins can increase blood pressure abruptly. Administration of local epinephrine-free anesthetic agents before fixation is critical, especially in patients with vascular lesions or with already increased intracranial pressure.

Determining the surgical approach and the size of the craniotomy is essential to prevent complications. Selection of the most appropriate approach should ensure good visualization and surgical manipulation of the lesion to avoid excessive retraction of the surrounding neural tissue. Prolonged uncontrolled brain retraction causes small infarcts and hemorrhage in the white

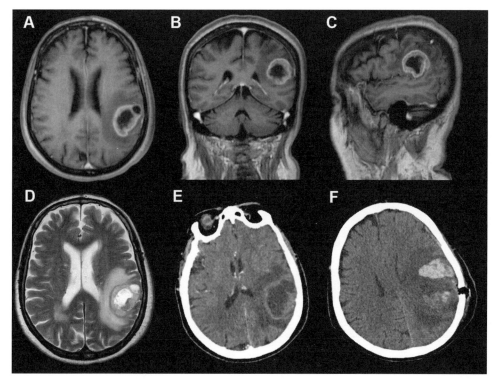

Figure 3.1 Grade IIIa complication posterior to a stereotactic biopsy procedure in an 81-year-old female with a Karnofsky ≤70 and a left fronto-temporal glioblastoma. (A), (B), and (C) demonstrate axial, coronal, and sagittal views, respectively, on a T1 enhanced MRI. (D) shows perilesional edema on axial T2 view. (E) represents a preoperative CT contrast scan. (F) shows a postoperative CT demonstrating intra- and peritumoral bleeding.

matter, venous congestion, and associated edema. In this stage, systemic hypertension can induce diffuse vasogenic edema and, where an abnormal extracellular environment prevails, it can cause cytotoxic edema owing to secondary metabolic brain damage. If this procedure is conducted on previously edematous tissue, the probability of ischemic damage is even higher. Spatulas should be used cautiously on previously contused tissue because they can cause hemorrhage in neural tissue under pressure, and extend initial contusions.

Development of ischemic or hemorrhagic lesions increases proportionally to the time that the spatula is in use, and varies largely according to the patient's age. In young patients, brain tolerance to large retraction is higher than in elderly patients as a consequence of elasticity, an older brain being less elastic and more likely to suffer contusions, intracerebral hematoma, or increased cerebral edema than a young one when exposed to this type of procedure.

External lumbar drainage, ventriculostomy, and the microsurgical opening of cisterns and fissures enable a controlled release of CSF thereby avoiding or minimizing the use of a spatula for a good exposure of the surgical area. By raising the patient's head, CBF and ICP decrease thus improving venous flow and relaxing brain tissue.

An excessively large craniotomy needlessly exposes healthy brain tissue and increases the likelihood of brain injuries during therapeutic surgical maneuvers. A small craniotomy in an edematous brain can cause neural tissue herniation as a result of the bone defect produced during the procedure, and may result in ischemic or hemorrhagic lesions in the cortex beneath the craniotomy edges as well as compromise the cortical venous drainage, which would increase the underlying edema further. After the craniotomy has been made, an excessive coagulation of the cortex to approach subcortical lesions can lead to necrosis and adjacent edema. An interhemispheric approach can cause acute thrombosis in the superior sagittal sinus (SSS), with varying clinical impact depending on localization. Surgical occlusion of the SSS is well tolerated when performed in the anterior third, i.e., anteriorly to the confluence of the Rolandic vein. Posterior anastomotic veins such as the vein of Trolard should be recognized and preserved. Closure

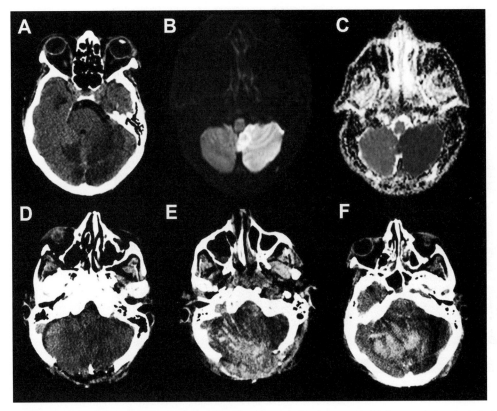

Figure 3.2 Grade IV complication in a 49-year-old male with a posterior fossa stroke. (A) shows an ischemic stroke in the left cerebellum hemisphere. (B) and (C) show diffusion and (A), (C), and (D) map views demonstrating the ischemic lesion. (D) shows a postoperative CT with the decompressive craniectomy. (E) and (F) represent hemorrhagic transformation of the ischemic lesion on CT scan.

of the SSS distal to the drainage of Rolandic veins is not commonly well tolerated, with bilateral ischemic venous infarction tending to be the norm rather than the exception. Improved quality of preoperative imaging and intraoperative image-guided navigation enable a better localization of subcortical lesions and help in limiting incisions of the cerebral cortex.

Closure-related complications

Closure is a vital stage in surgery as this time is characterized by frequent complications. A tidy hemostasis in the surgical site and Valsalva maneuvers previous to closure can reduce the development of hematoma within the surgical lodge. Decompression following excision of large lesions, e.g., tumor removal, can lead to superficial neural tissue sliding down into the resulting cavity. This downward shift of tissue can drag small epidural and subdural veins and cause EDH and/or SDH. These complications can be avoided by tacking up the dura to the craniotomy edges and by filling up the residual cavity with saline solution.

Intracranial hypertension that cannot be treated during surgery can become an obstacle for bone flap replacement. Management of this situation includes raising the patient's headrest, ensuring a good jugular venous return (it may be necessary to unlock the fixation headrest and rotate the patient's head to a more neutral position), and performing anesthesiological maneuvers (mannitol, hyperventilation, and cerebral suppression) to prevent cortical lacerations and increased edema because of compression of the superficial venous system. Should these maneuvers fail, an alternative would be enlarging the craniotomy to turn the approach into a decompressive craniectomy and a wide duroplasty, leaving the replacement of the bone flap for a subsequent second surgical procedure (Figure 3.3).

Complications associated with trauma surgery

Surgery after traumatic brain injury may be indicated to manage different conditions, such as acute or

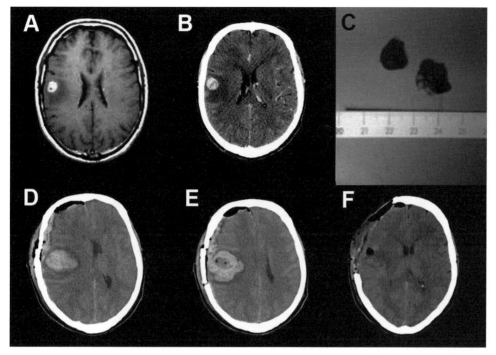

Figure 3.3 Grade IIIb complication in a 59-year-old male with a right frontal melanoma. (A) shows a hyperintense tumor on axial T1 weight contrast MRI. (B) demonstrates contrast on axial CT for neuronavigation. (C) shows the removed dark-colored tumor, 1 cm size. (D) and (E) demonstrate 48 hours postoperative lodge hematoma. (F) shows decompressive craniectomy and hematoma drainage.

chronic SDH, EDH, ICH, fractures, and edema refractory to medical treatment. Surgical management of chronic SDH is frequent in neurosurgery; as a consequence of sudden decompression, rapid evacuation of large SDH can result in traction of bridging veins and development of an acute ipsilateral or contralateral SDH (Figure 3.4). To avoid this, the opening of the dura must be as small as possible, and the SDH evacuated in a controlled manner. In a contused brain, evacuation of an acute traumatic SDH can lead to sudden reperfusion and cause venous or arterial hemorrhage as a result of the tamponade effect being released [11]. Dural tacking-up points and gradually paused decompression can prevent venous hemorrhage secondary to dural separation from the bone. Decompressive craniectomy may be indicated in malignant intracranial hypertension, which is generally associated with hemorrhagic contusions, brain herniation, and edema. This treatment per se is not associated with the postoperative development of new contusions or the growth of primary ones, and can be a life-saving procedure [12,13].

Complications associated with brain aneurysm surgery

The aim of surgical clipping or embolization of a brain aneurysm is to prevent its rupture or rebleeding, which have incidence rates in the case of ruptured aneurysm of 4% for the first day, 50% for the first six months, and 3% per year thereafter with an annual mortality of 2% [14]. Brain tissue reacts to subarachnoid hemorrhage (SAH) with vascular permeability changes, potentially leading to impaired autoregulation and vascular reactivity, which contribute to the development of cerebral edema. In this scenario, surgical maneuvers (deep retraction, transitory clipping, clip misplacement leading to relative arterial occlusion, manipulation causing vasospasm) are predisposing factors for late ischemia. In order to avoid excessive brain retraction, which is usually necessary in anterior communicating artery and basilar tip aneurysms, surgical maneuvers (ventriculostomy, external lumbar drainage, and opening of fissures and cisterns) or medical maneuvers (hyperventilation, mannitol or

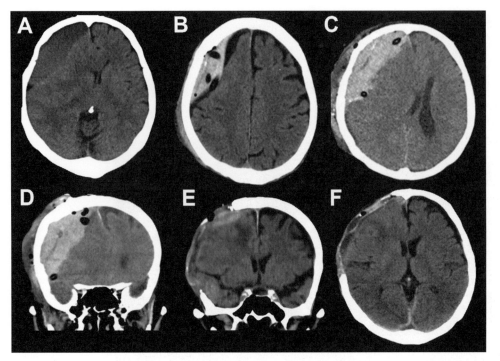

Figure 3.4 Grade IIIa complication in an 83-year-old male with a subacute subdural hematoma and thrombocytopenia. (A) shows a right frontal subacute hematoma on a CT scan. (B) represents a burr-hole evacuation, subdural drainage, and postoperative hemorrhage. (C) and (D) demonstrate progression of the acute postoperative subdural hematoma. (E) and (F) show coronal and axial CT views of a decompressive craniotomy performed to treat the SDH.

furosemide) should be used for cerebral relaxation, although several studies argue that these could increase the risk of rebleeding [15–17].

The intraoperative aneurysmatic rupture rate stands at 18% to 40% in old series, with frequency increasing during early surgical management [18,19]. This complication can be managed by applying small pieces of cotton, double suction, low-intensity bipolar coagulation, transitory clipping, and access to the internal carotid artery in the neck or partial frontal-temporal resections to gain proximal control, depending on aneurysm size, rupture, localization, and surgical stage (Figure 3.5).

Transitory clipping offers improved exposure of the aneurysm neck to fix or reposition the definitive clip; however, where the procedure extends beyond a given limit, ischemia can occur in the supplied territory. The clip can also cause mechanical damage to the vascular endothelium with progressive thromboembolic vascular occlusion occurring at clip removal. Even though it has not yet been proven in well designed multicenter studies, neuroprotecting agents (such as calcium channel blockers, free radical scavengers, mannitol, etc.), could be considered during this maneuver to minimize the toxic effects of ischemia without reducing the cerebral metabolic rate of oxygen consumption. Cerebral metabolic demand can be decreased by reducing neuronal electrical activity (with barbiturates, isoflurane). In a similar way, maintenance of neuronal energy could be decreased through alternatives such as hypothermia.

Postoperative ischemic or hemorrhagic complications following a misclipped aneurysm or occlusion of the afferent vessel or neighboring vessels can be prevented through routine intraoperative angiography.

Complications in arteriovenous malformation (AVM) surgery

Arteriovenous malformations (AVMs) are composed of a central nidus of abnormal vessels, wherein the arterial blood flows directly into draining veins with no capillary interposition. These vessels are angiographically, physiologically, and histologically different; they have a large lumen and extremely thin walls as a consequence of their adaptive and structural variation related to a chronic ischemic vascular bed. Prevalence is approximately 0.14%, with an

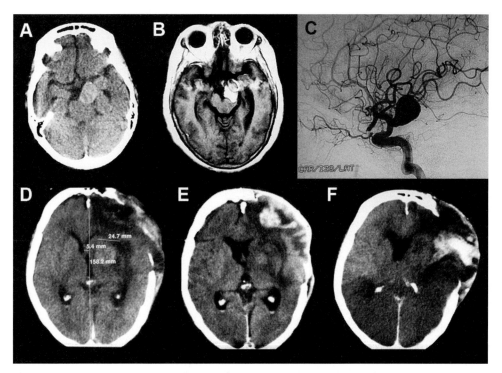

Figure 3.5 Grade IV complication in a 73-year-old female operated from a left posterior communicating artery (PoCA) aneurysm. (A) preoperative CT demonstrating an unruptured PoCA aneurysm. (B) and (C) represent an angio-MRI and angiography, respectively, showing the anatomical relationships and size of the aneurysm. (D) immediate postoperative CT obtained after aneurysm rupture and transitory proximal and distal clipping (20 minutes) during surgery. (E) and (F) show decompressive craniectomy and evolution of postoperative ischemia with hemorrhagic transformation and cerebral tissue herniation.

annual bleeding rate standing at 2% to 4% [20,21]. Therapeutic options include observation for unruptured AVMs, microsurgery for small malformations in non-eloquent areas, stereotactic radiosurgery for <3.5-cm deep lesions (although complete obliteration takes one to three years during which radiation necrosis edema and hemorrhage can occur), and embolization alone or combined with surgical management [22].

After excision of the arteriovenous shunt, the volume of some of the previously dilated vessels is reduced. However, in several cases, the vessels remain unchanged or even dilate and cause edema, hyperemia, and swelling of the hypoperfused area as a consequence of the resolution of the blood theft caused by the malformation. Most of the AVM feeding arteries are reactive to vasoactive substances (5TH, NT, PGE2) whereas a small subgroup shows no response or contraction in response to mechanical stimuli during surgical manipulation. Normal perfusion pressure breakthrough syndrome is a complication in most patients with this type of vessel. It is characterized by postoperative edema and hemorrhage secondary to impaired autoregulation [23]. Preoperative administration of propranolol 20 mg PO QID for three days can lower the risk of this postoperative adverse event. Occlusive hyperemia is another common complication resulting from the coagulation of draining veins in adjacent brain tissue or late thrombosis, which results in hemorrhagic or ischemic phenomena [24]. Partial excision of the vascular nidus considerably increases the risk of rebleeding, which can be reduced through exhaustive microsurgical revision, and intra- and postoperative angiographic monitoring.

Compared with microsurgery, radiosurgery alone and radiosurgery combined with previous embolization is associated with a higher risk of bleeding and complications [22].

Tumor surgery complications

Expansion of brain tissue after excision of large lesions can cause perilesional edema and increased intracranial pressure, which can be even higher than the hypertension caused by the tumor itself. This can be due to local acidosis in the tissue around the lesion causing vasomotor paralysis and subsequent impaired self-regulation, specifically after rapid surgical decompression. In this scenario, decompression followed by reperfusion of chronic ischemic tissue can lead to near or distant hemorrhagic infarcts. The residual cavity also includes an area of increased risk prone to postoperative hemorrhage because small vessels with transient vasospasm following surgical manipulation or narrow vessels may be excluded from hemostasis maneuvers after lesion removal. Procedures such as gradual excision of large tumor lesions, Valsalva maneuvers, and bringing systemic blood pressure up to the values the patient had before anesthetic induction while the surgical lodge is microscopically controlled can help reduce the probability of postoperative hematomas.

Intra- and postoperative stroke

The sensitivity for postoperative stroke depends largely on the effectiveness and thoroughness in the reporting of these adverse events. The assessment of surgical complications is an important tool in neurosurgical practice because it can improve safety and quality of patient care. The different views and definitions of what is considered a complication, coupled with the absence of a widely accepted classification of postoperative adverse events, may lead to a subjective interpretation of surgical negative outcomes.

We developed a classification of these adverse events focused on general postoperative morbidity. Complications were classified according to a four-grade severity scale based on the therapy administered to treat the adverse event [25] (Table 3.1). Grade I or mild complications were defined as any non-life-threatening deviation from the normal postoperative course that could be treated without invasive procedures. Grade I adverse events were divided into two subgroups based on the drug treatment required: Grade Ia complications included events with spontaneous resolution, requiring no drug treatment; Grade Ib complications included events requiring drug therapy. Grade II or moderate complications included adverse postoperative events requiring invasive management such as surgical, endoscopic, and/or endovascular procedures. Grade II events were also classified into two subgroups, depending on the need for general anesthesia: Grade IIa comprised complications treated without general anesthesia whereas Grade IIb comprised postoperative adverse events treated under general anesthesia. Grade III

Table 3.1 Classification of neurosurgical complications.

Grade I – Mild	Any non-life-threatening deviation from normal postoperative course, not requiring invasive treatment
Grade Ia	Complication requiring no drug treatment
Grade Ib	Complication requiring drug treatment
Grade II – Moderate	Complication requiring invasive treatment such as surgical, endoscopic, or endovascular interventions
Grade IIa	Complication requiring intervention without general anesthesia
Grade IIb	Complication requiring intervention with general anesthesia
Grade III – Life-threatening	Complications requiring management in intensive care unit
Grade IIIa	Complication involving single organ failure
Grade IIIb	Complication involving multiple organ failure
Grade IV	Complication resulting in death
Suffix "T" (transient)	New neurologic deficit improving within 30 days of surgical procedure; can be added to each grade of complication
Suffix "P" (persistent)	New neurologic deficit extending beyond 30 days of surgical procedure; can be added to each grade of complication

complications referred to life-threatening adverse events requiring treatment and care in a more complex hospital area, such as an intensive care unit (ICU). These adverse events were classified into Grade IIIa, which included single organ dysfunction, and Grade IIIb, which included multiple organ dysfunctions, a condition of severe morbidity constituting a most frequent cause of death. Grade IV included death as a result of complications.

This classification also enabled the diagnosis of new focal neurological findings (potential cerebral ischemic events), which were classified as "transient" – where improvement was achieved within 30 days after the procedure – and "persistent" – where they extended beyond that time period. The series of 2,431 neuro-surgeries considered for this study was conducted at the Hospital Italiano de Buenos Aires between 2008 and 2011. The global rate of complications of this series stood at 13.03% (n = 317). Stroke was a complication in 2.05% of the total number of procedures, hemorrhagic events being the most common (1.19%), followed by ischemic events (0.45%), and edematous events (0.41%). These adverse phenomena rarely appear in a pure form but rather in association, although we classified them separately according to their origin for description. Out of the total number of stroke-originated complications, 6% were mild or Grade 1, 10% moderate, 62% severe, and 22% of the patients died.

Postoperative care requires a multidisciplinary approach, which includes not only health personnel but also the patient and his/her family. Any adverse postoperative event must be managed jointly as a medical team, with one given spokesperson who communicates the health condition, the examinations performed and their results, or further procedures to be conducted. Early recognition and management of complications is the best chance to prevent further deterioration of the patient's clinical condition and to potentially achieve a quick and complete recovery.

References

1. Walker A E, Robins M, Weinfeld F D. The National Survey of Stroke: Clinical findings. *Stroke.* 1981; 12:13–44.

2. Kalfas I H, Little J R. Postoperative hemorrhage: a survey of 4992 intracranial procedures. *Neurosurgery.* 1988; 23: 343–7.

3. Palmer J D, Sparrow O C, Iannotti F I. Postoperative hematoma: A 5-year survey and identification of avoidable risk factors. *Neurosurgery.* 1994; 35: 1061–5.

4. MacMahon S, Rodgers A. Blood pressure, antihypertensive treatment and stroke risk. *J Hypertens Suppl.* 1994; 12: S5–14.

5. Cohen Y C, Djulbegovic B, Shamai-Lubovitz O, Mozes B. The bleeding risk and natural history of idiopathic thrombocytopenic purpura in patients with persistent low platelet counts. *Arch Intern Med.* 2000; 160: 1630–8.

6. Biller J, Feinberg W M, Castaldo J E, *et al.* Guidelines for carotid endarterectomy: A statement for healthcare professionals from a special writing group of the Stroke Council, American Heart Association. *Circulation.* 1998; 97: 501–9.

7. Feinberg W M, Albers G W, Barnett HJ, *et al.* Guidelines for the management of transient ischemic attacks. From the Ad Hoc Committee on Guidelines for the Management of Transient Ischemic Attacks of the Stroke Council of the American Heart Association. *Circulation.* 1994; 89: 2950–65.

8. Korinth M C. Low-dose aspirin before intracranial surgery – results of a survey among neurosurgeons in Germany. *Acta Neurochir.* 2006; 148: 1189–96.

9. Benveniste R, Germano I M. Evaluation of factors predicting accurate resections of high-grade gliomas by using frameless image-guided stereotactic guidance. *Neurosurgical Focus.* 2003; 14: e5.

10. Martin A, Rojas S, Chamorro A, *et al.* Why does acute hyperglycemia worsen the outcome for transient focal cerebral ischemia? Role of corticosteroids, inflammation, and protein O-glycosylation. *Stroke.* 2006; 37: 1288–95.

11. Nadig A S, King A T. Traumatic extradural haematoma revealed after contralateral decompressive craniectomy. *Br J Neurosurg.* 2012. www.ncbi.nlm.nih .gov/pubmed/22762248

12. Sturiale C L, De Bonis P, Rigante L, *et al.* Do traumatic brain contusions increase in size after decompressive craniectomy? *J Neurotrauma.* 2012; 29: 2723–26.

13. Walcott B P, Nahed B V, Sheth S A, *et al.* Bilateral hemicraniectomy in non-penetrating traumatic brain injury. *J Neurotrauma.* 2012; 29: 1879–85.

14. Winn H R, Richardson A E, Jane JA. The long-term prognosis in untreated cerebral aneurysm: A 10-year evaluation of 364 patients. *Ann Neurolog.* 1977; 1: 358–70.

15. Voldby B, Enevoldsen E M. Intracranial pressure changes following aneurysm rupture. Part 3: Recurrent hemorrhage. *J Neurosurg.* 1982; 56: 784–9.

16. Connolly E S Jr, Kader A A, Frazzini V I, Winfree C, Solomon R A. The safety of intraoperative lumbar drainage for acutely ruptured intracranial aneurysm: Technical note. *Surg Neurol.* 1997; 48: 338–44.

17. Rosenorn J, Westergaard L, Hansen P H. Mannitol induced rebleeding from intracranial aneurysm: Case report. *J Neurosurg.* 1983; 59: 529–30.

18. Graf C J, Nibbelink D W. Randomized treatment study: Intracranial surgery. In Sahs A L and Nibbelink D W, eds. *Aneurysm Subarachnoid Hemorrhage: Report of the Cooperative Study.* Baltimore: Urban and Schwarzenburg. 1981; 145–202.

19. Schramm J, Cedzich C. Outcome and management of intraoperative aneurysm rupture. *Surg Neurol.* 1993; 40: 26–30.

20. Ondra S L, Troupp H, George E D, Schwab K. The natural history of symptomatic arteriovenous malformations of the brain: A 24-year follow-up assessment. *J Neurosurg.* 1990; **73**: 387–91.

21. Kondziolka D, McLaughlin M R, Kestle J R W. Simple risk predictors for arteriovenous malformations hemorrhage. *Neurosurgery.* 1995; **37**: 851–5.

22. Baijim van Beijnum J, van der Worp H B, Buis D R, *et al.* Treatment of brain arteriovenous malformations: a systematic review and meta-analysis. *JAMA.* 2011; **306**: 2011–19.

23. Spetzler R F, Wilson C B, Weinstein P, *et al.* Normal perfusion pressure breakthrough theory. *Clin Neurosurg.* 1978; **25**: 651–72.

24. al-Rodhan N R, Sundt T M, Piepgras D G, *et al.* Occlusive hyperemia: A theory of the hemodynamic complications following resection of intracerebral arteriovenous malformations. *J Neurosurg.* 1993; **78**: 167–75.

25. Landriel Ibañez F A, Hem S, Ajler P, *et al.* A new classification of complications in neurosurgery. *World Neurosurg.* 2011; **75**: 709–15.

Vasospasm and delayed cerebral ischemia in aneurysmal subarachnoid hemorrhage

Fernando D. Goldenberg, Mario D. Terán and Federico Landriel

Introduction

It is known that patients with aneurysmal subarachnoid hemorrhage (aSAH) may develop neurological deficits due to focal or global ischemia of varying degrees secondary to delayed vasospasm. When the cerebral blood flow is insufficient to provide an adequate oxygen supply to the demanding brain tissue cell metabolism fails and if the availability of oxygen is not quickly restored cell death may occur due to ischemia. Because of this, one of the most important predictors of poor neurological outcome in patients suffering aSAH is delayed cerebral ischemia (DCI) mostly secondary to vasospasm [1].

Ecker and Riemenschneider described for the first time almost 50 years ago cerebral vasospasm after aneurysmal rupture by tracking patients with aSAH for about 30 days with serial imaging studies. The findings were widely accepted and it is now known that the development of cerebral vasospasm following aSAH is associated with high mortality and disability constituting one of the most important prognostic factors for outcome after aSAH. This complication occurs in up to 70% of affected patients with aSAH; however, it gives rise to clinical symptoms in only about 20% of patients with vasospasm diagnosed by cerebral angiography. Treatment of this condition has evolved dramatically and clinicians now have a wide arsenal of drugs and devices to treat this complication.

Traditionally, DCI has been attributed to a low-flow state secondary to proximal arterial spasm at the level of the circle of Willis. However, there are some findings that challenge this relatively simple concept: brain tissue infarct can be observed even in the absence of significant proximal spasm and despite successful early treatment of significant angiographic

vasospasm some patients may eventually develop cerebral ischemia [2]. Based on some of these apparently contradicting findings, the notion of simple proximal arterial spasm as the only cause of brain infarction and clinical deterioration may not be enough. Instead, the development of DCI and consecutive neurological impairment is most likely to be multifactorial.

In recent years, two important mechanisms occurring in the pre-vasospasm period of patients have been identified: early brain direct injury and diffuse cortical ischemia. Clinical observations and animal models have shown the presence, in varying degrees, of transient diffuse brain ischemia early after the bleeding [3,4] in the concurrent presence of oxyhemoglobin in the subarachnoid space. In addition to that, the blood–brain barrier disruption and the presence of early transient acute vasoconstriction with impaired cerebral perfusion may also be contributors to DCI in association with the already known proximal arterial spasm in aSAH [5].

Definition of vasospasm and delayed cerebral ischemia

Late neurological worsening in patients with aSAH has been classically associated with the presence of vasospasm; however, it can also be due to completely different mechanisms. On this basis it is important to define some concepts: DCI is a clinical diagnosis of new focal or global brain ischemia, or radiological evidence of recent cerebral ischemia not attributed to any other identified cause. This picture can be clinically silent especially in patients with poor-grade aSAH. Some series have reported up to 20% of patients with aSAH having evidence of ischemic lesions on brain computed tomography (CT) scan even though this was not even suspected clinically [6,7].

Treatment-Related Stroke, ed. Alexander Tsiskaridze, Arne Lindgren and Adnan Qureshi. Published by Cambridge University Press. © Cambridge University Press 2016.

Delayed cerebral ischemia may develop in the presence or absence of angiographic vasospasm and in many cases it may present with transient neurological deficit responding favorably to various treatments and thereby not resulting in an ischemic stroke.

Cerebral vasospasm is defined as a late (typically starting at or after day 4 after the onset of the bleeding) narrowing of cerebral arteries, predominantly in and around the circle of Willis. It may be associated with clinical or radiological signs of cerebral ischemia in the territories perfused by the involved vessels.

Angiographic vasospasm is present in about 70% of patients with aSAH, it typically starts after day 4 following the initial bleeding, reaches its peak between days 7 to 10 and may remit after two to three weeks, although 10% of the patients may show very early (within the first three days after the bleeding) vasospasm already present in the diagnostic angiogram [8]. Focal or global neurological deficits attributed to vasospasm occur in only half of patients with angiographic vasospasm, and of these, only 20% will evolve into an ischemic stroke.

Pathophysiology of arterial spasm and DCI in SAH

Delayed cerebral ischemia secondary to vasospasm in aSAH is the final event of a series of pathophysiological mechanisms occurring in the cerebral arterial vasculature. The main known involved factors include:

Oxyhemoglobin

Ferrous ions released from the oxyhemoglobin present in the blood clot in the subarachnoid space, which leads to delayed arterial spasm by multiple mechanisms. These include neuronal apoptosis [9], nitric oxide reduction [10], increased endothelin-1 levels [11], direct oxidative stress damage to the vascular smooth muscle [5], production of free radicals, peroxidation of cell membrane lipids [12], and modification of the calcium and potassium channels [13] among the most important.

In recent times, the role of oxidative stress has been emphasized as a major cause of vasospasm, probably by causing direct activation of calcium channels in the vascular smooth muscle. Oxygen free radicals acting on the arachidonic acid generate vasoactive lipids that will eventually constrict the smooth muscle [14]. Products generated by oxidative stress-induced oxidation of bilirubin may also promote vasoconstriction, but this mechanism is not entirely clear.

Oxidative stress in the subarachnoid space activates protein kinase C and Rho kinase, both with positive effects on the constriction of smooth muscle, cell proliferation, and generation of vascular smooth muscle hypertrophy leading to arterial remodeling as observed in vasospasm [15].

Endothelin-1

Endothelin-1 is a potent vasoconstrictor peptide; several studies have demonstrated the presence of high levels of this peptide in the cerebrospinal fluid of humans and animals with vasospasm secondary to aSAH [11,16]. The increase in endothelin-1 is mediated by several factors including the presence of oxyhemoglobin and leukocytes in the subarachnoid space and an increase in the synthesis of this peptide by astrocytes [17].

Nonetheless, arterial vasoconstriction can be observed in the absence of elevated levels of endothelin-1 and this mechanism would be mediated by an increase in the sensitivity of the endothelin-1 receptor in arteries. A recently published phase III clinical trial explored the use of a selective antagonist of endothelin-1 receptors (clazosentan) in patients with aSAH. Although a significant reduction in the incidence of angiographic vasospasm was noted, no significant difference in the clinical outcome as measured by disability and dependence by the modified Rankin scale was achieved [18].

Nitric oxide

Inhibition of vascular smooth muscle relaxation also contributes to vasospasm in aSAH and this is where the role of nitric oxide (NO) becomes important. Specifically in aSAH there is inhibition of neuronal NO synthase, dysfunction of endothelial NO synthase in cerebral arteries, and greater affinity of NO by the hemoglobin's *heme* molecule. These factors contribute to the NO "depletion" as a key pathophysiological component of vasospasm in aSAH [10]. Numerous studies have been undertaken, mainly in animals, with therapies based on the contribution of NO through genetic therapy [19], intrathecal, intra-arterial, and intravenous infusion of NO among others [20–22].

The important role of statins in NO regulation has been described recently; they increase the expression of endothelial NO synthase, the mechanism probably mediated by an increase in the activity of the endothelial synthase's mRNA after treatment with statins, which results in an increased synthesis of NO and improvement of the cerebral blood flow (CBF) [23]. In a retrospective study, patients receiving statins for at least one month before presenting with aSAH had a significantly lower incidence of vasospasm [24]. Another prospective, randomized study showed a lower incidence of vasospasm in patients treated with statins within 14 days of having suffered an aSAH [25].

Role of erythrocytes in the subarachnoid space

The decomposition products of erythrocytes dispersed into the subarachnoid space have been associated with the development of vasospasm in aSAH. The risk of vasospasm is related to the amount of blood in the subarachnoid space observed in the initial scan, and the time of initiation of the arterial narrowing coincides with the time of hemolysis of erythrocytes in the subarachnoid space, approximately four days. These metabolites generate an indirect inhibition of potassium channels, which promotes the entry of calcium into the intracellular space, increased synthesis of endothelin-1, and decreased synthesis of NO [4, 26].

Vascular cell membrane

The small diameter of the cerebral arteries (<200 μm) plays an important role in CBF autoregulation.

In aSAH, calcium channels encoded from a gene (CaV 2.3), called R-type voltage-dependent channels, are expressed, which leads to an increased passage of calcium to the intracellular space with subsequent vasoconstriction [27]. Another mechanism that increases intracellular calcium after aSAH is the depolarization of the cell membrane caused by the presence of oxyhemoglobin in the subarachnoid space, generating the suppression of voltage-dependent potassium channels, referred to as KV, that exchange potassium by calcium, and an increase in the production of a metabolite of the P450 cytochrome named 20-hydroxyarachidonic acid [28].

Membrane depolarization favored by the above-mentioned factors and an increased expression of calcium channels that facilitate the entry of the ion to the intracellular space generate vasoconstriction. At the same time, the decreased expression of L-type calcium channels restricts the usefulness of agents such as nimodipine, which are acting exactly on these channels for the treatment of vasospasm.

Early brain injury in aSAH

One of the most important developments in recent years is the recognition of early brain injury after aSAH generated by the impact of the initial bleeding and its detrimental effect on patient outcomes.

The term "early cerebral damage" refers to the diffuse brain injury that happens within the first 72 hours after bleeding, i.e., before the development of vasospasm. This injury includes a rise in intracranial pressure, overall reduction of CBF, impaired blood–brain barrier, cerebral edema, and eventually neuronal death [29].

The decrease in cerebral perfusion pressure that occurs after the aneurysm rupture has been described by Nornes in the past [3]; however, its negative impact on the final outcome of affected patients has been better understood recently. Many times, after aneurysmal rupture, transient circulatory arrest can ensue due to severe intracranial hypertension and lead to diffuse transient cerebral ischemia with a potentially lethal effect. If the patient survives this stage, a second ischemic insult may result from the alteration of the blood–brain barrier leading to development of global cerebral edema, increased intracranial pressure, decreased CBF, and neuronal death [5].

Cortical spreading depression

Cortical spreading depression (SD) can be described as a low-voltage electrical negative variation that starts as a transient depolarization in the ischemic core followed by spreading through the metabolically compromised ischemic penumbra, heading towards the surrounding healthy tissue. It usually occurs as a temporal cluster of repeated events, lasting for eight to ten minutes and traveling at a speed of 2 to 3 mm/minute.

During experimentally induced SD there is an increase in the CBF to compensate for high metabolic demands. Cortical spreading depression causes neuronal damage by increasing the mismatch between energetic demands and O_2 availability, exacerbating ischemia.

By applying to animals a biological fluid similar to cerebrospinal fluid obtained from animals with SAH on the subarachnoid space, Dreier [26] showed the presence of depolarization waves diffusely throughout the cortex with subsequent generation of microvascular spasm followed by ischemia and resulting in diffuse cortical necrosis. This finding was similar to that observed in histopathological studies of brain tissue obtained at autopsy from patients who died of aSAH [30].

Another prospective multicenter study by Dreier in patients with aSAH showed the presence of diffuse cortical depolarization waves that were associated with the presence of DCI. These recordings were obtained by electrocorticography through subdural electrodes placed during the operation. These depolarization waves were more frequent within the first seven days of bleeding and the analysis of these results showed that the diffuse cortical necrosis was present in early stages of the disease [31].

Microthrombosis

There is a growing interest in the role that platelets and the coagulation system play in DCI. Platelet aggregation can produce micro infarcts and compromise distal cerebral blood flow and this has been shown in postmortem studies in patients with aSAH [32].

Apoptosis

Endothelial cell apoptosis seems to be a mechanism linked to the rupture of the blood–brain barrier,

development of cerebral edema, and secondary lesions associated with aSAH [33].

Predictors of vasospasm in aSAH

Scores based on initial CT findings, such as the original Fisher scale, were developed in order to predict the risk of cerebral vasospasm following aSAH. Three commonly used scales for prediction of vasospasm and DCI in aSAH are shown in Table 4.1.

There is a relationship between vasospasm and subarachnoid blood volume and lately an association between intraventricular blood volume and vasospasm has also been described. Other factors that may increase the incidence of vasospasm include: age less than 60 years, poor initial neurological status, fever, hypovolemia, dehydration, electrolyte imbalance, hypotension, and the location of the aneurysm [7].

Diagnosis and monitoring of cerebral vasospasm

The gold standard method for identification of cerebral vasospasm has been cerebral digital subtraction angiography (DSA), an invasive method, relatively expensive and not always available immediately. It entails some risk of contrast-induced nephropathy, vascular injury, and eventually stroke, therefore the

Table 4.1 Three commonly used scales for prediction of vasospasm and delayed cerebral ischemia (DCI) in aneurysmal subarachnoid hemorrhage (SAH).

Grade	Fisher [34]	Kistler [35]	Claasen [36]
0	–	–	Neither SAH nor IVH. **Very low risk of DCI.**
1	No blood seen on CT. **Low risk of VSP.**	No blood seen on CT.	Minimal SAH or thin, diffuse SAH without IVH. **Low risk of DCI (12%).**
2	Diffuse SAH (vertical layers <1 mm thickness). **Low risk of VSP.**	Diffuse SAH (vertical layers <1 mm thickness).	Minimal SAH with IVH in both lateral ventricles. **Intermediate risk of DCI (21%).**
3	Localized clot and/or thick vertical layers of blood (>1 mm thickness). **High risk of VSP.**	Clot bigger than 1 mm thickness in the vertical plane or bigger than 5 × 3 m in the horizontal plane. **High risk of VSP.**	Thick cisternal clot without IVH. **Intermediate risk of DCI (19%).**
4	Diffuse SAH or no blood but with IVH or intraparenchymal clot. **Low risk of VSP.**	Diffuse SAH with intraparenchymal clot or IVH, without blood in the basal cisterns.	Thick cisternal clot with IVH in both lateral ventricles. **High risk of DCI (40%).**

IVH: intraventricular hemorrhage.

detection and monitoring of cerebral vasospasm can be relatively complicated. It is clear that not all patients with aSAH should undergo serial cerebral DSA for the detection and monitoring of vasospasm and some recently issued guidelines have addressed the proper monitoring of those patients who develop vasospasm [37,38].

Transcranial Doppler ultrasonography (TCD)

This method was developed in the 1980s for the detection and monitoring of cerebral vasospasm. It utilizes the Doppler effect and can indirectly infer the vessel diameter and calculate the velocity of blood flow through transcranial ultrasonographic insonation of the major intracranial arteries of the base of the skull. Due to the fact that it is an indirect method, the measurement of the vessel diameters and flow rates may be altered or influenced by various features of the patient or the operator's experience.

Roughly 30% of the patients may have anatomical characteristics such as the thickness of the bone or the soft tissue that may compromise the correct insonation. Apart from these caveats, TCD is a very useful method for the detection and monitoring of cerebral vasospasm.

It is estimated that this method has a sensitivity of 38% to 91%, a specificity of 94% to 100%, a positive predictive value of 83% to 100%, and a negative predictive value of 29% to 98% for the detection of vasospasm [37]. Based on this it is important to understand that isolated TCD measurements can have good specificity but poor sensitivity and it is therefore appropriate to perform serial measurements to obtain a trend of values [39].

Since 2004, the criteria established by the American Academy of Neurology (AAN) for the diagnosis of cerebral vasospasm by TCD have been used: mean flow velocity greater than 120 cm/second, a rising flow velocity above 50 cm/second between two consecutive measurements, and a Lindegaard Index of greater than 6. The Lindegaard Index refers to the relationship between the mean flow velocity of the middle cerebral artery on one side and the mean flow velocity of the extracranial portion of the ipsilateral internal carotid artery [40] (Table 4.2).

As mentioned above, isolated TCD measurements can lead to incorrect results and inadequate interpretations. Often the diagnosis of vasospasm is made by this method when patients have presented any signs of neurological impairment due to hypoperfusion or ischemia, so that serial measurements in patients with

Table 4.2 Transcranial Doppler and CT perfusion criteria for vasospasm.

Modality	Criteria
Transcranial Doppler	Mean middle cerebral artery (MCA) flow velocity <120 cm/s is consistent with absence of vasospasm. Mean MCA flow velocity >120 cm/s is consistent with vasospasm. Lindegaard Index (MCA/internal carotid artery ratio) >6 is consistent with vasospasm. Rapid rise in MCA mean flow velocity (>50 cm/s increase between measurements[a]) is consistent with vasospasm.
CT perfusion	**Mean transit time > 6.4 s may be additive to CT angiography predicting DCI.**

Data from [38,40].
[a] It is common to perform measurements with about 12 to 24 hour intervals.

a high clinical suspicion of vasospasm are necessary for evaluation of findings obtained by using this method.

Digital cerebral angiography

Cerebral DSA has constituted the gold standard method for the diagnosis of cerebral vasospasm. As already mentioned it is, however, invasive, relatively expensive, and not always available immediately. Its use for the diagnosis of vasospasm should be reserved for those patients who have high clinical suspicion of vasospasm and for those in which other diagnostic techniques are not sufficient for some other reason (Figure 4.1). It is noteworthy that in patients with aSAH who develop new neurological deficits, DSA can confirm the diagnosis of vasospasm and also offer in situ therapeutic alternatives.

CT angiography and CT brain perfusion

The methods for measurement of cerebral perfusion and arterial diameter by CT are relatively new and less invasive techniques (in comparison with DSA) and can serve as tools for the diagnosis and monitoring of cerebral vasospasm and risk for developing brain

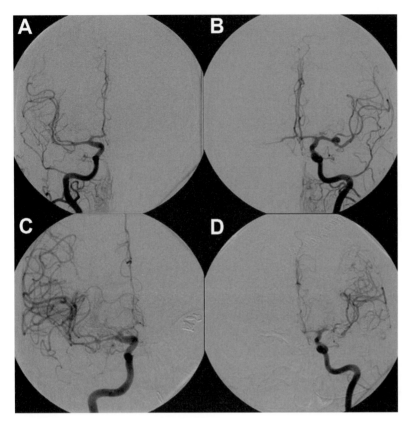

Figure 4.1 Cerebral digital subtraction angiography. (A) and (B) demonstrate right and left internal carotid artery injections at day 1 after rupture of a left middle cerebral artery bifurcation aneurysm. (C) and (D) show the same arterial injections at day 8 after bleeding with signs of significant angiographic vasospasm at both right and left proximal middle and anterior cerebral arteries.

ischemia. A recent meta-analysis evaluating the accuracy of CT angiography [41] as a method for cerebral vasospasm detection and tracking showed a sensitivity of about 80% and a specificity of 93%. However, the utility of this method in predicting the development of vasospasm-associated cerebral ischemia was limited [42].

Computed tomography perfusion requires iodinated contrast infusion to calculate cerebral blood flow (CBF), mean transit time (MTT), time to peak (TTP), and cerebral blood volume (CBV) in the cerebral hemispheres. Brain ischemia and areas of hypoperfusion can be detected by comparisons between the hemispheres and by measuring absolute values of CBF, MTT, and CBV (see Table 4.2). In a meta-analysis by Greenberg [42], CT perfusion showed a sensitivity of 74% and a specificity of 93% for the diagnosis of cerebral vasospasm and brain ischemia in SAH (Figure 4.2). Like CT angiography, the predictive value of delayed cerebral ischemia with perfusion CT is still uncertain.

From a practical standpoint, CT angiography and perfusion CT are useful tools for the diagnosis and management of cerebral vasospasm in patients where conventional methods such as TCD have non-specific or dubious results or when the new neurological deficits cannot be adequately explained.

In the vast majority of cases of aSAH, the affected vessels are the ones comprising the circle of Willis, and vasospasm usually arises in these arteries. Nonetheless there are times when vasospasm occurs diffusely or even affects distal, second, and third order arterial branches. In these cases the value of TCD and CT angiography for its diagnosis may be limited.

Monitoring DCI

While radiological examinations are important for the diagnosis and monitoring of cerebral vasospasm, their usefulness to predict the development of DCI is uncertain. Radiologic studies offer a temporal snapshot of the vascular diameters and (in the case of CT perfusion) cerebral perfusion. Therefore the clinical examination remains the best tool for the diagnosis and monitoring of cerebral ischemia as well as to assess the clinical response when some therapy is implemented.

Unlike imaging studies, clinical assessments can be carried out in a serial manner and provide real-time information on each intervention. In patients with good-grade aSAH (Hunt & Hess grade 1–2), frequent neurological examination allows early detection of new neurological deficits or clinical signs that can indicate the presence of cerebral vasospasm and ischemia. In those with poor-grade aSAH

Table 4.3 Potential signs of incipient delayed cerebral ischemia.

New focal neurologic deficit.
Unexplained global decline in Glasgow Coma Scale.
Unexplained increase in mean arterial pressure.
Increasing TCD flow velocities.
Unsuspected evidence of stroke on CT or MRI.
Angiographic worsening of known vasospasm.
EEG signs of new focal ischemia.
Focal signs of brain tissue hypoxia or metabolic failure on multimodal intracranial monitoring.

Data from [43].

(Hunt & Hess grade 3–5) the sensitivity of the clinical examination for the detection of DCI is lower, especially for those who are comatose. In these patients multimodal neurological monitoring may be needed to detect a worsening of the patient's condition (Table 4.3).

Currently there are various forms of neurological monitoring that include continuous electroencephalography, brain tissue oximetry, cerebral microdialysis, thermal diffusion flowmetry, near-infrared spectroscopy, and more. Although the literature of each of these forms of monitoring is emerging, current evidence is insufficient to recommend their use on a routine basis [44].

Prevention of DCI

Aneurysmal subarachnoid hemorrhage is often accompanied by specific endocrine disorders. The most frequently observed complication is hypovolemic hyponatremia; this condition called cerebral salt wasting syndrome (CSWS) was, until several years ago, confused with the syndrome of inappropriate secretion of antidiuretic hormone (SIADH) and was therefore sometimes treated with fluid restriction. These patients when treated with water restriction

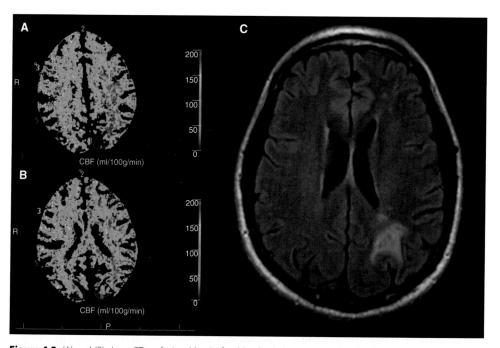

Figure 4.2 (A) and (B) show CT perfusion (day 9 after bleeding) showing significantly reduced cerebral blood flow (CBF) in most of the left middle cerebral artery distribution territory due to vasospasm. (C) demonstrates brain MRI, FLAIR sequence (day 20 after bleeding), showing a small residual subcortical infarct in the left parietal lobe after successful medical treatment with induced arterial hypertension.

far more often had DCI with a subsequent worse prognosis. Based on these findings, one of the pillars for the prevention of DCI has been the prevention of hypovolemia and maintenance of a euvolemic state.

Several pharmacological agents have been studied for the prevention of vasospasm especially for antagonizing smooth muscle contraction. Of these, nimodipine is currently the only agent approved in the United States by the Food and Drug Administration (FDA) for the prevention of cerebral vasospasm in aSAH.

Nimodipine

Calcium antagonists have been extensively studied as neuroprotection agents and for the prevention of cerebral vasospasm and DCI in aSAH. In clinical studies, blocking calcium channels inhibits vascular smooth muscle contraction. However, in these studies there was not a significant decrease of angiographic vasospasm in patients receiving oral nimodipine.

Despite these findings, patients receiving oral nimodipine have been shown to have better clinical results and outcome [45].

The recommended nimodipine dose is 60 mg PO every 4 hours for 21 days or for shorter time if the patient is discharged earlier [46]. For patients who present with hypotension or hemodynamic disturbances associated with its administration, an alternative is to give 30 mg PO every 2 hours if tolerated.

Permissive arterial hypertension

Once the aneurysm is excluded from the cerebral circulation, the therapeutic approach is focused on the prevention of DCI and maintenance of an adequate cerebral perfusion pressure. A sudden, unexplained increase in blood pressure can be an early sign of vasospasm or cerebral ischemia. While blood pressure targets should be tailored to each patient's background, it is not recommended to use antihypertensive agents in aSAH patients with vasospasm unless the blood pressure is extremely high or there is evidence of end-organ damage [43]. In patients chronically receiving beta-blockers for the management of blood pressure, abrupt discontinuation of these agents is not recommended unless they present with severe hypotension. Use of vasopressor drugs prophylactically in patients without evidence of vasospasm or cerebral ischemia has not shown better results and should not be used [47,48].

Prevention of hypovolemia

Depletion of intravascular volume in patients with aSAH is harmful. Multiple studies have shown that hypovolemia is associated with an increased incidence of cerebral ischemia and higher risk of late mortality [49]. Taking into account the negative effects of pronounced hypervolemia and hypovolemia, current clinical practice focuses on maintaining euvolemia. However, the determination of intravascular volume status is difficult to assess in critically ill patients. Maintaining an adequate and strict intake–output fluid balance and taking into account insensible fluid losses related to fever and tachypnea are important.

There are multiple non-invasive cardiac output monitoring devices commercially available but their routine use for the prevention of DCI in patients without significant hemodynamic compromise has not been proved.

Other measures to prevent DCI

There are very active ongoing research efforts regarding prevention of DCI associated with aSAH. Examples are the use of continuous intravenous infusion of magnesium acting as a blocker of calcium channels to inhibit vascular smooth muscle contraction. There have been some early promising results [50] but a recent randomized trial did not show improved results with its use [51].

Statins have also been broadly studied but recent data have not shown a convincing association between early initiation of statins therapy and reduced incidence of DCI [52]. As previously mentioned, a study using clazosentan, a selective antagonist of endothelin receptors, did not show better clinical outcomes when compared with placebo [18].

Another clinical trial using prophylactic mechanical angioplasty in the proximal segment of the cerebral arteries showed less need for subsequent treatment of vasospasm but an unacceptably high incidence of complications associated with the procedure and therefore prophylactic angioplasty for the prevention of DCI is not recommended [38,53].

Treatment of DCI

A main goal of treatment is to prevent DCI, the main determinant of long-term outcome after aSAH. Reaching this goal depends on an adequate assessment and interpretation of early symptoms and signs that precede the development of cerebral ischemia. Their

Table 4.4 Suggested treatment of delayed cerebral ischemia. For details, please see text.

Recommendation	Class of evidence	Level of evidence
Oral nimodipine is indicated to reduce poor outcome related to aneurysmal subarachnoid hemorrhage.	I	A
Induction of hypertension unless blood pressure is elevated at baseline or cardiac status precludes it.	I	B
Cerebral angioplasty or selective intra-arterial vasodilator therapy is reasonable in patients with symptomatic cerebral vasospasm, particularly those who are not rapidly responding to hypertensive therapy.	IIa	B
Alternatively, cerebral angioplasty and/or selective intra-arterial vasodilator therapy may be reasonable after, together, or in place of triple-H therapy, depending on the clinical scenario.	IIb	B

Triple-H: hypervolemia, hypertension, and hemodilution.
Adapted from the American Heart Association recommendations [37].

timely and proper recognition allow for adequate selection of therapeutic strategies for the prevention of ischemic stroke (see Table 4.4).

Delayed cerebral ischemia prophylaxis in asymptomatic patients with measures such as induced hypervolemia, hypertension, and prophylactic angioplasty have shown a high rate of complications and no significant clinical benefit [53].

It is essential to reserve aggressive treatments for patients with signs or symptoms of cerebral vasospasm and ischemia, such as the presence of new neurological deficits, sudden and unexplained increase in blood pressure coupled with a significant increase in mean flow velocities measured by TCD, or worsening of angiographic vasospasm [43].

Hemodynamic management

The classical treatment of vasospasm known as "triple-H" (hypervolemia, hypertension, and hemodilution), despite its popularity, has controversial evidence regarding effectiveness.

The focus of this strategy is to optimize cerebral perfusion pressure (CPP) by increasing the preload to the right chambers of the heart (hypervolemia), increasing the mean arterial pressure with vasopressor agents (hypertension), and improving the rheological properties of the blood (hemodilution). It is currently known that excessive intravenous fluid intake may worsen cerebral edema and increase the risk of fluid overload with consequent lung injury, and that uncontrolled hemodilution can trigger

ischemia by reducing the ability for transporting oxygen [54].

The induction of hypertension is the main component for the treatment of vasospasm and for the prevention of DCI. When cerebral autoregulation is intact, the brain is able to maintain a stable CBF even within a wide variation of mean arterial blood pressure. However in vasospasm, cerebral autoregulation is impaired and in a substantial proportion of patients is abolished to a large extent. Under these circumstances the relationship between CBF and mean arterial blood pressure or CPP becomes linear, i.e., increases in mean arterial blood pressure generate a secondarily increased CBF, whereas declines in mean arterial blood pressure lead to decreased CBF elevating the risk of cerebral ischemia [55].

The recommended target value of mean arterial blood pressure varies widely in the literature, and differs considerably between treating physicians. While some prefer to accept standardized numerical values (e.g., systolic blood pressure between 180 and 220 mmHg and mean arterial blood pressure between 110 and 140 mmHg) others opt for a percentage increase of blood pressure above a baseline (e.g., mean arterial blood pressure 10% or 20% above baseline) [56].

In patients with a ruptured aneurysm that also have other aneurysm(s) that have not bled, augmentation of the blood pressure for treating vasospasm seems to be safe once the ruptured aneurysm has been excluded from the circulation [57].

The Neurocritical Care Society consensus recommends the induction of hypertension in patients with aSAH (once the ruptured aneurysm has been excluded) who develop cerebral vasospasm, with a target blood pressure based on the patient's clinical response while carefully watching for the appearance of treatment-related adverse effects. They also recommend considering the temporary suspension of nimodipine if it interferes with the patient's positive clinical response to induced hypertension [38].

Regarding the vasopressor agents used for blood pressure augmentation, there is a wide range of possibilities including dopamine, noradrenaline, phenylephrine, and epinephrine. The choice of agent depends on the clinical characteristics of each particular patient. The peripheral vasoconstrictor activity of these drugs is associated with a variable inotropic effect. The medical team must quickly identify the patient's hemodynamic status and choose the most appropriate vasoactive agent to use.

Until recently, hypervolemia was a mainstay in the treatment of cerebral vasospasm and numerous observational studies focused on the effect of hypervolemia on CBF and the reversal of neurological deficits. However, the results obtained were variable and although there was an increase of CBF, the volume of fluids needed to achieve this status was significantly high. Probably parts of the unwanted responses observed in these studies could be explained by variations in the pretreatment hemodynamic status of the patients: as an example, the response to volume expansion with a fixed amount of fluids was probably suboptimal in previously volume-depleted patients. Because of the potential adverse effects of hypervolemia, euvolemia is currently recommended as a therapeutic target.

Another very important parameter to consider is the cardiac index (cardiac output in relation to body surface area). In normal conditions, the cerebral autoregulation will maintain a stable CBF even with significant variations in cardiac index. However, as mentioned earlier, in most cases of SAH cerebral autoregulation is severely compromised and as with mean arterial blood pressure changes, the relationship between the cardiac index and CBF then becomes linear. Inotropic support, through augmenting the cardiac index, may increase the CBF in those cases where only blood pressure elevation is insufficient [54]. Dobutamine and milrinone are inotropic agents that can be used if necessary. From a practical point of view inotropic support may be a valid strategy for the treatment of cerebral vasospasm and for the prevention of DCI mainly in the following groups of patients: (a) euvolemic patients with poor baseline systolic heart function (congestive heart failure, history of cardiomyopathy, and acute neurogenic heart failure), (b) patients who are already spontaneously hypertensive with simultaneous normal-low cardiac index, (c) patients who do not improve clinically despite induced arterial hypertension, and (d) those with a ruptured but not treated or partially treated aneurysm in which inducing arterial hypertension could lead to an increased risk of aneurysm re-rupture and therefore increasing the cardiac index without significantly elevating the blood pressure could be a reasonable option.

Although hemodilution is a strategy that is part of the classic triple-H, anemia is independently associated with worse outcomes in aSAH [58]. The hemoglobin concentration needed to ensure a proper balance between blood viscosity and oxygen-carrying capacity is not well defined. In a recent study a hemoglobin level between 10 and 11.5 g/dL was associated with better outcomes. Although the study was not designed to determine the optimal hemoglobin concentration, patients with the previously mentioned values had a lower incidence of ischemic stroke [59].

The Neurocritical Care Society recommends maintaining a hemoglobin concentration between 8 and 10 g/dL; however, in patients who develop severe vasospasm and are at high risk of DCI the target value should be slightly higher [38].

Pharmacological treatment and angioplasty

The precise timing of initiation of therapy for treatment of arterial vasospasm has not yet been clearly defined. A retrospective study demonstrated that an adequate clinical response to medical treatment within two hours of initiation of the clinical deterioration was independently associated with lower mortality and better functional outcomes in aSAH patients with vasospasm [60]. Another retrospective study evaluated early endovascular treatment response. Corresponding results were obtained and patients with signs of cerebral ischemia associated with vasospasm receiving endovascular treatment within two hours of onset of symptoms, had better outcome compared with patients in whom endovascular therapy was initiated later on [61].

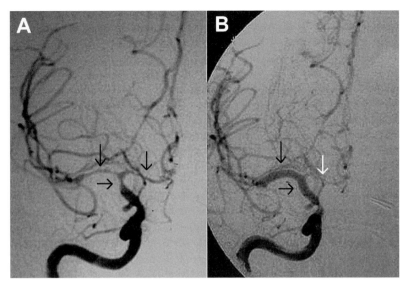

Figure 4.3 Cerebral digital subtraction angiography, right internal carotid artery injection. (A) Shows severe vasospasm in the terminal internal carotid artery (ICA), proximal middle cerebral artery (MCA), and anterior cerebral artery (ACA) (black arrows). (B) Same projection post balloon angioplasty showing very significant caliber improvement of the terminal ICA and proximal MCA (black arrows). Severe vasospasm remains in the proximal ACA where angioplasty was not performed (white arrow).

The above results indicate that patients who do not respond to medical treatment in a reasonable period of time (of about two hours) should be considered candidates for endovascular treatment.

Similarly, patients who have a contraindication to receive a complete and aggressive medical treatment should be considered for early endovascular treatment.

Intra-arterial injection of vasodilators requires an angiographic study to identify regions of significant cerebral vasospasm that match the patient's clinical deficit. Intra-arterial infusion of vasodilators can be used in the presence of symptomatic diffuse, or multi-vessel, or distal vasospasm.

Papaverine, a vasodilator alkaloid, was earlier widely used for endovascular treatment of vasospasm; however, its short duration of action requires repeated infusions and therefore increased risk of complications associated with repeated cerebrovascular instrumentations [61] and risk of inducing intracranial hypertension during the infusions.

Although there is no drug currently approved by the FDA for intra-arterial treatment of cerebral vasospasm, calcium channel blockers such as nicardipine and verapamil are frequently used for this purpose.

Verapamil, an L-type calcium channel blocker, is intra-arterially administered in aliquots. Despite its intra-arterial administration, verapamil enters the systemic circulation and may cause increased intracranial pressure, reduced blood pressure, and heart rate decrease. These effects are more frequent during rapid infusions and may last several hours [62].

Nicardipine, a dihydropyridine calcium channel blocker, is also infused in aliquots [63]. It has less effect on intracranial pressure but generates hypotension more often than verapamil. Intra-arterial infusion of milrinone has demonstrated a vasodilator effect in patients with cerebral vasospasm and has been tested primarily in diffuse or distal vasospasm, but evidence of its results is limited [64].

Percutaneous transluminal balloon angioplasty is probably the most durable intervention that increases the vascular diameter (Figure 4.3). The associated risks of arterial dissection, arterial rupture, and distal embolization are relatively high and their consequences can be potentially devastating. This procedure is indicated for proximal and sometimes regional vasospasm and is most commonly used on the intracranial internal carotid artery and middle cerebral artery [65].

Although there can be re-stenosis of the treated vessels by angioplasty, the incidence of this phenomenon is low and the need for re-interventions is uncommon.

Duration of treatment

It is known that the period of time in which a patient with aSAH can develop serious complications often extends until about day 21 and also that many of these patients do not require aggressive therapy throughout this whole period. Often determining the right time to begin phasedown of treatments already in place is more difficult than defining when to initiate them.

Conclusions

As described in this chapter, one of the main goals of treatment in aSAH besides excluding the ruptured aneurysm from the circulation is to prevent the development of cerebral ischemia and avoid poor outcomes in this serious medical condition. Surprisingly there is little literature that specifically guides the clinician in the stepwise reduction of therapeutic measures. This fact may sometimes lead to overtreatment or unnecessarily prolonged hospitalization.

Frequent detailed neurological examination, critical thinking, and judicious use of ancillary tests help the clinician in determining the optimal timing of initiation and de-escalation of therapies. Very frequent reassessment of the clinical results obtained after treatment changes is essential to guide the next step.

References

1. Rosengart A J, Schultheiss K E, Tolentino J, Macdonald R L. Prognostic factors for outcome in patients with aneurysmal subarachnoid hemorrhage. *Stroke.* 2007; **38**: 2315–21.

2. Rabinstein A A, Weigand S, Atkinson J L, Wijdicks E F. Patterns of cerebral infarction in aneurysmal subarachnoid hemorrhage. *Stroke.* 2005; **36**: 992–7.

3. Nornes H. The role of intracranial pressure in the arrest of hemorrhage in patients with ruptured intracranial aneurysm. *J Neurosurg.* 1973; **39**: 226–34.

4. Dreier J P, Ebert N, Priller J, et al. Products of hemolysis in the subarachnoid space inducing spreading ischemia in the cortex and focal necrosis in rats: A model for delayed ischemic neurological deficits after subarachnoid hemorrhage? *J Neurosurg.* 2000; **93**: 658–66.

5. Ostrowski R P, Colohan A R, Zhang J H. Molecular mechanisms of early brain injury after subarachnoid hemorrhage. *Neurol Res.* 2006; **28**: 399–414.

6. Vergouwen M D, Vermeulen M, van Gijn J, et al. Definition of delayed cerebral ischemia after aneurysmal subarachnoid hemorrhage as an outcome event in clinical trials and observational studies: Proposal of a multidisciplinary research group. *Stroke.* 2010; **41**: 2391–5.

7. Schmidt J M, Wartenberg K E, Fernandez A, et al. Frequency and clinical impact of asymptomatic cerebral infarction due to vasospasm after subarachnoid hemorrhage. *J Neurosurg.* 2008; **109**: 1052–9.

8. Baldwin M E, Macdonald R L, Dezheng H, et al. Early vasospasm on admission angiography in patients with aneurysmal subarachnoid haemorrhage is a predictor for in-hospital complications and poor outcome. *Stroke.* 2004; **35**: 2506–11.

9. Cahill J, Calvert J W, Zhang J H. Mechanisms of early brain injury after subarachnoid hemorrhage. *J Cereb Blood Flow Metab.* 2006; **26**: 1341–53.

10. Pluta R M. Delayed cerebral vasospasm and nitric oxide: Review, new hypothesis, and proposed treatment. *Pharmacol Ther.* 2005; **105**: 23–56.

11. Seifert V, Loffler B M, Zimmermann M, Roux S, Stolke D. Endothelin concentrations in patients with aneurysmal subarachnoid hemorrhage. Correlation with cerebral vasospasm, delayed ischemic neurological deficits, and volume of hematoma. *J Neurosurg.* 1995; **82**: 55–62.

12. Sehba F A, Bederson J B. Mechanisms of acute brain injury after subarachnoid hemorrhage. *Neurol Res.* 2006; **28**: 381–98.

13. Turner C P, Bergeron M, Matz P, et al. Heme oxygenase-1 is induced in glia throughout brain by subarachnoid hemoglobin. *J Cereb Blood Flow Metab.* 1998; **18**: 257–73.

14. Dietrich H H, Dacey R G, Jr. Molecular keys to the problems of cerebral vasospasm. *Neurosurgery.* 2000; **46**: 517–30.

15. Nishizawa S, Laher I. Signaling mechanisms in cerebral vasospasm. *Trends Cardiovasc Med.* 2005; **15**: 24–34.

16. Zimmermann M, Seifert V. Endothelin and subarachnoid hemorrhage: An overview. *Neurosurgery.* 1998; **43**: 863–75.

17. Fassbender K, Hodapp B, Rossol S, et al. Endothelin-1 in subarachnoid hemorrhage: An acute-phase reactant produced by cerebrospinal fluid leukocytes. *Stroke.* 2000; **31**: 2971–5.

18. Macdonald R L, Higashida R T, Keller E, et al. Randomized trial of clazosentan in patients with aneurysmal subarachnoid hemorrhage undergoing endovascular coiling. *Stroke.* 2012; **43**: 1463–9.

19. Luders J C, Weihl C C, Lin G, et al. Adenoviral gene transfer of nitric oxide synthase increases cerebral blood flow in rats. *Neurosurgery.* 2000; **47**: 1206–14.

20. Clatterbuck R E, Gailloud P, Tierney T, et al. Release of a nitric oxide donor for the prevention of delayed cerebral vasospasm following experimental subarachnoid hemorrhage in nonhuman primates. *J Neurosurg.* 2005; **103**: 745–51.

21. Tierney T S, Pradilla G, Wang P P, Clatterbuck R E, Tamargo R J. Intracranial delivery of the nitric oxide donor diethylenetriamine/nitric oxide from a controlled-release polymer: Toxicity in cynomolgus monkeys. *Neurosurgery.* 2006; **58**: 952–60.

22. Pluta R M, Dejam A, Grimes G, Gladwin M T, Oldfield E H. Nitrite infusions to prevent delayed cerebral vasospasm in a primate model of subarachnoid hemorrhage. *JAMA.* 2005; **293**: 1477–84.

23. McGirt M J, Lynch J R, Parra A, *et al.* Simvastatin increases endothelial nitric oxide synthase and ameliorates cerebral vasospasm resulting from subarachnoid hemorrhage. *Stroke.* 2002; **33**: 2950–6.

24. McGirt M J, Pradilla G, Legnani F G, *et al.* Systemic administration of simvastatin after the onset of experimental subarachnoid hemorrhage attenuates cerebral vasospasm. *Neurosurgery.* 2006; **58**: 945–51.

25. Tseng M Y, Czosnyka M, Richards H, Pickard J D, Kirkpatrick P J. Effects of acute treatment with pravastatin on cerebral vasospasm, autoregulation, and delayed ischemic deficits after aneurysmal subarachnoid hemorrhage: A phase II randomized placebo-controlled trial. *Stroke.* 2005; **36**: 1627–32.

26. Dreier J P, Korner K, Ebert N, *et al.* Nitric oxide scavenging by hemoglobin or nitric oxide synthase inhibition by n-nitro-l-arginine induces cortical spreading ischemia when K^+ is increased in the subarachnoid space. *J Cereb Blood Flow Metab.* 1998; **18**: 978–90.

27. Ishiguro M, Wellman T L, Honda A, *et al.* Emergence of a R-type Ca^{2+} channel (CAV 2.3) contributes to cerebral artery constriction after subarachnoid hemorrhage. *Circ Res.* 2005; **96**: 419–26.

28. Pluta R M, Hansen-Schwartz J, Dreier J, *et al.* Cerebral vasospasm following subarachnoid hemorrhage: Time for a new world of thought. *Neurol Res.* 2009; **31**: 151–8.

29. Kusaka G, Ishikawa M, Nanda A, Granger D N, Zhang J H. Signaling pathways for early brain injury after subarachnoid hemorrhage. *J Cereb Blood Flow Metab.* 2004; **24**: 916–25.

30. Birse S H, Tom M I. Incidence of cerebral infarction associated with ruptured intracranial aneurysms. A study of 8 unoperated cases of anterior cerebral aneurysm. *Neurology.* 1960; **10**: 101–6.

31. Dreier J P, Woitzik J, Fabricius M, *et al.* Delayed ischaemic neurological deficits after subarachnoid haemorrhage are associated with clusters of spreading depolarizations. *Brain.* 2006; **129**: 3224–37.

32. Stein S C, Levine J M, Nagpal S, LeRoux P D. Vasospasm as the sole cause of cerebral ischemia: how strong is the evidence? *Neurosurg Focus.* 2006; **21**: E2.

33. Park S, Yamaguchi M, Zhou Z, *et al.* Neurovascular protection reduces early brain injury after subarachnoid hemorrhage. *Stroke.* 2004; **35**: 2412–17.

34. Fisher C M, Kistler J P, Davis J M. Relation of cerebral vasospasm to subarachnoid hemorrhage visualized by computerized tomographic scanning. *Neurosurgery,* 1980; **6**: 1–9.

35. Kistler J P, Crowell R M, Davis K R. The relation of cerebral vasospasm to the extent and location of subarachnoid blood visualized by CT scan: A prospective study. *Neurology,* 1983; **33**: 424–36.

36. Claassen J, Bernardini G L, Kreiter K *et al.* Effect of cisternal and ventricular blood on risk of delayed cerebral ischemia after subarachnoid hemorrhage: The Fisher scale revisited. *Stroke.* 2001; **32**: 2012–20.

37. Connolly E S, Jr., Rabinstein A, Carhuapoma J R, *et al.* Guidelines for the management of aneurysmal subarachnoid hemorrhage: A statement for healthcare professionals from a special writing group of the stroke council, American Heart Association. *Stroke.* 2012; **43**: 1711–37.

38. Diringer M N, Bleck T P, Claude Hemphill J, 3rd, *et al.* Critical care management of patients following aneurysmal subarachnoid hemorrhage: Recommendations from the Neurocritical Care Society's multidisciplinary consensus conference. *Neurocrit Care.* 2011; **15**: 211–40.

39. Washington C W, Zipfel G J. Detection and monitoring of vasospasm and delayed cerebral ischemia: A review and assessment of the literature. *Neurocrit Care.* 2011; **15**: 312–17.

40. Sloan M A, Alexandrov A V, Tegeler C H, *et al.* Assessment: Transcranial Doppler ultrasonography: Report of the therapeutics and technology assessment subcommittee of the American Academy of Neurology. *Neurology.* 2004; **62**: 1468–81.

41. Harrigan M R, Magnano C R, Guterman L R, Hopkins L N. Computed tomographic perfusion in the management of aneurysmal subarachnoid hemorrhage: New application of an existent technique. *Neurosurgery.* 2005; **56**: 304–17.

42. Greenberg E D, Gold R, Reichman M, *et al.* Diagnostic accuracy of CT angiography and CT perfusion for cerebral vasospasm: A meta-analysis. *Am J Neuroradiol.* 2010; **31**: 1853–60.

43. Stocchetti N. Triggers for aggressive interventions in subarachnoid hemorrhage. *Neurocrit Care.* 2011; **15**: 324–8.

44. Hanggi D. Monitoring and detection of vasospasm II: EEG and invasive monitoring. *Neurocrit Care.* 2011; **15**: 318–23.

45. Dorhout Mees S M, Rinkel G J, Feigin V L, *et al.* Calcium antagonists for aneurysmal subarachnoid hemorrhage. *Stroke.* 2008; **39**: 514–15.

46. Philippon J, Grob R, Dagreou F, *et al.* Prevention of vasospasm in subarachnoid haemorrhage. A controlled study with nimodipine. *Acta Neurochirurgica.* 1986; **82**: 110–14.

47. Treggiari M M, Walder B, Suter P M, Romand J A. Systematic review of the prevention of delayed ischemic neurological deficits with hypertension, hypervolemia,

and hemodilution therapy following subarachnoid hemorrhage. *J Neurosurg.* 2003; **98**: 978–84.

48. Rinkel G J, Feigin V L, Algra A, van Gijn J. Circulatory volume expansion therapy for aneurysmal subarachnoid haemorrhage. *Cochrane Database Syst Rev.* 2004; CD000483.

49. Hasan D, Vermeulen M, Wijdicks E F, Hijdra A, van Gijn J. Effect of fluid intake and antihypertensive treatment on cerebral ischemia after subarachnoid hemorrhage. *Stroke.* 1989; **20**: 1511–15.

50. Wong G K, Poon W S, Chan M T, *et al.* Intravenous magnesium sulphate for aneurysmal subarachnoid hemorrhage (IMASH): A randomized, double-blinded, placebo-controlled, multicenter phase III trial. *Stroke.* 2010; **41**: 921–6.

51. Dorhout Mees S M, Algra A, *et al.* Magnesium for aneurysmal subarachnoid haemorrhage (MASH-2): A randomised placebo-controlled trial. *Lancet.* 2012; **380**: 44–9.

52. Tseng M Y. Summary of evidence on immediate statins therapy following aneurysmal subarachnoid hemorrhage. *Neurocrit Care.* 2011; **15**: 298–301.

53. Zwienenberg-Lee M, Hartman J, Rudisill N, *et al.* Effect of prophylactic transluminal balloon angioplasty on cerebral vasospasm and outcome in patients with Fisher grade III subarachnoid hemorrhage: Results of a phase II multicenter, randomized, clinical trial. *Stroke.* 2008; **39**: 1759–65.

54. Diringer M N, Axelrod Y. Hemodynamic manipulation in the neuro-intensive care unit: Cerebral perfusion pressure therapy in head injury and hemodynamic augmentation for cerebral vasospasm. *Curr Opin Crit Care.* 2007; **13**: 156–62.

55. Lee K H, Lukovits T, Friedman J A. "Triple-H" therapy for cerebral vasospasm following subarachnoid hemorrhage. *Neurocrit Care.* 2006; **4**: 68–76.

56. Meyer R, Deem S, Yanez N D, *et al.* Current practices of triple-H prophylaxis and therapy in patients with subarachnoid hemorrhage. *Neurocrit Care.* 2011; **14**: 24–36.

57. Platz J, Guresir E, Vatter H, *et al.* Unsecured intracranial aneurysms and induced hypertension in cerebral vasospasm: Is induced hypertension safe? *Neurocrit Care.* 2011; **14**: 168–75.

58. Le Roux P D. Anemia and transfusion after subarachnoid hemorrhage. *Neurocrit Care.* 2011; **15**: 342–53.

59. Naidech A M, Shaibani A, Garg R K, *et al.* Prospective, randomized trial of higher goal hemoglobin after subarachnoid hemorrhage. *Neurocrit Care.* 2011; **13**: 313–20.

60. Frontera J A, Fernandez A, Schmidt J M, *et al.* Clinical response to hypertensive hypervolemic therapy and outcome after subarachnoid hemorrhage. *Neurosurgery.* 2010; **66**: 35–41.

61. Kimball M M, Velat G J, Hoh B L. Critical care guidelines on the endovascular management of cerebral vasospasm. *Neurocrit Care.* 2011; **15**: 336–41.

62. Stuart R M, Helbok R, Kurtz P, *et al.* High-dose intra-arterial verapamil for the treatment of cerebral vasospasm after subarachnoid hemorrhage: Prolonged effects on hemodynamic parameters and brain metabolism. *Neurosurgery.* 2011; **68**: 337–45.

63. Tejada J G, Taylor R A, Ugurel M S, *et al.* Safety and feasibility of intra-arterial nicardipine for the treatment of subarachnoid hemorrhage-associated vasospasm: Initial clinical experience with high-dose infusions. *Am J Neuroradiol.* 2007; **28**: 844–8.

64. Shankar J J, dos Santos M P, Deus-Silva L, Lum C. Angiographic evaluation of the effect of intra-arterial milrinone therapy in patients with vasospasm from aneurysmal subarachnoid hemorrhage. *Neuroradiology.* 2011; **53**: 123–8.

65. Jestaedt L, Pham M, Bartsch A J, *et al.* The impact of balloon angioplasty on the evolution of vasospasm-related infarction after aneurysmal subarachnoid hemorrhage. *Neurosurgery.* 2008; **62**: 610–17.

Chapter 5

Stroke occurring on medical wards

David J. Blacker

Introduction

In-hospital stroke (IHS) occurring in patients on medical wards is an important subset of IHS, comprising 40% of one large prospective IHS registry [1], and 3.5% of the total population of one consecutive series [2] of ischemic stroke. Such patients are often elderly, and commonly have numerous medical problems including vascular risk factors, and established vascular pathology. Embolism from a cardiac source is a common mechanism. The mortality rate is often high. The illnesses prompting the hospital admission often include cardiac events and malignancy [1,3]. Infectious and inflammatory pathologies may contribute to a prothrombotic milieu [4], predisposing to arterial and venous ischemic events. Dehydration, fever, leucocytosis, interruption of antithrombotic medication, and fluctuations in blood pressure (possibly related to pain), may be other contributing factors [2,4]. Paradoxical embolism from lower extremity venous thrombosis in patients with a patent foramen ovale is another possible but rare mechanism, particularly in immobile patients. Other patients may be at risk for haemorrhagic stroke due to antithrombotic medications or coagulopathy related to hematological illnesses, malignancy, or hepatic or renal dysfunction. In-hospital stroke occurring in the complex medical patient might also be a trigger for the treating physicians to change medical care to a palliative approach.

The following sections cover the links between stroke and various medical illnesses (arranged by body system), and discuss acute and early secondary prevention management issues.

Stroke on the cardiology wards and coronary care unit

Cardiovascular illnesses account for the most common admission diagnosis in IHS [1,3], and cardiac embolism is cited as the most frequent mechanism of IHS. Stroke is a relatively uncommon complication of acute coronary syndromes (ACS), occurring in only 0.9% of ACS patients during hospitalization in one large registry [5]. However, because of the great number of ACS patients, the overall contribution to IHS is large. In the era prior to routine use of thrombolytic therapy for ACS, there were high rates of mainly ischemic stroke, in the order of 1.7 to 3.2% of acute myocardial infarction (MI) patients [6]. In the modern era, the rate of ischemic stroke is lower (0.1–1.3%), but intracranial hemorrhage (ICH) has emerged as an infrequent (0.07–1.5%), but very important issue [6]. The greatest risk for stroke is during the first six days of hospitalization [5]. Acute coronary syndrome patients with ST-segment MI (STEMI) are at a greater risk, compared with non-ST-segment MI (NSTEMI) or unstable angina. Coronary artery bypass surgery (CABG), atrial fibrillation (AF), previous stroke, initial enzyme elevation, and advanced age are the important risk factors for IHS in ACS patients [5]. Importantly, the stroke-related mortality is over 30%, and ACS patients remain at risk for fatal stroke for many months following hospital discharge [5]. One of the major risks for stroke in ACS patients is AF. One registry noted that only 55% of hospitalized patients who had AF, many of whom were at very high risk for stroke, were anticoagulated [7]. There is thus

Treatment-Related Stroke, ed. Alexander Tsiskaridze, Arne Lindgren and Adnan Qureshi. Published by Cambridge University Press. © Cambridge University Press 2016.

a large and important group of hospitalized patients whose stroke risk is probably being undertreated. Decisions in these patients are often complicated because of the concurrent use of antiplatelet agents for other coronary indications such as stents (see further discussion later in this section).

Treatments for ACS such as CABG and percutaneous coronary interventions are additional risks and mechanisms for stroke; these are covered elsewhere in Chapter 9.

Another complex situation occurring on cardiology wards is stroke in patients with infective endocarditis (IE). Cerebrovascular complications, including embolic infarction, intraparenchymal and subarachnoid hemorrhage complicate up to 40% of patients with IE [8]. Embolism is more common with mitral, compared with aortic, valve involvement, and with vegetations that are mobile or larger than 10 mm [8]. Hemorrhage may be due to septic arteritis, transformation of ischemic infarction, use of anticoagulation, or rupture of a mycotic aneurysm.

Acute stroke treatment issues

Acute therapy for ACS patients who suffer an IHS may be complicated by the logistical issues common to other forms of stroke, i.e., delayed recognition, and difficult access to urgent neuro-imaging [3]. Moving a cardiac patient out of a monitored environment for brain CT or MRI may be an important issue. While portable monitoring equipment can be used, performing an MRI on an unstable cardiac patient may be problematic. Recent MI has long been listed as a relative contraindication for tissue-plasminogen activator (t-PA) [9], mainly out of concerns for the possibility of hemopericardium, or fragmentation and embolization of intracardiac thrombus. Concurrent use of antithrombotic and anticoagulant medication is also an issue. More recently, a review [10] suggested that the time window for use of t-PA might be safely reduced from three months, as recommended in some guidelines [9] to seven weeks after AMI. This is no help for the early IHS situation, and no mention is made of any difference between STEMI and NSTEMI patients. It is possible that NSTEMI patients are at less risk of the above possible complications. Treating clinicians and patients need to consider these issues and make a decision on the risks and benefits in this situation.

Blood pressure management in cardiac patients suffering an acute stroke is a common issue for discussion between the attending stroke physician and the cardiologist. Recent studies [11,12] have provided good data to support the long-held concerns about rapid lowering of blood pressure in acute ischemic stroke patients; however, cardiologists are typically worried about hypertension during and immediately following ACS. Many medications routinely used in ACS (nitrates, beta-blockers, morphine, and ACE inhibitors) will acutely lower blood pressure. A balance between these competing concerns must be reached on an individual patient basis.

Acute stroke in patients with IE presents a very difficult management dilemma. Septic embolism has been listed as a contraindication for thrombolytic therapy, because of concerns regarding risk of hemorrhage. However, it has been suggested that thrombolysis could be considered in this situation following case reports [13] of successful treatment with t-PA in patients with IE, as well as endovascular stroke treatment [14]. With increasing access to acute brain and vascular imaging, especially CT angiography, the presence of concurrent vascular lesions at risk for bleeding can be identified rapidly.

Significant ICH in an ACS patient is a grave situation, with anesthesia and neurosurgical intervention being very difficult in the setting of medication-related coagulopathy and unstable cardiac status. Reversal of anticoagulation is a high priority, but problematic because of the risk for thrombotic complications. It should be noted that the Factor Seven for Acute Hemorrhagic Stroke (FAST) trial [15] of factor VII for ICH showed a significant increase in myocardial infarcts in ICH patients treated with this agent. On the other hand, rates of thrombotic complications in anticoagulation-related ICH patients, in an observational series [16], where most underwent intensive reversal of anticoagulation, were quite low. This issue is covered further in Chapter 24.

Secondary prevention issues

The medical therapies used for secondary prevention following ACS, and for ischemic heart disease (IHD), are very similar to those prescribed for ischemic cerebrovascular disease. An important difference is that the long-term use of combination antiplatelet therapy shows no benefit (except for aspirin plus dipyridamole vs. aspirin), but proven harm from excess hemorrhage, in the setting of cerebrovascular disease. In stroke and TIA patients, the combination of aspirin plus clopidogrel vs. aspirin [17], and aspirin plus clopidogrel vs. clopidogrel [18] were both shown to confer no long-term advantage, and had excessive rates of systemic and intracranial hemorrhage. A more recent Chinese study [19] suggested that commencement of the combination within 24 hours of minor ischemic stroke or TIA, and continuation for 90 days was more effective than aspirin alone, and had low rates of hemorrhagic complications.

A common and difficult dilemma is the combination of antiplatelet therapy and anticoagulants in patients with IHD and AF. One recent review [20] suggests that the common practice of combining anticoagulants and antiplatelet agents for patients with IHD and AF is actually unnecessary and dangerous. Note was made of older studies demonstrating equivalence between anticoagulants and antiplatelet agents for IHD (in patients without AF). Thus anticoagulation alone, without the addition of an antiplatelet agent, is reasonable. Observational data described in the above review [20] confirms high rates of hemorrhagic complications in patients on combination antithrombotics, particularly "triple therapy", namely aspirin, clopidogrel, and warfarin. This typically is used when the patient with AF also has coronary stents. It may be reasonable to accept the high risk of hemorrhagic complications during the minimal time period required for such antithrombotic therapy, according to the nature of the stent, before reverting to "dual therapy", in discussion with the interventional cardiologist.

Acute coronary syndrome patients who suffer an IHS may be found to have a concurrent high-grade extracranial carotid stenosis. This is not surprising, since ACS patients commonly have a vascular profile predisposing them to both coronary and carotid atherosclerosis, typically Caucasian male smokers. Such patients are at high risk of early stroke recurrence, but are also at a high risk for periprocedural stroke and cardiac events. The question thus arises how to best manage a patient with a recent stroke and concurrent ACS, where revascularization of either the carotid or coronary arteries (or both) may be indicated. Data from "purely" stroke studies [21] have shown that the risk of recurrent stroke related to high-grade symptomatic carotid stenosis is probably as high as 18% within the first month after the qualifying event. It is uncertain if this figure is similar in patients with the combination of stroke and ACS. Data from trials of carotid endarterectomy (CEA) suggest that the maximal benefit is obtained by surgery within the

first two weeks of the qualifying stroke [22], but this does not account for patients with a concurrent ACS. When no coronary revascularization is indicated, carotid angioplasty and stenting (CAS) may be the preferred option, based upon a large trial [23] showing less risk of NSTEMI related to CAS compared with CEA, but it should be noted that periprocedural stroke is more common with CAS than CEA, particularly in older patients. The other consideration for carotid surgery in patients with an ACS is the use of concurrent dual antiplatelet therapy, which may be of concern for the surgeon.

The situation is even more complicated where revascularization of both carotid and coronary circulations is indicated. Patients with recent coronary conditions face a major risk of MI, heart failure, and death following non-cardiac surgery such as CEA. Patients with recent stroke, particularly large infarcts, may be at risk from surgery and anesthesia exacerbating the ischemia due to hemodynamic instability, or hemorrhagic transformation related to hypertension and antithrombotic medications. Rates of stroke and death are more than doubled in patients undergoing combined CEA and CABG, compared with CABG alone [24]. The strategy of combining CAS with CABG seems attractive; however, a meta-analysis [25] of the cumulative results of different revascularization strategies found no major differences. It should be noted that much of this data is based on patients with asymptomatic rather than active carotid disease. One review [26] suggested that revascularization of asymptomatic carotid lesions prior to CABG is only rarely indicated, usually in the setting of bilateral high-grade lesions, or where there is a high-grade stenosis combined with a contralateral occluded artery. Thus there is some importance in determining if the carotid lesion is indeed symptomatic, especially since the cardiac pathology may be an alternative mechanism leading to the stroke. This is where expert neurological input may be helpful. Indeed some guidelines [27] have emphasized the need for individual patient assessment with neurologist input in these difficult cases, and in fact list this as the major recommendation. The occurrence of TIA prior to stroke (and the cardiac lesion), may suggest that the carotid stenosis is the culprit lesion. Multiple strokes in different vascular territories implies a cardiac source. Other clues include an analysis of the blood pressure, and distribution of cerebral infarcts on imaging. In addition to clinical evaluation, there may be a role in the future for advanced vascular imaging that looks closely at a carotid lesion, possibly detecting plaque inflammation as well as transcranial ultrasound examination for identifying multiple microembolic signals from a symptomatic carotid artery stenosis.

Another group of cardiology patients with IHS where a difficult decision on surgery is required are those with IE who require urgent cardiac valve surgery. Concerns regarding the potential for deterioration of the neurological state need to be balanced against the patient's cardiac condition. Anesthesia and cardiopulmonary bypass (CPB) have the potential to create hemodynamic instability, which in the setting of poststroke impaired autoregulation, may potentially exacerbate the neurological injury. One review [25] suggested deferring any surgery under general anesthesia for stroke patients for at least a month, because of these reasons. An observational study [28] of IE patients with cerebral infarction found the risk of neurological deterioration to be 20% when surgery was performed within the first three days, 20 to 50% between days three and fourteen, falling to <10% after fourteen days, and then <1% after a month. The authors [28] concluded that valve surgery should be deferred for a month in such patients, unless severe heart failure mandates early operation. Another issue is concurrent heparinization during CPB, and the concern for hemorrhage.

Cardiac patients who survive an ICH are a complex group of patients, with treatment decisions made by cardiologists and stroke physicians needing to balance the risk of recurrent cardiac and cerebral ischemic events with the risk of recurrent ICH. These are not equivalent events. While the risk of ischemic events, especially in AF patients, is higher, the significance of an ICH (especially if anticoagulated) is often more profound, with a high mortality rate. One increasingly frequent dilemma is the combination of AF with a high CHADS$_2$ score, and great risk of recurrent ischemic stroke, in patients who have had an ICH related to anticoagulation. The circumstances and pathology of the ICH are probably worth considering in the decision process. A "provoked" hemorrhage, e.g., an incidental trauma in a patient with an elevated INR resulting in a subdural hematoma, may be of less concern for recommencement of anticoagulation than a spontaneous ICH in a patient with documented good control of the INR. A deep ICH, probably related to hypertension, seems to have a low

risk of recurrence, and a theoretical risk model [29] suggests that recommencement of anticoagulants might be reasonable in this situation, and another review [30] recommends that recommencement of anticoagulation after about ten weeks might be reasonable. Lobar hemorrhage, with underlying amyloid angiopathy, is a more concerning situation, because the recurrence rate is substantial, and the model advises against recommencing anticoagulation in these cases. With the increasing use of MRI, cerebral microhemorrhages are being increasingly identified, and frequently these are commonly asymptomatic. When seen in patients who have had a combination of AF-related ischemic stroke and anticoagulation-related ICH, a difficult dilemma arises, although currently available data do not support the use of MRI to exclude anticoagulation in patients with AF [30]. One potential option when the ICH risk is high in a patient with AF and a high CHADS$_2$ score, might be the use of left atrial appendage (LAA) occlusion devices. Most thrombi in AF form in the LAA. The rationale for LAA occlusion is to exclude these from the circulation, thereby possibly reducing the risk of embolism, without the requirement for long-term anticoagulation. Early data [31] from a trial comparing LAA occlusion with warfarin suggest this could provide one of the few therapeutic options for such patients. The role of the direct thrombin inhibitors or factor Xa inhibitors such as dabigatran, apixaban, or rivaroxaban in this situation is yet to be defined. Although these agents seem to result in lower rates of ICH compared with warfarin for patients in AF [32–35], this does not prove that they are a treatment alternative in patients that have had an anticoagulant-related ICH. There are additional concerns about increased coronary ischemic events with the use of some of these agents, as well as the fact that there is no easy way to rapidly reverse the effect. While dialysis for removing the substance from the circulation is possible, this is not a rapidly available or feasible treatment in a patient with an acute ICH.

Stroke on the neurology ward

Early recurrent stroke, in patients already on a stroke unit admitted because of a stroke or TIA, is an important issue, but not the focus of this chapter. But stroke sometimes also occurs in patients with other neurological conditions.

Patients hospitalized with illnesses such as seizures or demyelination would not seem to be at any extra risk for stroke, although there seems to be no literature about this. Stroke, particularly venous thrombosis, may be a potential complication of encephalitis and other conditions that raise intracranial pressure. Neurology patients with Guillain–Barré syndrome (GBS) or other conditions receiving treatment with intravenous immune globulin (IVIG) may also be at risk for thrombotic complications, and there is a small case series [36] of stroke in this setting. The posterior reversible encephalopathy syndrome may also be seen related to IVIG, and this may enter the differential of acute stroke in such patients [37]. Paradoxical emboli through a PFO may be a potential issue in GBS patients who are frequently immobilized and at risk of deep venous thrombosis for lengthy periods of time.

Acute stroke treatment issues

Acute therapies, particularly thrombolysis, may have to take into account the fact that neurology patients may have recently had a lumbar puncture, where thrombolysis should be avoided for at least a week, possibly longer.

Secondary prevention issues

In terms of early secondary prevention, anticoagulant interactions with medications including anticonvulsants might need to be considered. In the longer term, unstable seizures may well be a relative contraindication for anticoagulation of stroke patients.

Stroke on the renal unit

Renal failure is an additional risk for atherosclerosis, beyond the contribution of traditional risk factors [38]. It is also a risk for hemorrhage, likely related to poorly functioning platelets and hypertension. Dialysis patients are at a greatly increased risk for stroke, with one study [39] finding a five- to ten-fold increased risk compared with controls. A transcranial Doppler ultrasound study [40] showed increased mean blood flow velocities in dialysis patients compared with controls, possibly related to the anemia of chronic renal failure. This alteration of cerebral hemodynamics, especially when combined with the blood pressure and volume fluctuations of dialysis, may well be factors predisposing the renal dialysis patient to stroke. Extracranial carotid atherosclerosis, when severe, could also contribute to compromised cerebral hemodynamics. There is currently great interest in the role of blood pressure fluctuation as a trigger for stroke in non-dialysis patients [41], so this may well be very important. These fluctuations, combined with the heparin used in dialysis, could also be important predisposing factors for hemorrhage.

Acute stroke treatment issues

One issue that commonly arises acutely in the assessment of acute stroke patients with renal impairment is the use of intravenous contrast agents in acute imaging, particularly CT angiography. Imaging should not be delayed pending the results of blood tests, since most acute decisions can be made with a non-contrast CT. Dialysis may be required later for patients who undergo diagnostic or therapeutic angiographic procedures. Thrombolysis in patients with renal failure has been reported in a small case series [42] of 20 patients with an estimated glomerular filtration rate (eGFR) <60 mL/min/1.73 m^2, and did not seem to be associated with adverse outcomes, particularly ICH. Another study [43] also suggested no increased risk with "any" level of renal impairment, but for "severe" impairment, with eGFR <30 ml/min/1.73 m^2, rates of hemorrhagic transformation were significantly higher, in the order of 15%. There is scant data about treating dialysis patients with t-PA. At one forum [44], a panel of stroke experts was interviewed regarding their experience and views regarding the treatment of hemodialysis patients with t-PA for acute stroke. About a dozen experts expressed a preference for using mechanical clot extraction.

Secondary prevention issues

Anticoagulation with warfarin in renal failure patients is problematic, with significant risk of hemorrhagic complications. For a patient with AF and renal failure and risk of thrombo-embolic stroke, the risk/benefit ratio is quite different to usual, and it has been suggested [45] that even in AF, renal failure patients should not be treated with anticoagulation. Direct thrombin inhibitors or factor Xa inhibitors have not been recommended for patients with estimated creatinine clearance of <30 mL/min, but the situation may be different for those with an eGFR of 30 to 49 mL/min if an adjusted dose is used [46–49]. The renal transplant patient is also at risk of stroke, not only because of the underlying renal issues, but also the atherogenic long-term side effects of immunosuppression.

Stroke on the oncology ward

Underlying malignancy was a factor in 13% of patients in one IHS registry [1]. Stroke is relatively common in cancer patients, with up to 15% suffering thromboembolism [50]. With improvements in cancer treatment resulting in prolonged survival, there may be greater numbers of cancer patients experiencing stroke. The underlying stroke mechanism may either be "conventional" (i.e., atherosclerotic, cardiac embolism etc.), cancer related, or related to the treatment of cancer. Malignancy may predispose to arterial and venous ischemic stroke related to alteration in clotting factors and dehydration. Adenocarcinoma-derived cytokines, tumor-necrosis factor, and direct vessel compression or infiltration may contribute to thrombosis. Non-bacterial thrombotic endocarditis and paradoxical embolism from DVT and patent foramen ovale are potential cardiac embolic sources. Hemorrhagic cerebral metastases are classically seen in patients with disseminated melanoma, as well as renal cell carcinoma, thyroid tumors, and rarely with other malignancies. Coagulopathic states related to leukemia, bone marrow infiltration, or liver metastases may result in hemorrhagic stroke. Also irradiation therapy as well as pharmacological treatment of cancer has been related to stroke risk – for details on this please see Chapter 11 for stroke after irradiation therapy, Chapter 22 for medication-induced stroke, and Chapter 23 for cerebral venous thrombosis in relation to cancer therapeutic regimens. In-hospital stroke may well be a final event prompting palliative management in cancer patients.

Acute stroke treatment issues

Current guidelines do not exclude cancer patients from thrombolytic therapy for ischemic stroke. Acutely there may be concerns about coagulopathy and thrombocytopenia related to liver metastases, bone marrow infiltration or suppression, or medications. This typically requires waiting for the results of relevant blood tests before the commencement of thrombolysis. A recently presented series [51] of sequentially admitted patients with the diagnosis of acute ischemic stroke and malignancy included 18 treated with intravenous thrombolysis. Compared with age- and gender-matched control stroke patients also undergoing thrombolysis, there was no significant

difference in efficacy or safety; however, the in-hospital mortality was higher in the cancer patients: 3/18 (17%) vs. 1/27(4%). This might be related to decisions to withdraw medical care because of the combination of stroke-related disability and malignancy.

Secondary prevention issues

Venous thrombosis is a well known association of malignancy, and prophylactic and therapeutic regimens typically with low molecular weight heparins are described [52], often in preference to oral anticoagulants. There is less information pertaining to arterial thrombo-embolic events.

Stroke on the hematology ward

Probably the most concerning situation is the risk of ICH in the setting of hematological disorders effecting platelet or coagulation function. Intracranial hemorrhage is a common form of death in patients with leukemia, and is a potential problem in patients with idiopathic thrombocytopenic purpura (ITP), and myelodysplastic disorders. Treatments such as bone marrow transplantation and myelosuppressive chemotherapy also place patients at risk of hemorrhagic complications. Almost 3% of patients with bone marrow transplants in one series [53] were found to have strokes, usually hemorrhage related to thrombocytopenia, or as a complication of fungal infection.

Prothrombotic states such as presence of lupus anticoagulant or anticardiolipin antibodies may be potentially easier to treat, but "mixed states" with a risk for bleeding and thrombosis such as thrombotic thrombocytopenic purpura (TTP) may be extremely difficult states to manage.

Stroke on the respiratory ward

There is increasing recognition of infection as a trigger for vascular events, including stroke, and respiratory infections are commonly identified. Additionally, patients with chronic airflow limitation (CAL) commonly have cardiovascular risk factors that predispose them to stroke, and CAL itself is considered an independent risk factor for cardiovascular disease [54]. Coughing may be a trigger for embolic stroke [55], related to raising intrathoracic pressure, and there is also a report [56] of coughing causing a carotid dissection with subsequent stroke.

Pneumonia is a major risk factor for death after stroke, thus if stroke occurs in a patient already hospitalized with the pneumonia, the situation is likely to be grave. There is some data to suggest that prophylactic antibiotic treatment for patients with stroke may be beneficial in reducing pneumonia [57].

There should not be specific concerns regarding acute and preventive therapies for respiratory patients, although the issue of sedation or anesthesia for acute endovascular interventions may be relevant in this group.

Stroke on the gastroenterology ward

The foremost concern for stroke on the gastroenterology ward relates to the potential for hemorrhage related to coagulopathy. Stroke complicates up to 6.5% of liver transplantations [58]. The majority of these strokes are hemorrhagic, with a very high case fatality rate. Age and concurrent systemic infection were possible risk factors. Patients hospitalized because of inflammatory bowel condition such as ulcerative colitis [59] or Crohn's disease may be a group at risk for arterial and venous thrombotic complications [60]. Inflammatory bowel disease was reported to be present in 2.3% of patients with cerebral venous thrombosis in one series [61]. One population-based case control study [62] did not find any overall risk for ischemic stroke in patients with Crohn's disease, but suggested that there may be an increased risk for younger patients (less than 60 years of age). A recent systematic review and meta-analysis found that inflammatory bowel disease (IBD) is associated with a modest increase in the risk of cardiovascular morbidity [63].

Acute stroke treatment issues

Stroke may be difficult to recognize in the setting of hepatic encephalopathy, and there is a report [64] of reversible focal neurological signs occurring in this condition, mimicking stroke. Because of concerns regarding hemorrhagic risk related to gastric, hepatic, and hematological pathology, it would seem that potential for use of thrombolysis in such patients is limited. There is a report [65] of successful intra-arterial thrombolysis in a patient with Crohn's disease who had a middle cerebral artery occlusion, and the authors suggested that technique as the preferred option for treatment of stroke in this setting.

Secondary prevention issues

Antiplatelet agents and anticoagulants are problematic in gastroenterology patients with gastric and hepatic pathology. Similarly, lipid-lowering agents, particularly statins, are problematic in patients with liver dysfunction.

Stroke in hospitalized diabetic patients

Diabetes mellitus is obviously a well-recognized risk factor for stroke, but the patient hospitalized for diabetic ketoacidosis (DKA), or hyperosmolar non-ketotic coma (HONK), is at particular risk for this [66]. There are numerous reports of ischemic stroke complicating DKA, especially in the pediatric literature [67], with a number of reports of such strokes being complicated by massive cerebral edema. Patients with HONK are at particular risk of cerebral venous thrombosis, possibly related to the hyperviscosity of that condition. Concurrent focal neurological signs may be difficult to recognize due to the altered conscious state. Hypoglycemia may result in focal neurological signs and thus be a stroke mimic.

Acute stroke treatment issues

Marked hyperglycemia is a risk for poor outcome and hemorrhagic transformation after thrombolysis [68]. The combination of diabetes mellitus and prior stroke was an exclusion criterion for one large study [69] of stroke thrombolysis in the 3- to 4.5-hour time window. It would thus seem that the glycemic state is a factor to consider in the risk/benefit ratio of thrombolytic therapy.

The other issue to consider is control of the glycemic state immediately after stroke. Intuitively, it might be expected that "tight" glycemic control might favorably affect the observed adverse outcomes, and several studies have examined the hypothesis that using insulin infusions to target a set glycemic range after stroke may be beneficial compared with standard care. However, a Cochrane review [70] of seven such trials including 1,296 participants found no difference in the outcome of death or disability, and found that treatment with intravenous insulin was associated with a greater incidence of hypoglycemia.

Secondary prevention issues

Long-term survival rates in patients with type 1 diabetes who suffer a stroke are very poor. One series [71] found that at one, five, and ten years after the incident stroke, survival rates were only 80.6%, 45.2%, and 9.6%. This ten-year survival figure is about half that seen in a general stroke population (that included diabetic stroke patients). The secondary prevention issues are similar to those in non-diabetic patients.

Stroke on the psychiatry ward

Several conditions that may lead to inpatient admission to a psychiatry ward may potentially predispose to IHS. These include drug-induced psychosis, schizophrenia, and depression. Amphetamines and cocaine may cause psychosis resulting in admission, and predispose to cerebral vasculopathies with resultant ischemic and hemorrhagic stroke. Rates of nicotine and marijuana use are high in psychiatric populations, and both drugs have vasospastic actions, which likely predispose to stroke. There may be a possible link between the use of various antipsychotic medications and cardiovascular events [72,73]. It is possible that fluctuations in blood pressure in the setting of other psychiatric conditions, including attempted suicide, could be a factor in precipitating stroke. Younger schizophrenic patients in one study [74] were at twice the risk for developing stroke compared with controls, during a five-year period after hospitalization. Lifestyle factors such as unhealthy diet, obesity (possibly related to antipsychotic medications), and smoking were thought to explain some, but not all of the increased risk. Another study [75] showed depression to be an additional risk factor for stroke.

Acute stroke treatment issues

The recognition of stroke symptoms may well be difficult in hospitalized psychiatric patients, and it is possible that medical staff may erroneously consider acute neurological symptoms in such patients to be due to conversion disorder. Conversion disorder is a not uncommon stroke mimic, and at least one series [76] found no hemorrhagic complications among such patients treated with intravenous thrombolysis. The physical layout of a psychiatry ward is often different to the typical medical ward or emergency department, creating a challenge (for example locating equipment) for acute stroke clinicians in assessing patients. Mental status and competency issues may provide a challenge in obtaining consent for acute procedures, although the psychiatry team should be able to provide support for this.

Secondary prevention issues

Ongoing compliance with secondary preventive medication, and smoking cessation, may be difficult issues in this patient population.

Stroke on other medical wards

Stroke occurring on the general medical wards, particularly in patients with multiple comorbidities, may pose a substantial challenge. Advanced age and concurrent illnesses such as dementia may lead to a somewhat nihilistic approach. Non-stroke specialists might tend to overestimate the severity of stroke, and be less optimistic regarding the potential for recovery. This could impact on overall management decisions, sometimes leading to premature withdrawal of care, or palliative management. Consultation with a stroke specialist is therefore advisable.

References

1. Vera R, Lago A, Fuentes B, et al. In-hospital stroke: a multi-centre prospective registry. *European J Neurology.* 2011; **18**:170–6.

2. Nadav L, Gur A Y, Korczyn A D, Bornstein N M. Stroke in hospitalized patients: are there special factors? *Cerebrovasc Dis.* 2002; **13**:127–31.

3. Farooq M U, Reeves M J, Gargano J, et al. In-hospital stroke in a statewide stroke registry. *Cerbrovasc Dis.* 2008; **25**:12–20.

4. Blacker D J. In-hospital stroke. *Lancet Neurol.* 2003; **2**: 741–6.

5. Budaj A, Flasinska K, Goer J M, et al. Magnitude of and risk factors for in-hospital and postdischarge stroke in patients with acute coronary syndromes: Findings from a Global Registry of Acute Coronary Events. *Circulation.* 2005; **111**:3242–7.

6. Mahaffey K W, Granger C B, Sloan M A, et al for the GUSTO-1 Investigators. Risk factors for in-hospital nonhemorrhagic stroke in patients with acute myocardial infarction treated with thrombolysis. *Circulation.* 1998; **97**:757–64.

7. Waldo A L, Becker R C, Tapson V F, Colgan K J for the NABOR steering committee. Hospitalized patients with atrial fibrillation and a high risk of stroke are not being provided with adequate anticoagulation. *J Am Coll Cardiol.* 2005; **46**:1729–36.

8. Habib G. Management of infective endocarditis. *Heart.* 2006; **92**:124–30.

9. Adams H P, del Zoppo G, Alberts M J, et al. Guidelines for the early management of adults with ischemic stroke. *Stroke.* 2007; **38**:1655–711.

10. De Sliva D A, Manzano J J F, Chang H M, Wong M C. Reconsidering recent myocardial infarction as a contraindication for IV stroke thrombolysis. *Neurology.* 2011; **76**:1838–40.

11. Sandset E C, Bath P M, Boysen G, *et al.* The angiotensin-receptor blocker candesartan for treatment of acute stroke (SCAST): a randomised, placebo-controlled, double blind trial. *Lancet.* 2011; **377**:741–50.

12. Beer C, Blacker D, Bynevelt M, Hankey G J, Puddey I B. A randomised placebo controlled trial of early ischemic stroke with atorvastatin and irbesartan. *Int J Stroke.* 2012; **7**:104–11.

13. Sontineni S P, Moos A N, Andukari V G, Schima S M, Esterbrooks D. Effectiveness of thrombolytic in acute embolic stroke due to infective endocarditis. *Stroke Res Treat.* 2010; **2010**:841797.

14. Dabeabneh H, Hedna VS, Ford J, *et al.* Endovascular intervention for acute stroke due to infective endocarditis: a case report. *Neurosurg Focus.* 2012; **32**: E1.

15. Diringer M N, Skolnick B E, Mayer S A, *et al.* Thromboembolic events with recombinant factor VII in spontaneous intracerebral hemorrhage: results from the Factor Seven for Acute Hemorrhagic Stroke (FAST) trial. *Stroke.* 2010; **41**:48–53.

16. Phan T G, Koh M, Wijdicks E F. Safety of discontinuation of anticoagulation in patients with intracranial hemorrhage at high thromboembolic risk. *Arch Neurol.* 2000; **57**:1710–13.

17. Diener H C, Bogousslavsky J, Brass L M, *et al.* Aspirin and Clopidogrel Compared with Clopidogrel Alone after Recent Ischaemic Stroke or Transient Ischaemic Attack in High-risk Patients (MATCH): Randomised, double-blind, placebo-controlled trial. *Lancet.* 2004; **364**:331–7.

18. Bhatt D L, Fox K A, Hacke W, *et al.* Clopidogrel and aspirin versus aspirin alone for the prevention of atherothrombotic events. *N Engl J Med.* 2006; **354**: 1706–17.

19. Wang Y, Wang Y, Zhao X, *et al.* Clopidogrel with aspirin in acute minor stroke or transient ischemic attack. *N Engl J Med.* 2013; **369**:11–19.

20. Fisher M, Loscalzo J. The perils of antithrombotic therapy and potential resolutions. *Circulation.* 2011; **123**:232–5.

21. Petty G W, Brown R D, Whisnant J P, *et al.* Ischemic stroke subtypes: a population–based study of functional outcome, survival and recurrence. *Stroke.* 2000; **31**:1062–8.

22. Rothwell P M, Eliasziw M, Gutnikov S A, Warlow C P, Barnett H J. Carotid Endarterectomy Trialists Collaboration. Endarterectomy for symptomatic carotid stenosis in relation to clinical subgroups and timing of surgery. *Lancet.* 2004; **363**:915–24.

23. Brott T G, Hobson R W 2nd, Howard G, *et al.* Stenting versus endarterectomy for treatment of carotid-artery stenosis. *N Engl J Med.* 2010; **363**:11–23.

24. Hill M D, Shrive F M, Kennedy J, Feasby T E, Ghali W A. Simultaneous carotid endarterectomy and coronary artery bypass surgery in Canada. *Neurology.* **64**:1435–7.

25. Naylor A R, Mehta Z, Rothwell P M. A systematic review and meta-analysis of 30-day outcomes following staged carotid artery stenting and coronary bypass. *Eur J Vasc Endovasc Surg.* 2009; **37**:379–84.

26. Blacker D J, Flemming K D, Link M J, Brown R D. The pre-operative cerebrovascular consultation: common cerebrovascular questions before general or cardiac surgery. *Mayo Clin Proc.* 2004; **79**:223–9.

27. Tendera M, Aboyans V, Bartelink M, *et al.* ESC Guidelines on the diagnosis and treatment of peripheral artery diseases. *European Heart Journal.* 2011; **32**:2851–906.

28. Anstwurm K, Borges A C, Halle E, *et al.* Timing the valve replacement in infective endocarditis involving the brain. *J Neurol.* 2004; **251**:1220–6.

29. Eckman M H, Rosand J, Knudsen K A, Singer D E, Greenberg S M. Can patients be anticoagulated after intracerebral hemorrhage? A decision analysis. *Stroke.* 2003; **34**:1710–16.

30. Paciaroni M, Agnelli G. Should oral anticoagulants be restarted after warfarin-associated cerebral haemorrhage in patients with atrial fibrillation? *Thrombosis and Haemostasis.* 2014; **111**:14–18.

31. Holmes D R, Reddy D Y, Turi Z G, *et al.* Percutaneous closure of the left atrial appendix versus warfarin therapy for prevention of stroke in patients with atrial fibrillation: a randomised non-inferiority trial. *Lancet.* 2009; **374**:534–42.

32. Connolly S J, Ezekowitz M D, Yusuf S, *et al.* Dabigatran versus warfarin in patients with atrial fibrillation. *N Engl J Med.* 2009; **361**:1139–51.

33. Granger C B, Alexander J H, McMurray J J, *et al.* Apixaban versus warfarin in patients with atrial fibrillation. *N Engl J Med.* 2011; **365**:981–92.

34. Patel M R, Mahaffey K W, Garg J, *et al.* Rivaroxaban versus warfarin in nonvalvular atrial fibrillation. *N Engl J Med.* 2011; **365**:883–91.

35. Hankey G J. Intracranial hemorrhage and novel anticoagulants for atrial fibrillation: What have we learned? *Curr Cardiol Rep.* 2014; **16**:480.

36. Caress J B, Cartwright M S, Donofrio P D, Peacock J D. The clinical features of 16 cases of stroke associated with the administration of IVIG. *Neurology.* 2003; **60**: 1822–4.

37. Incecik F, Herquner M O, Altunbasak S, Yildizdas D. Reversible posterior encephalopathy syndrome due to intravenous immunoglobulin in a child with Guillain-Barre syndrome. *J Paediatr Neurosci.* 2011; 6:138–40.

38. Townsend R R. Stroke in chronic kidney disease: prevention and management. *Clin J Am Soc Nephrol.* 2008; 33:S11–S16.

39. Seliger S L, Gillen D L, Longstreth W T, Kestenbaum B. Stehman-Breen C O. Elevated risk of stroke among patients with end-stage renal disease. *Kidney International.* 2003; 64:603–9.

40. Farhoudi M, Azar S A, Abdi R. Brain hemodynamics in patients with end-stage renal disease between hemodialysis sessions. *IJKD.* 2012; 6:110–13.

41. Rothwell P M. Does blood pressure variability modulate cardiovascular risk? *Curr Hypertens Rep.* 2011; 13:177–86.

42. Agrawal V, Rai B, Fellows J, McCullough P A. In-hospital outcomes with thrombolytic therapy in patients with renal dysfunction presenting with acute ischemic stroke. *Nephrol Dial Transplant.* 2010; 25:1150–7.

43. Tutuncu S, Ziegler A M, Scheitz J F, et al. Severe renal impairment is associated with symptomatic intracerebral hemorrhage after thrombolysis for ischemic stroke. *Stroke.* 2013; 44:3217–19.

44. Palacio S, Gonzales N R, Sangha N S, Birnbaum L A, Hart R G. Thrombolysis for acute stroke in hemodialysis: international survey of expert opinion. *Clin J Am Soc Nephrol.* 2006; 1:1357–9.

45. Bennett W M. Should dialysis patients ever receive warfarin and for what reasons? *Clin J Am Soc Nephrol.* 2006; 1:1357–9.

46. Verheugt F W, Granger C B. Oral anticoagulants for stroke prevention in atrial fibrillation: Current status, special situations, and unmet needs. *Lancet.* 2015; 386:303–10.

47. Ng K P, Edwards N C, Lip G Y, Townend J N, Ferro C J. Atrial fibrillation in CKD: Balancing the risks and benefits of anticoagulation. *American Journal of Kidney Diseases.* 2013; 62:615–32.

48. Kruger T, Brandenburg V, Schlieper G, Marx N, Floege J. Sailing between scylla and charybdis: Oral long-term anticoagulation in dialysis patients. *Nephrology, Dialysis, Transplantation.* 2013; 28:534–41.

49. Camm A J, Lip G Y, De Caterina R, et al. Focused update of the ESC guidelines for the management of atrial fibrillation: An update of the 2010 ESC guidelines for the management of atrial fibrillation. Developed with the special contribution of the European Heart Rhythm Association. *Eur Heart J.* 2012; 33:2719–47.

50. Bang O Y, Seok J M, Kim S G, et al. Ischemic stroke and cancer: stroke severely impacts cancer patients, while cancer increases the number of strokes. *J Clin Neurol.* 2011; 7:53–9.

51. Schwarzbach C J. Systemic thrombolysis in cancer patients: is it safe and effective? *Cerebrovasc Dis.* 2012; Supp 2:64.

52. Khorana A A. Cancer and thrombosis: implications of published guidelines for clinical practice. *Annals of Oncology.* 2009; 20:1619–30.

53. Coplin W M, Cochran M S, Levine S R, Crawford S W. Stroke after bone marrow transplantation. Frequency, aetiology and outcome. *Brain.* 2001; 124:1043–51.

54. Finkelstein J, Cha E, Scharf S. Chronic obstructive pulmonary disease as an independent risk factor for cardiovascular morbidity. *International Journal of COPD.* 2009; 4:337–49.

55. Seok H Y, Seo W, Eun M, et al. Transient increase in intrathoracic pressure as a contributing factor to cardioembolic stroke. *J Clin Neurol.* 2010; 6:212–15.

56. Tan S, Humphrey G, Miles P. Stroke due to carotid artery dissection. *Postgrad Med J.* 1991; 67:588–9.

57. Harms H, Prass K, Meisel C, et al. Preventive antibacterial therapy in acute ischemic stroke: A randomised controlled trial (PATHERIS). *PLoS ONE.* 2008; 3(5):e2158.

58. Ling L, He X, Zeng J, Lian G Z. In-hospital cerebrovascular complications following orthotopic liver transplantation: A retrospective study. *BMC Neurology.* 2008; 8:52.

59. Joshi D, Dickel T, Aga R, Smith-Laing G. Stroke in inflammatory bowel disease: A report of two cases and review of the literature. *Thrombosis Journal.* 2008; 6:2.

60. Moris G. Inflammatory bowel disease: An increased risk factor for neurologic complications. *World Journal of Gastroenterology.* 2014; 20:1228–37.

61. Cognat E, Crassard I, Denier C, Vahedi K, Bousser M G. Cerebral venous thrombosis in inflammatory bowel diseases: eight cases and literature review. *Int J Stroke.* 2011; 6:487–92.

62. Andersohn F, Waring M, Garbe E. Risk of ischemic stroke in patients with Crohn's disease: A population-based nested case-control study. *Inflamm Bowel Dis.* 2010; 16:1387–92.

63. Singh S, Singh H, Loftus E V, Jr., Pardi D S. Risk of cerebrovascular accidents and ischemic heart disease in patients with inflammatory bowel disease: A systematic review and meta-analysis. *Clinical Gastroenterology and Hepatology.* 2014; 12:382–93.

64. Yamamoto Y, Nishiyama Y, Katsura K, Yamazaki M, Katayama Y. Hepatic encephalopathy with reversible focal neurologic signs resembling acute stroke: case report. *J Stroke Cerebrovasc Dis.* 2011; 20:377–80.

65. Brosch J R, Janicki M J. Intra-arterial thrombolysis as an ideal treatment for inflammatory bowel disease

related thromboembolic stroke: A case report and review. *Int J Neurosci.* 2012; **122**:541–4.

66. Chen H, Wang C, Lee H, *et al.* Short-term case fatality rate and associated factors among inpatients with diabetic ketoacidosis and hyperglycaemic hyperosmolar state: A hospital-based analysis over a 15 year period. *Inter Med.* 2010; **49**:729–37.

67. Foster J R, Morrison G, Fraser D D. Diabetic ketoacidosis-associated stroke in children. *Stroke Research and Treatment.* 2011; doi:10.4061/2011/219706.

68. Wahlgren N, Ahmed N, Eriksson N, *et al.* Multivariable analysis of outcome predictors and adjustment of main outcome results to baseline data profile in randomised controlled trials. Safe Implementation of Thrombolysis in Stroke Monitoring Study (SITS-MOST). *Stroke.* 2008; **39**:3316–22.

69. Hacke W, Kaste M, Bluhmki E, *et al.* Thrombolysis with alteplase 3 to 4.5 hours after acute ischaemic stroke. *N Engl J Med.* 2008; **359**:1371–29.

70. Bellolio M F, Gilmore R M, Stead L G. Insulin for glycaemic control in acute ischaemic stroke. *Cochrane Database Syst Rev.* 2011; **9**:CD005346.

71. Hardie K, Hankey G J, Jamrozik K, Broadhurst R J, Anderson C. Ten year survival after first-ever stroke in the Perth community stroke study. *Stroke.* 2003; **34**: 1842–6.

72. Douglas I J, Smeeth L. Exposure to antipsychotics and risk of stroke: self controlled case series study. *BMJ.* 2008; 337a1277, doi:10.1136/bmj.a1277.

73. Wang S, Liknkletter C, Dore D, *et al.* Age, antipsychotics, and the risk of ischemic stroke in the veterans health administration. *Stroke.* 2012; **43**:28–31.

74. Lin H C, Hsiao F H, Pfeiffer S, Hwang Y T, Lee H S. An increased risk of stroke among young schizophrenia patients. *Schizophrenia Research.* 2008; **101**:234–41.

75. Pan A, Okereke O I, Sun Q, *et al.* Depression and incident stroke in women. *Stroke.* 2011; **42**:2770–5.

76. Chernyshev O Y, Martin-Schild S, Albright KC, *et al.* Safety of tPA in stroke mimics and neuroimaging-negative cerebral ischemia. *Neurology.* 2010; **74**:1340–5.

Stroke in trauma patients

David J. Blacker

Introduction

Stroke occurring in patients hospitalized because of trauma is a substantial diagnostic and management challenge. It is sometimes possible that stroke may be the cause of an accident leading to a trauma. The trauma patient may actually have stroke symptoms before reaching hospital, but the dramatic and sometimes life-threatening nature of trauma-related injury may mean that less attention is paid to the neurological symptoms (by the patient themselves, and medical staff). Stroke caused by the trauma may also be delayed in onset. In many of these scenarios, stroke occurring in the trauma patient is not recognized until the patient is already in hospital. In a state-wide registry [1] of in-hospital stroke, 7% of patients had an admission diagnosis of trauma or an orthopedic problem. In patients with multiple trauma or head injury the diagnosis can be difficult and delayed. In many situations, the stroke treatment options are extremely limited. The outcome, particularly in the multitrauma patient, is frequently poor.

Stroke mechanisms in acute trauma patients

Most attention has been paid to arterial injury to the great vessels of the head and neck in trauma patients, but it should not be forgotten that there are other potential mechanisms.

Arterial injury

A hospital-based series [2] described the characteristics of patients suffering stroke in the context of polytrauma (defined as at least two injuries, one involving a major vital organ such as lung or liver). Traumatic craniocervical arterial dissection (TCAD) was the most commonly identified mechanism, and skull or facial fractures were a possible marker for this, with most of the patients with dissection also having these injuries. TCAD has also been referred to as blunt cerebrovascular injury (BCVI). Motor vehicle accidents are a common cause of BCVI to the carotid or vertebral arteries, but other injuries including falls, near hangings, biking and snow sports accidents are potential causes. There are a number of likely direct causative mechanisms for the vascular injury [3], including acceleration/deceleration resulting in shearing forces to the vessel wall, and direct compression of the artery against hard bony structures during flexion/extension and rotational head movements. The carotid artery may be compressed between the spine and the mandible. The vertebral artery is commonly dissected at the C1–C2 level by rotational forces, and can be directly traumatized when there is fracture or dislocation of facet joints or transverse processes. The arterial injury creates a nidus for platelet aggregation [3] with subsequent distal embolization being the more common mechanism for ischemic stroke, rather than arterial occlusion causing infarction due to hypoperfusion, according to the pattern of infarct distribution observed in one study [4]. There is often a "silent period" between the injury, and the onset of stroke symptoms, typically between 10 and 72 hours [3].

Attempts have been made to predict the likelihood of BCVI, particularly with a view to identifying and potentially treating and preventing stroke. Combinations of injury patterns, symptoms and signs have been the basis of screening criteria for BCVI [3]. Mid-facial, base of skull, and cervical spine fractures may be markers of risk for BCVI [3,5] and are likely to be associated with shearing and torsional stresses sufficient to damage the

---

Treatment-Related Stroke, ed. Alexander Tsiskaridze, Arne Lindgren and Adnan Qureshi. Published by Cambridge University Press. © Cambridge University Press 2016.

arteries [2]. A prospective study [6] used a number of clinical criteria derived from the literature to select trauma patients for four-vessel angiography. Criteria included the presence of neurological symptoms or signs suggesting stroke or TIA or a Horner's syndrome, signs of local soft tissue injury to the neck, and specific injuries, such as skull base, mid-face and cervical spine fractures, and major thoracic injuries such as first rib or sternal fractures, flail chest, and pulmonary contusions. In 325 patients undergoing angiography, 100 (30.8%) had positive findings, ranging from minor luminal irregularities in 21 (6.5%) through to occlusion in 11 (3.4%), and transection in 3 (0.9%). Dissection with greater than 25% reduction of the intraluminal diameter, intraluminal thrombus, or a raised intimal flap was found in 44 (13.5%), and pseudoaneurysm in 21 (6.5%). The latter two groups (i.e., 20% of the patients), were treated with heparin if there were no contraindications due to other injuries, or aspirin if there were. The injuries most likely to be associated with significant angiographic abnormalities were mid-face and cervical spine fractures, where almost 31% of patients in each category had a major vascular lesion. The yield in patients with thoracic or soft tissue neck injuries was much lower (10% and zero). The authors [6] recommended that screening was not indicated in the latter two groups of patients, although with the current availability of non-invasive CT or MR angiography, the decision to image the cervical vessels is now substantially easier. These non-invasive techniques have been shown to have very similar accuracy to digital subtraction angiography in trauma patients, are substantially easier to perform, and are also cheaper [7].

Blunt thoracic aortic injury is a major cause of death from trauma [8]. Associated with this, injury to the intrathoracic origin of the craniocervical arteries may result in stroke. Less severe trauma has been reported [9] to cause stroke due to embolism from protruding atheroma of the aortic arch.

Cardiac emboli

Another potential mechanism is atheroembolism from a cardiac source. Within the series of stroke in polytrauma patients [2], four had strokes related to a cardiac source. Two were likely due to direct cardiac blunt injury resulting in documented regional wall motion abnormalities, and two patients developed atrial fibrillation. Paradoxical embolism via a patent foramen ovale may be of particular concern in immobilized patients with lower limb or pelvic injuries.

Other miscellaneous causes

In the subacute, recovery phase, multitrauma patients, in a similar way as complex medical patients, may be predisposed to arterial and venous ischemic events because of the potential prothrombotic milieu as discussed in Chapter 5. Withdrawal of antithrombotic medications because of trauma-causing hemorrhagic complications has been implicated in at least one patient with a delayed onset in-hospital thrombotic stroke following trauma [2]. A hypertensive hemorrhage occurring in hospital after trauma has also been reported [2], possibly linked to pain related to the trauma-induced injuries, and consequent blood pressure elevations and fluctuations. The issue of fat embolism is also mentioned in Chapter 13.

It should be mentioned that stroke patients are at substantially increased risk of fractures [10], related to falls, and localized osteoporosis. Given that prior risk of stroke places patients at increased risk for subsequent stroke, such patients when hospitalized for trauma are a high-risk population.

Time course and recognition of stroke after trauma

The precise time of stroke onset may be difficult to identify, particularly in polytrauma patients with impaired consciousness related to cerebral injury, or the use of sedating medications. Limb fractures may also make hemiparesis difficult to recognize. Many patients are recognized to have stroke symptoms within the first 48 hours post trauma [2,3], but stroke may occur days to weeks later, particularly if indirect mechanisms are implicated. Stroke occurring during the months after trauma is discussed later in this chapter.

Acute therapy for stroke in trauma patients

In terms of acute therapy, multitrauma and head-injured patients pose great management dilemmas. Significant head trauma within the previous three months is listed as an exclusion criterion, and serious trauma within 14 days is listed as a relative exclusion criterion to intravenous tissue-plasminogen activator (t-PA) in the American Heart Association (AHA)

Stroke guidelines [11]. A series [12] of five patients with simple limb fractures who were treated with intravenous t-PA has recently been reported. In four of the five patients a stroke resulted in a fall, causing the fracture. Two of the patients had their fractures reduced and placed in a backslab (plaster applied only on one side of the limb), prior to treatment with intravenous t-PA, all less than three hours after symptom onset. Apart from some minor bruising and swelling at the fracture site, there were no major hemorrhagic complications, and no late fracture problems. There are dramatic case reports [13,14] of mechanical clot extraction and intra-arterial thrombolytic therapy in a few patients with acute stroke related to trauma, usually in the context of arterial dissection, with distal embolization and major arterial occlusion. Recent trials demonstrating significant benefits of mechanical thrombectomy combined with intravenous t-PA, compared with intravenous therapy alone [15], are likely to stimulate the expansion of interventional neuroradiology services to provide mechanical thrombectomy. It is highly likely that major centers receiving trauma patients will also have access to this form of stroke therapy. Recommendation number five in a focused update to the 2013 AHA stroke guidelines [16] states that in carefully selected patients who have contraindications to intravenous t-PA, endovascular therapy with stent retrievers within six hours of stroke onset is reasonable. This may well be applicable to some trauma patients.

There has been substantial discussion in the trauma literature regarding the use of antithrombotic medications for the treatment of BCVI, particularly during the latent period, after the injury, with a view to preventing ischemic stroke as a complication. There appears to be no good randomized data, and such studies would be extremely difficult to perform in this group of patients. Observational data [17,18] have suggested that more than a third of trauma patients with BCVI were unsuitable for any form of antithrombotic therapy because of the hemorrhagic nature of other injuries. Ischemic stroke rates were as high as 57% in these patients [19], but this does not infer that treatment with anticoagulants improves neurological outcome in BCVI [3]. Older small series [17–21] from the surgical literature commonly recommended anticoagulation with heparin, although some [22,23] advised aspirin as an alternative. Endovascular repair using stents has also become more common [24], although some reports [25] have found higher rates of occlusion and other complications with stenting compared with medical therapy alone. Given that we know from large randomized studies [26] in atheroembolic stroke that there is no benefit for early anticoagulation to reduce the risk of early recurrent stroke, it would seem unlikely that anticoagulation would be of significant overall benefit to BCVI patients, who may well be at great risk from systemic hemorrhagic complications due to other injuries. Even antiplatelet therapy (which is also required intensively following stenting procedures) may have hazards in trauma patients. Following on from the recent advances regarding mechanical thrombectomy as an acute therapy option, perhaps an alternative could be to put less emphasis on the use of anticoagulation or even antiplatelet therapy in this group of patients, and more emphasis on ensuring that the patient is in a setting where endovascular stroke therapy could be undertaken should stroke symptoms develop. This might require transfer of the patient to another facility where interventional radiology services are available.

Stroke in the months after trauma

In one study, 2.9% of patients with traumatic brain injury (TBI) suffered a stroke within the first three months [27], a time when many may still have been inpatients in tertiary hospitals or rehabilitation facilities. This rate was more than ten-fold increased compared with controls, and the increased risk of stroke was also found at one-year (4.6-fold increase), and at five-year (2.3-fold increase) follow up. The presence of a skull fracture was the strongest marker for stroke risk. Traditional risk factors such as hypertension and atrial fibrillation were considered and adjusted for, but the authors noted that hypertension and sleep apnea are common complications after TBI, so these may partially account for increased stroke risk [27]. In addition to the well recognized mechanism of direct arterial injury the authors propose that TBI might potentially "loosen" clots formed within atherosclerotic vessels. They also proposed an additional possible cause of stroke in TBI patients: the use of antipsychotic medication. These agents, particularly the increasingly used atypical neuroleptic agents, have been recognized to potentially increase stroke risk [28]. It is also possible that pain-related blood pressure fluctuations, and the use of NSAID medications for analgesia [29], may play a role in increasing stroke risk.

Another group of hospitalized trauma patients, typically on rehabilitation wards, who appear to be at an approximately three-fold increased risk for stroke, are spinal cord injury (SCI) patients. A nationwide cohort study [30] from Taiwan used a comprehensive database to examine the risk of stroke in SCI patients. Stable SCI patients were matched with controls of similar age, gender, and similar cardiovascular risk-factor profiles. The overall hazard ratio for stroke in the SCI group was 2.85, with a higher rate of ischemic than hemorrhagic stroke. The authors [30] speculate that SCI patients may develop additional risk for stroke beyond the traditional cardiovascular risks including obesity, dyslipidemia, diabetes mellitus, and reduced exercise (all of which are prominent in SCI patients). These other, less recognized stroke risk factors may include infection, inflammation, and hypercoagulability. Additionally, SCI patients may be vulnerable to fluctuations of blood pressure, particularly in the presence of autonomic dysreflexia. Blood pressure variability may well be an important trigger of stroke [31].

Concluding remarks

It is likely that a collaborative approach between trauma unit and stroke unit staff is the best way to manage trauma patients who suffer a stroke. Vigilance to the development of stroke symptoms is critical, and close observation of "at-risk" patients is important. Stroke physicians should be in the best position to balance the complexities of acute treatment decisions, in discussion with surgical and interventional radiology colleagues. Endovascular therapy may become an increasingly available therapeutic option. The expertise of stroke unit nursing and allied health staff [32] is also very important, and there are specific details of stroke care that they can assist trauma unit and intensive care staff with.

References

1. Farooq M U, Reeves M J, Gargano J, et al. In-hospital stroke in a statewide registry. Cerebrovasc Dis. 2008; 25:12–20.

2. Blacker D J, Wijdicks E F. Clinical characteristics and mechanisms of stroke after polytrauma. Mayo Clin Proc. 2004; 79:630–5.

3. Cothren C C, Moore E E. Blunt cerebrovascular injuries. Clinics. 2005; 60:489–96.

4. Lucas C, Moulin T, Deplanque D, Tatu L, Chavot D. Stroke patterns of internal carotid artery dissection in 40 patients. Stroke. 1998; 29:2646–8.

5. Mokri B, Piepgras D G, Houser O W. Traumatic dissections of the extracranial internal carotid artery. J Neurosurg. 1988; 68:189–97.

6. Ringer A J, Matern E, Parikh S, Levine N B. Screening for blunt cerebrovascular injury: selection criteria for use of angiography. J Neurosurg. 2010; 112: 1146–9.

7. Wang A C, Charters M A, Thawani J P, et al. Evaluating the use and utility of noninvasive angiography in diagnosing traumatic blunt cerebrovascular injury. J Trauma Acute Care Surg. 2012; 72:1601–10.

8. Clancy T V, Gary M J, Covington D L, Brinker C C, Blackman D. A statewide analysis of level I and II trauma centers for patients with major injuries. J Trauma. 2001; 51:346–51.

9. Corti R, Alerci M, Tosi C, et al. Images in cardiovascular medicine. Cerebral arterial embolism from a protruding atheroma of the aortic arch after a nonpenetrating chest trauma. Circulation. 1999; 100: 1009–10.

10. Dennis M S, Lo K M, McDowall M, West T. Fractures after stroke. Stroke. 2002; 33:728–34.

11. Jauch E C, Saver J L, Adams H P, et al. Guidelines for the early management of patients with acute ischemic stroke: a guideline for healthcare professionals from the American Heart Association/American Stroke Association. Stroke. 2013; 44:870–947.

12. Ahmad N, Ward E, Natarajan I, Roffe C. Intravenous stroke thrombolysis in the presence of traumatic bone fractures. Cerebrovasc Dis. 2012; Supp 2:83.

13. Cohen J E, Gomori J M, Grigoriadis S, et al. Intra-arterial thrombolysis and stent placement for traumatic carotid dissection with subsequent stroke: A combined simultaneous endovascular approach. J Neurol Sciences. 2008; 269:172–5.

14. Sugrue P A, Hage Z A, Surdell D L, et al. Basilar artery occlusion following C1 lateral mass fracture managed by mechanical and pharmacological thrombolysis. Neurocritical Care. 2009; 11:255–60.

15. Furlan A J. Endovascular therapy for stroke: it's about time. N Engl J Med. 2015; 45:35–8.

16. Powers W J, Derdeyn C P, Biller J, et al. AHA/ASA focused update of the 2013 guidelines for the early management of patients with acute ischemic stroke regarding endovascular treatment. Stroke. 2015; published before print June 29, 2015.

17. Stein D M, Boswell S, Sliker C W, Lui F Y, Scalea T M. Blunt cerebrovascular injuries: does treatment always matter? J Trauma. 2009; 66:132–43.

18. Cothren C C, Biffl W L, Moore E E, Kashuk J L, Johnson J L. Treatment for blunt cerebrovascular injuries: equivalence of anticoagulation and antiplatelet agents. *Arch Surg.* 2009; **144**:685–90.

19. Callcut R A, Hanseman D J, Solan P D, *et al.* Early treatment of blunt cerebrovascular injury with concomitant hemorrhagic neurological injury is safe and effective. *J Trauma Acute Care Surg.* 2012; **72**: 338–45.

20. Davis J W, Holbrook T L, Hoyt D B, *et al.* Blunt carotid dissection: incidence, associated injuries, screening and treatment. *J Trauma.* 1990; **30**:1514–17.

21. Anson J, Cromwell R M. Cervicocranial arterial dissection. *Neurosurgery.* 1991; **29**:89–96.

22. Wahl W L, Brandt M M, Thompson B G, Taheri P A, Greefield L J. Antiplatelet therapy: an alternative to heparin for blunt carotid injury. *J Trauma.* 2002; **52**:896–901.

23. Cothren C C, Moore E E, Biffl W L, *et al.* Anticoagulation is the gold standard therapy for blunt carotid injuries to reduce stroke rate. *Arch Surg.* 2004; **139**:545–6.

24. DiCocco J M, Fabian T C, Emmett K P, *et al.* Optimal outcomes for patients with blunt cerebrovascular injury (BCVI): tailoring treatment to the lesion. *J Am Coll Surg.* 2011; **212**:547–9.

25. Cothren C C, Moore E E, Ray C E, *et al.* Carotid artery stents for blunt cerebrovascular injury: risks exceed benefits. *Arch Surg.* 2005; **140**:480–5.

26. International Stroke Trial Collaborative Group. The International Stroke Trial (IST): a randomised trial of aspirin, subcutaneous heparin, both or neither among 19 435 patients with acute ischaemic stroke. *Lancet.* 1997; **349**:1569–81.

27. Chen Y H, Kang J H, Lin H C. Patients with traumatic brain injury. Population-based study suggests increased risk of stroke. *Stroke.* 2011; **42**:2733–9.

28. Glenn M B. Sudden cardiac death and stroke with use of antipsychotic medications: Implications for clinicians treating individuals with traumatic brain injury. *J Head Trauma Rehabil.* 2010; **25**:68–70.

29. Blacker D J. NSAIDS and stroke risk. *Med J Aust.* 2011; **41**:488.

30. Wu J C, Chen Y C, Liu L, *et al.* Increased risk of stroke after spinal cord injury. *Neurology.* 2012; **78**: 1051–7.

31. Rothwell P M. Does blood pressure variability modulate cardiovascular risk? *Curr Hypertens Rep.* 2011; **13**:177–86.

32. Weinhardt J, Jacobson K. Stroke assessment in the perioperative patient. *Orthop Nurs.* 2012; **31**:21–6.

Chapter

7

Stroke associated with endovascular procedures

Nabeel A. Herial, Mushtaq H. Qureshi and Adnan I. Qureshi

Introduction

An estimated 35,000 to 75,000 in-hospital stroke (IHS) cases occur each year in the United States [1] and one out of every five acute ischemic stroke patients treated with thrombolytics is receiving treatment for IHS [2]. As many as 15% of all acute strokes treated in hospitals are related to strokes occurring in patients admitted to hospital. The majority of these cases have a cardiovascular admission diagnosis (approximately 40%), followed by a neurological or neurosurgical diagnosis [3]. Nearly 68% of IHS patients had an invasive diagnostic, surgical, or other endovascular procedure undertaken prior to the stroke. Cerebrovascular ischemic or hemorrhagic complications are unwanted but frequently encountered circumstances surrounding endovascular procedures.

In this chapter we elaborate on the pathophysiology underlying thrombosis, identify the endovascular procedures frequently associated with an increased risk for stroke, explore the mechanisms, and explain the characteristics of a stroke after such endovascular procedures.

Pathophysiology underlying thrombosis and endothelial repair

The endothelium is a cellular layer that surrounds the blood vessels and provides protection to the luminal contents from collagen and other thrombogenic materials such as von Willebrand factor and tissue factor. Disruption of the endothelial layer triggers platelet activation, adhesion, and aggregation. Additionally, activation of the coagulation cascade is also noted. A correlation between the extent of endothelial damage and thrombosis has been established [4–95].

Platelet adhesion

Glycoproteins (GPs) present on the platelet surface are responsible for adhesion of platelets to the vessel wall following tissue injury (Figure 7.1). Activation of platelets is the subsequent step in the thrombotic process that follows adhesion and involves several chemical processes. Adenosine diphosphate (ADP), thromboxane A2, and serotonin are known chemicals that further facilitate platelet activation [4–44]. Platelet activation further leads to increased expression of GP IIb/IIIa receptors on the platelet surface [4–78]. The GP IIb/IIIa receptors then bind to fibrinogen and trigger platelet aggregation. Tissue factor that is exposed following injury to the vessel wall binds to coagulation factors VII and subsequently stimulates factor X. The sequence of events involved in the coagulation process is discussed in the next section.

Coagulation cascade

The coagulation pathway is a sequence of enzymatic events that ultimately leads to formation of a thrombus (Figure 7.2). It includes an intrinsic and extrinsic pathway that culminate in a common last enzymatic reaction that produces factor X. The intrinsic pathway is more important, but a slower process compared to the extrinsic pathway and is triggered when the sub-endothelial surface is exposed after tissue damage. Activation of factor XII occurs after binding of this molecule to the exposed surface of the vessel wall. Through mechanisms of auto-activation of factor XII, and forward activation

Treatment-Related Stroke, ed. Alexander Tsiskaridze, Arne Lindgren and Adnan Qureshi. Published by Cambridge University Press. © Cambridge University Press 2016.

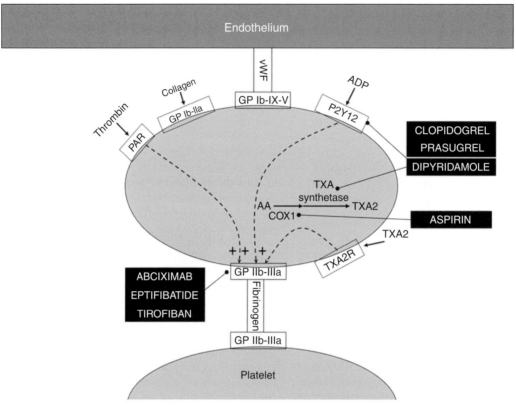

Figure 7.1 Platelet activation and targets for antiplatelet agents. Antiplatelet agents listed at the point of their mechanism of action. Note the positive feedback provided by ADP and thrombin released by activated platelets. (Source: Hussein H M, *et al. Am J Neuroradiol.* 2013; 34:700–6).

of the intrinsic pathway, factor X is ultimately activated. Factor VIII is implicated in the activation of factor X.

The extrinsic pathway is an alternative and rapid mechanism of thrombus formation following tissue injury. Activation of factor X occurs almost instantaneously, when tissue factor or factor III binds to factor VII, which is then activated to form a complex of tissue factor, activated factor VII, calcium, and a phospholipid. This complex then rapidly activates factor X, which is essential for the common final pathway leading to formation of thrombin (factor IIa).

Formation of a thrombus through activation of the coagulation cascade depends on the degree of tissue factor and thrombin production, which reportedly continues for nearly 24 hours after the arterial injury [4–47,95]. The thrombin levels in the plasma remain elevated for about three days after initial vascular insult, but it is the persistent activation of thrombin that is responsible for several thrombotic complications surrounding endovascular procedures [4–47]. Acetylsalicylic acid (ASA) counters these late

effects of thrombin reportedly via factor Xa/Va activity [4–119]. Antithrombin III counteracts thrombin and factors IX and X [4–128].

Repair

The process of endothelial repair is dependent on the intact endothelial cells adjacent to the site of injury and is typically complete in about a two-week duration [4–89]. However, the architecture and alignment of the renewed cellular layer is altered, and endothelial function is impaired for about four weeks [4–42]. Endothelial tissue growth over foreign bodies, such as metallic stents, a process frequently referred to as endothelialization, typically takes about four weeks [4–122].

Antithrombotic agents

Two major pathways exist in the formation of intravascular thrombus. One involves platelet adhesion and aggregation, and the other tissue factor directed

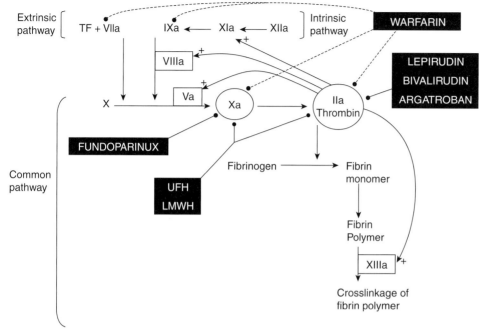

Figure 7.2 Diagram of coagulation cascade and anticoagulant targets of action. Intrinsic, extrinsic, and common pathways are depicted. (Source: Hussein H M, *et al. Am J Neuroradiol*. 2012; 33:1211–20.)

coagulation cascade. In the next section we discuss currently available pharmacological agents used in the prevention of thrombosis.

Platelet adhesion and aggregation

Agents frequently referred to as antiplatelets are extensively used in cardiovascular and cerebrovascular diseases. Molecular targets of these agents include inhibition of thromboxane A2, or ADP release, or via the GP IIb/IIIa receptor blockade.

Aspirin

The antiplatelet effects of aspirin are via an irreversible inhibition of the cyclo-oxygenase-1 pathway and production of thromboxane A2 [4–104]. Complete inhibition of thromboxane A2 production is noted with an aspirin dose of 100 mg [4–96]. The antiplatelet effect of aspirin is typically immediate and lasts for several days. Although it is argued that higher doses of aspirin are more effective [34], known evidence suggests no significant difference between different daily doses.

Aspirin is a weak platelet inhibitor and does not inhibit platelet aggregation by thromboxane A2-independent pathways or affect platelet adhesion or secretion [103]. Therefore aspirin has no effect on

thrombin, which is thought to play a major role in acute ischemic syndromes. Aspirin, unlike the newer antiplatelet agents, does not affect platelet secretion and thus has no effect on local accumulation of platelet-derived mitogenic factors [103]. These mitogenic factors promote cellular proliferation and lead to re-stenosis and accelerated atherosclerosis after angioplasty. Another limitation of aspirin therapy is that individual responses to aspirin vary unpredictably.

Ticlopidine and clopidogrel

Ticlopidine and clopidogrel are thienopyridine derivatives that inhibit platelet aggregation. Both are orally administered agents, metabolized in the liver, and have renal elimination of their active metabolites. Both ticlopidine and clopidogrel inhibit the binding of ADP to its platelet receptor (Figure 7.1). This ADP receptor blockade leads to direct inhibition of fibrinogen binding to the GP IIb/IIIa complex. The inhibition of platelet aggregation by both agents is concentration dependent. Adequate inhibition with ticlopidine (500 mg, daily) or clopidogrel (75 mg, daily) requires two to three days after the initiation of therapy [27]. Maximal inhibition occurs after four to seven days, and higher doses do not produce additional platelet impairment. The antiplatelet action is irreversible and lasts for eight to ten days. Concomitant aspirin use results in synergistic inhibition of platelet aggregation, presumably because of potentiation of the effect of aspirin on collagen-induced platelet aggregation [55]. Furthermore, the addition of aspirin to ticlopidine therapy reduces the delay observed in ticlopidine-induced platelet inhibition. Although ticlopidine and clopidogrel have not been compared, recent studies suggest that clopidogrel is more effective than either aspirin or ticlopidine in preventing coronary stent thrombosis caused by high shear stress [90]. However, in secondary stroke prevention, no increased benefit was noted between aspirin and Plavix (clopidigrel) monotherapy [129].

A major side effect of ticlopidine and clopidogrel is bleeding. Among patients with ischemic stroke enrolled in the Ticlopidine Aspirin Stroke Study and the Canadian American Ticlopidine Study, the rates of major hemorrhage and minor bleeding with ticlopidine were 0.2 to 0.5% and 6.5 to 9%, respectively [11,46,57]. In the Clopidogrel versus Aspirin in Patients at Risk for Ischemic Events Study, the frequency of major bleeding associated with clopidogrel was 1.4% [20]. In comparison, the rate of major bleeding associated with aspirin in the Ticlopidine Aspirin Stroke Study and the Clopidogrel versus Aspirin in Patients at Risk for Ischemic Events Study was 1.4 to 1.6% [11,20,57].

Cilostazol

Cilostazol is a selective phosphodiesterase-3 inhibitor used clinically for its antiplatelet effects [130]. There is evidence suggesting benefit from cilostazol in secondary stroke prevention [131] as an effective and safer alternative to aspirin [132,133]. Cilostazol prevents platelet aggregation by blocking platelet adenosine uptake and adenosine-induced platelet activation [134]. An increased benefit in patients with ischemic stroke and peripheral artery disease is proposed. A clinical trial evaluating safety and efficacy of dual antiplatelet agents, aspirin plus cilostazol, in comparison with aspirin alone is underway [135].

Platelet GP IIb/IIIa receptor-specific antibodies

Inhibition of GP IIb/IIIa receptors prevents binding of fibrinogen and thereby platelet aggregation irrespective of the triggering mechanism and represents the final common pathway in platelet aggregation [136].

Abciximab

Abciximab is a non-immunogenic modified human immunoglobulin that binds to the GP IIb/IIa receptors to demonstrate inhibition of platelet aggregation [82]. It is intravenously administered and is a short-acting agent with a half-life of 10 minutes, but its effects on platelets last for almost 48 hours.

Eptifibatide

Eptifibatide is an intravenously administered peptide inhibitor, more specifically targeting the GP IIb/IIIa receptors to carry out its pharmacological function. Non-peptide inhibitors of GP IIb/IIIa receptors are also available and include lamifiban and tirofiban. When 80% of the GP IIb/IIIa receptors are blocked, platelet aggregation is nearly completely eliminated, but the bleeding time is only mildly affected. Prolongation of bleeding time to 15 to 30 minutes is observed with 90% receptor blockade [25,29].

Tirofiban

Tirofiban is an intravenously administered non-peptide agent that prevents platelet aggregation by binding reversibly to the GP IIb/IIIa receptors. It has a fast-acting action and a half-life of about two hours. It is currently approved for treatment of acute coronary syndrome up to 48 hours after onset [137].

The optimal duration of treatment with drugs that inhibit GP IIb/IIIa receptors has not been determined. In the Evaluation of Abciximab for Prevention of Ischemic Complications Trial [38], a benefit was noted with drug administration one hour before the procedure and continued for 12 hours; this is currently the most accepted administration regimen. Currently there are no scientific data to support the use of GP IIb/IIIa antagonists in the management of acute stroke [138]. The Abciximab in Emergency Treatment of Stroke Trial (AbESTT) used abciximab in acute stroke management, but the trial was stopped due to high bleeding complications without an improvement of clinical outcome [139]. However, one study reported abciximab as safe and effective in the treatment of acute cerebral thromboembolic complications during neuroendovascular procedures [140]. A randomized clinical trial of tirofiban vs. placebo administered within 3 to 22 hours after symptom onset was safe in acute moderate stroke patients (with NIHHS 4 to 18) [141]. However, in a recent cohort study of tirofiban use in acute stroke patients that underwent endovascular thrombectomy, an increased risk of fatal intracerebral hemorrhage was reported [142].

Orally active inhibitors of GP IIb/IIIa receptors were also developed for possible use in long-term platelet aggregation. However, unlike the parenterally administered agents, the oral agents (orbofiban, roxifiban, sibrafiban, xemilofiban) were associated with increased hemorrhagic complications and no clear protection from ischemic events [143]. Mortality increased in each of the five trials (OPUS-TIMI 16, EXCITE, SYMPHONY, 2nd SYMPHONY, BRAVO, PURPOSE) [144–148]. A combined analysis using a sample size of 45,523 patients revealed a highly significant 35% relative increase in the risk of death and a two-fold increase in the risk of bleeding [149].

Inhibition of thrombin and fibrinogen activation

Tissue factor-induced activation of thrombin can be inhibited with use of any of the following agents: AT III-dependent inhibitors such as standard heparin, and low-molecular weight heparin (LMWH) preparations, direct thrombin inhibitors such as hirudin and its analogs bivalirudin and hirugen, or with indirect inhibitors such as warfarin.

Heparin

Intravenously administered heparin activates and modulates AT III activity, resulting in thrombin neutralization and inactivation of factors IXa, Xa, XIa, and XIIa [58]. Indirect actions that contribute to the anticoagulant effects of heparin include the specific inhibition of thrombin by heparin cofactor II and the restoration of endothelial surface electronegativity. Heparin also has antiplatelet effects in vivo, by preventing thrombin-induced platelet aggregation and inhibiting von Willebrand factor [94]. The anticoagulant effects of heparin are immediate and the half-life is approximately 1.5 hours.

Two major complications are associated with heparin treatment, i.e., hemorrhagic complications and idiosyncratic, immunologically induced thrombocytopenia [10]. Thrombocytopenia is observed 3 to 15 days after treatment initiation and usually resolves within 4 days after treatment cessation. Resistance to heparin may be encountered during treatment and effectiveness of heparin is usually correlated with degree of anticoagulation. Measurement of the activated coagulation time (ACT) is the preferred method for evaluation of responses to heparin due to its linear heparin dose–response curve. This relationship is maintained even at the higher doses of IV heparin used during interventional procedures [16]. Activated partial thromboplastin time (aPTT) is also a measure of heparin effectiveness; however, a non-linear, logarithmic response is noted at higher doses of heparin. Acute thrombosis immediately after coronary stent placement is correlated with low ACTs [12,41] and titration of IV heparin on the basis of ACT values, to ensure adequate antithrombin activity is recommended [12,41]. During the procedure, administration of a 10,000-unit bolus dose followed by repeated bolus doses to achieve an ACT of more than 300 seconds (HemoTec) or 350 seconds (Hemochron) is recommended. One study that evaluated ACT levels and procedural outcomes involving a carotid stenosis procedure reported an optimal peak procedural ACT time of 250 to 299 seconds [150]. On the contrary, use of IV heparin during the postprocedural period is controversial with no proven benefit in reducing thrombotic complications [36,43]. Furthermore, continuing heparin therapy after the procedure can increase the risk of bleeding from the site of the sheath [91].

Low molecular weight heparin

Heparin chains bind to endothelial cells and a variety of plasma proteins where the chains are rapidly cleaved by a saturable, dose-dependent mechanism [121]. This non-specific binding of heparin limits the amount of the same available to interact with AT III and decreases the anticoagulant effect of heparin. In contrast, LMWH preparations have lower affinity for both endothelial cells and the heparin-binding proteins observed in plasma [121]. The decreased non-specific binding of LMWH explains why LMWH has greater bioavailability at low doses and produces more predictable anticoagulant responses compared to standard heparin. In fact, the anticoagulant effects of weight-adjusted doses are so predictable that little or no laboratory monitoring is required.

Low molecular weight heparin, unlike standard unfractionated heparin, has little or no effect on coagulation tests. It retains the ability to inhibit thrombosis but is associated with fewer bleeding complications [14]. An additional advantage of LMWH is a lower risk of heparin-induced thrombocytopenia [120].

Two preparations, i.e., enoxaparin and dalteparin, have been approved for use in the United States. A double-blind, placebo-controlled clinical trial of high-risk coronary stenting that evaluated the effect of aspirin and ticlopidine vs. LMWH, aspirin, and ticlopidine, the High Risk Stent Trial, revealed no added benefit with the use of LMWH [151].

Direct inhibitors of thrombin

Low molecular weight heparin overcomes many of the pharmacokinetic limitations of standard heparin. However, both LMWH and standard heparin are relatively ineffective inhibitors of thrombin after its binding to fibrin [59,121]. In contrast, AT III-independent inhibitors of thrombin, such as hirudin and its analogs, are able to access and inactivate thrombin bound to fibrin [100,121]. Direct thrombin inhibitors seem to be promising adjunctive therapies in angioplasty [107]. They have no effect on platelets, eliminating the risk of heparin-induced thrombocytopenia [107]. In a dose-escalation study [107], bivalirudin was used instead of heparin for 291 patients undergoing coronary angioplasty. The rates of abrupt vessel closure and clinically important bleeding events with high doses of bivalirudin compared favorably with the rates observed when a similar patient group was treated with heparin. In a meta-analysis of several clinical trials with data on 30,446 patients, a higher risk of stent thrombosis but lower risk of major bleeding was observed with bivalirudin when compared to heparin. In a study evaluating dose response and effectiveness of bilavirudin, a high-dose protocol (target ACT 300–350) in neuroembolization procedures was considered a safe alternative to heparin [152].

Warfarin

Among the derivatives of naturally occurring lactones (coumarins), warfarin is the most widely used agent because of its pharmacodynamic profile. Coumarins modulate anticoagulant activity by retarding thrombin generation through inhibition of the vitamin K/epoxide reductase activity-dependent coagulation factors II, VII, IX, and X. Warfarin is rapidly absorbed from the gastrointestinal tract, with peak plasma values being reached within 90 minutes; its half-life is approximately 40 hours. Because the dose–response relationship for warfarin differs among individuals and many other drugs can interfere with its pharmacokinetics, close

monitoring is essential. The anticoagulant effects of warfarin appear when the normal clotting factors are cleared from the circulation (within 8 hours for factor VII but only after 72–96 hours for factors II, IX, and X). Loading doses of warfarin rapidly prolong the prothrombin time, but at a significant cost of increased risk of bleeding. Therefore loading doses are not recommended with warfarin. The thrombogenic potential may be higher at the initiation of therapy, because of the rapid depletion of vitamin K-dependent anticoagulant protein C (half-life, 6 hours). The major risk associated with warfarin use is bleeding. Low rates of intracranial hemorrhage (0.3% annually) or other major hemorrhage (1–2% annually) were documented in seven studies of stroke prevention using warfarin in cases of atrial fibrillation [111].

Use of antiplatelet vs. anticoagulant therapy in endovascular procedures

This question has been raised with respect to patients undergoing stent placement and angioplasty for treatment of coronary or cerebral vascular diseases. Patients were treated with a variety of anticoagulant agents in initial attempts to reduce the high risk of thrombosis associated with coronary artery angioplasty and stent placement. Between 1989 and 1993, the standard regimens consisted of aspirin, dipyridamole, dextran, heparin, and warfarin. These aggressive regimens produced considerable bleeding complications, especially hematomas at the insertion sites for femoral sheaths, at rates of 3 to 16% [83]. Furthermore, these anticoagulant regimens did not effectively prevent subacute thrombosis; the rate remained approximately 7% and was as high as 28% when stenting was used to salvage angioplastic procedures. Coupled with these disadvantages were prolonged hospital stays [69,153].

The high complication rates and the failure to prevent subacute thrombosis prompted a search for alternative antithrombotic regimens, with the emphasis on antiplatelet agents (aspirin and ticlopidine) rather than anticoagulants. This was supported by evidence suggesting that local platelet deposition and activation are the major factors in thrombosis after angioplasty and stent placement [64]. Initial research with attempts to identify regimens replacing anticoagulants with antiplatelet agents was successful [67]. The aspirin dose was lowered, heparin was administered only as a bolus dose and was followed by LMWH, ticlopidine was introduced, and dipyridamole, dextran, and warfarin were discontinued, all of which reduced the rate of bleeding complications by two-thirds and the frequency of subacute thrombosis was decreased to approximately one-eighth of the previous level (from 10.4% to 1.3–1.8%). In conclusion, during coronary artery stent deployment, the introduction of antiplatelet therapy (aspirin and ticlopidine), as opposed to anticoagulant therapy, has resulted in fewer bleeding complications, shorter hospital stays, and reduced stent thrombotic closure rates.

Combination antiplatelet therapy vs. monotherapy

Because of potential synergistic action, a combination of aspirin and ticlopidine has been evaluated for use for coronary stent placement. Initial non-randomized studies added ticlopidine (250 mg, twice daily, for one month) to the postprocedural regimen of aspirin and heparin or LMWH. In a French multicenter registry, 1,251 patients received ticlopidine, and the use of this agent led to a reduction in stent thrombosis from 10.4% to between 1.3 and 1.8%, with fewer bleeding complications [69]. In another study [26], 321 patients who underwent stent placement after high-pressure balloon expansion received aspirin (325 mg, once daily, for five days) and ticlopidine (250 mg, twice daily, for one month) or aspirin alone for one month. At six months, the rate of stent thrombosis was 0.8% for patients treated with aspirin and ticlopidine, compared with 1.4% for the group treated with aspirin alone [48,54]. In the larger Stent Antithrombotic Regimen Study, the incidence of MI, death, subsequent angioplasty, or coronary bypass at one month was reduced by 80% for the aspirin/ticlopidine group (compared with the patients treated with aspirin alone) [153]. Laboratory evidence supporting these clinical observations was also noted. A marked reduction in the deposition of platelets and fibrinogen on the stent surface in a baboon model of arterial thrombosis was seen when clopidogrel was used in combination with aspirin (compared with clopidogrel alone) [56].

Endovascular procedures and thrombogenic factors

Contrast agents

Angiographic contrast agents can be classified based on their osmolality as low-, iso-, or high-osmolar agents. Additionally, the contrast agents could be divided into ionic or non-ionic [98]. Risk of thrombus formation with contrast agents was basically derived from experiments measuring the rate of clot formation in syringes with a mixture of contrast and blood [42,67]. Contrast agents have been implicated in promoting blood clots in catheters and syringes used in angiography [51,61,97]. However, there is hardly any evidence from clinical studies supporting thromboembolic risk from contrast agents. In one prior study [45] non-ionic contrast agent use during coronary angioplasty was associated with higher risk of thrombosis particularly with prolonged exposure [98]. Contrast agents were noted to decrease platelet aggregation in laboratory studies and this effect was more with ionic agents [37,49]. Use of ionic contrast agents in place of non-ionic agents in cerebral angiography is of no real advantage, but for prolonged angiographic procedures ionic materials may be a consideration.

Angiographic devices

Catheters, microcatheters, and guide wires used in angiography may acts as nidi for thrombus formation [65,66] due to their surface properties and chemical composition [14,87,99,105]. Prior research has suggested a lower tendency of thrombus formation with use of polyurethane catheters due to their regular external surface [14]. Both polyurethane and polyethylene catheters have demonstrated smoother internal surfaces making them less thrombogenic. Heparin applied to the external surface of the catheters reduces incidence of thrombus deposition and adherence. This phenomenon is primarily due to the negative molecular charge of the heparin decreasing the interaction between catheter material and the blood [71]. Microcatheters with a hydrophilic coating that are currently available and more frequently used have significantly reduced the incidence of thrombosis. Research has shown greater advantage of hydrophilic catheters over non-hydrophilic or heparin-coated catheters [78]. Additionally, microcatheter material has also been implicated in thrombogenicity with polyvinylchloride as most thrombogenic [68].

Surfaces of the endovascular coils and stents are thrombogenic and when in contact with blood, a layer of platelets and fibrin is formed. The degree of thrombogenicity is directly dependent on the total surface area, surface charge, chemical properties, and the pattern of blood flow [8].

The endovascular coil embolization procedure for cerebral aneurysms is based on the principle of thrombogenicity. The coils are made of platinum and trigger electrothrombosis when in contact with platelets and fibrin in blood. Platinum coils carry a positive charge and are relatively more thrombogenic than stainless-steel, which is commonly used in the coil delivery system [17]. The effectiveness of the endovascular coils as thrombogenic agents is further enhanced by increasing the surface area and with improvements in coil design [17]. Newer coil technology that employs bioactive material such as polyglycolic acid (PGA) to obtain better angiographic occlusion and inflammatory response are currently available (Cerecyte, Micrus Endovascular, SanJose, CA; Matrix, HydroCoil, MicroVention, Aliso Viejo, CA; Nexus, Micro Therapeutics, Inc., Irvine, CA) and reportedly are not significantly different with regards to procedural and clinical outcomes compared to the bare platinum coils [154–157].

Embolic agents used in endovascular procedures such as microfibrillar collagen, gelfoam powder, and polyvinyl alcohol occlude the vessels and a thrombus typically forms within and around the embolic material. Distal migration of embolic agents causing obstruction of vessels is a potential complication that could be observed for up to four months [75].

Flow-diverting stents are relatively new devices designed for treatment of large intracranial aneurysms. These stents utilize the intravascular hemodynamics to assist in the restructure and obliteration of the aneurysms via thrombosis, inflammatory reaction, and endothelial growth [158]. Occlusion of the aneurysm is a process typically occurring over months and has a risk of occluding perforators arising from the parent vessel [159]. The flow-diverting devices characteristically have a large amount of metal coverage that is essential to impact flow diversion. The metal-covered area is typically thrombogenic and mandates use of pre- and post-stent antiplatelet therapy to prevent in-stent thrombosis [160–162].

A review of 206 intracranial aneurysms reported the following treatment complications with flow-diverting stents: stroke in 6.0%, in-stent thrombosis and stenosis in 4.9%, and death in 3.3%. Major complications with flow-diverting stents were related to perforator artery stroke, aneurysm re-rupture, and in-stent stenosis and thrombosis [163]. Two patients (3.5%) had asymptomatic in-construct stenosis of >50% [164]. The long-term clinical outcomes and incidence of complications related to flow-diverting stents remain to be seen.

Postprocedural incidence of major and minor stroke was reported as 0.46% and 0.38% respectively in a national prospective multicenter registry of 1,300 patients that underwent carotid stenting with proximal occlusion [165].

Fibrinolysis and thrombolytics

Fibrinolysis

Fibrinolysis is the intrinsic mechanism that halts the propagation of thrombus [4–13]. Plasminogen is a key fibrinolytic precursor compound present in the plasma and is triggered by the plasminogen activator [4–50]. Conversion of plasminogen then to plasmin is responsible for degradation of a fibrin clot [4–50]. Under normal homeostatic conditions, a balance between plasminogen activators in the body such as tissue-plasminogen activator (t-PA) and plasminogen activator inhibitors (PAIs) such as PAI-1 is noted. Both the plasminogen activators and the PAIs are synthesized and secreted by endothelial cells [4–80].

Thrombolytics

Dissolution of blood clots or thrombolysis could be achieved using intravenous (IV) or intra-arterial (IA) infusion of plasminogen activators that activate the fibrinolytic system. Agents available include streptokinase, prourokinase, urokinase, anisoylated plasminogen streptokinase activator complex, recombinant staphylokinase, and recombinant t-PA (alteplase or reteplase). In the clinical practice of endovascular surgery, the most frequently used thrombolytic agent is the recombinant t-PA. Thrombolysis is typically accomplished by conversion of proenzyme plasminogen into the active plasmin, which then breaks the fibrin-rich clots into soluble degradation products. Streptokinase and urokinase are known for their systemic action or non-clot specific action and on the contrary t-PA and pro-urokinase activate plasminogen with a clot-specific action [23]. In about 25% of cases that undergo thrombolysis, recanalization is limited with use of currently available thrombolytics and this is attributed to the composition of luminal thrombus [23]. Although fibrin dissolution is achieved, platelets and erythrocytes within a fibrin-rich clot are resistant to dispersion affecting the recanalization process [32].

The specific properties of applicable thrombolytic agents are discussed below.

t-PA

Activase and Retavase are two recombinant plasminogen activators available that are most effective in the presence of fibrin. The half-lives of Activase and Retavase are less than 5 minutes and 13 to 16 minutes, respectively. Studies have demonstrated that higher doses and faster administration are associated with more potent thrombolytic effects [106]. Because of the higher risk of bleeding complications associated with fixed-dose recombinant t-PA administration among patients with low body weights, weight adjustment of the dose is recommended [18]. Current guidelines recommend an Activase dose of 0.9 mg/kg (maximum of 90 mg) in eligible patients with acute ischemic stroke.

Urokinase

Urokinase, similar to streptokinase, lacks fibrin specificity and directly activates plasminogen, without forming an activator complex. The systemic thrombolytic effect of urokinase limits its use in endovascular surgery to local delivery.

Pro-urokinase

Pro-urokinase is a relatively fibrin-specific thrombolytic agent [30] and is rapidly cleared from plasma with an initial half-life of six to eight minutes. Intra-arterially administered pro-urokinase in the treatment of acute middle cerebral artery occlusion resulted in both a higher rate of recanalization and improved outcomes [31]. However, a higher rate of symptomatic intracranial hemorrhage was observed for patients who received pro-urokinase (10.2%, compared with 1.8% for patients treated with IV administered heparin).

Combination thrombolysis

Thrombolytic agents that target the fibrin component of the thrombus paradoxically increase thrombin activity and platelet activation [7]. Platelet activation releases a series of agonists, including PAI-1 [7]. Therefore after successful initial thrombolysis, a platelet-rich thrombus relatively more resistant to thrombolytic agents is formed. Antiplatelet agents, such as GP IIb/IIIa-specific antibodies, have a good potential for initial thrombolysis and also minimize reocclusion. A two-fold higher recanalization rate with the concurrent use of alteplase and integrilin in acute myocardial infarction patients is previously reported [110]. Similarly, the Thrombolysis in Myocardial Infarction investigators [7] reported that complete recanalization was achieved with a combination of low-dose alteplase and abciximab for patients with acute MIs. However, a similar approach in the management of cerebrovascular diseases is yet to be proven effective.

Intracranial or extracranial hemorrhage is the most important complication of thrombolysis. Risk is typically higher with simultaneous use of more than one thrombolytic. In ischemic stroke treated with intravenous thrombolytic agents (recombinant t-PA, urokinase, or streptokinase), a high incidence of early symptomatic (10%) or fatal (6%) intracranial hemorrhaging has been reported [119]. In circumstances of significant bleeding from thrombolytic therapy the suggested approach includes discontinuation of heparin therapy immediately and administration of protamine, cryoprecipitate, and fresh frozen plasma as indicated.

No clear advantage of using antithrombotic combination therapy with aspirin and heparin as a routine adjunct to thrombolysis has been demonstrated. Both aspirin and heparin have limited effects on the rate of coronary thrombolysis and do not consistently prevent reocclusion. These results are attributed to aspirin's non-selective inhibition of the synthesis of both proaggregatory and antiaggregatory prostaglandins and the ineffectiveness of heparin in the inhibition of clot-associated thrombin. Because of a lack of confirmatory evidence supporting the use of heparin to maintain vessel patency after thrombolysis, no widely accepted guidelines for combination therapy exist. In a meta-analysis, the early use of aspirin with intravenous thrombolytic therapy for ischemic stroke treatment was associated with higher odds of death than observed in trials that tended to avoid early aspirin use (odds ratio, 2.06 vs. 1.01) [119].

Treatment monitoring and point of care testing (POC)

Thromboembolic risk surrounding endovascular procedures is often minimized using antiplatelet therapy. However, the response to antiplatelet agents may be different in certain patients affecting the level of platelet inhibition. Measuring the degree of platelet inhibition identifies non- or low responders and treats them accordingly. Point of care testing quickly provides information on platelet inhibition that is critical for interventionalists and we discuss different POC devices and their clinical utility.

VerifyNow (Accumetrics, San Diego, California) is a test based on the phenomenon of platelet aggregation as measured by light transmittance through whole blood or plasma. If platelets are not inhibited, the activation process will ensue with subsequent platelet aggregation. The device measures change in the optical signal intensity secondary to platelet aggregation and quantifies platelet inhibition. The device measures the effects of GP IIb/IIIa inhibitors, aspirin, clopidogrel, and prasugrel [166,167].

In the VerifyNow aspirin assay, arachidonic acid is the platelet agonist used. If aspirin has produced the expected antiplatelet effect i.e., inhibiting cyclooxygenase, arachidonic acid will not be converted to thromboxane A2 and platelets will exhibit minimal aggregation around beads. Results are interpreted on the basis of the extent of platelet aggregation reported in aspirin reaction units (ARUs). A preclinical trial conducted by the manufacturer suggested that in patients who are on aspirin, a value of <550 ARU demonstrates an aspirin effect, while a value of ≥550 ARU indicates no platelet dysfunction (i.e., cyclooxygenase resistance) with 91% sensitivity and 100% specificity.

The VerifyNow P2Y12 assay is used to measure the effect of P2Y12 ADP-receptor inhibitors clopidogrel and prasugrel [168]. The assay provides results in P2Y12 reaction units (PRU), with low PRU (or higher percentage inhibition) indicating high P2Y12-receptor inhibition and good response to clopidogrel or prasugrel. Results may be affected by GP IIb/IIIa inhibitor drugs and cilostazol, but aspirin and other non-steroidal anti-inflammatory drugs have no effect.

VerifyNow GP IIb/IIIa assay uses iso-thrombin-receptor-activating peptide as an activator. The assay reports patient results in platelet aggregation units (PAU), which indicate the amount of iso-thrombin-receptor-activating peptide-mediated activation of GP IIb/IIIa receptors involved in platelet aggregation. Expected values are in the range of 0 to 330 PAU and no differences in baseline PAU values between patients with and without the following medications: aspirin, ticlopidine, clopidogrel, heparin, warfarin, acetaminophen, non-steroidal anti-inflammatory drugs, beta-blockers, calcium channel blockers, statins, and nitrates [169].

Plateletworks (Helena Laboratories, Beaumont, Texas) is a simple assay that uses standard cell-counting principles. Two values are obtained, baseline count and another count after adding a platelet agonist. In the presence of an agonist, platelets aggregate; therefore they exceed the threshold limitations for platelet size and are no longer counted as platelets. The difference in the platelet count between the two samples provides a measurement of platelet aggregation and is reported as percentage aggregation. Currently three different assays are available based on the agonists: collagen, ADP, and arachidonic acid. The arachidonic acid assay is specifically designed to measure the antiplatelet activity of aspirin, while both the collagen and ADP assays can be used to measure the antiplatelet effects of GP IIb/IIIa inhibitors, clopidogrel, prasugrel, and ticlopidine [170].

Clot Signature Analyzer (CSA) (Xylum, Scarsdale, New York) is a global hemostasis screen for assessing both platelet function and fibrin clot formation under shear stress. The device uses non-anticoagulated whole blood and provides a collagen-induced thrombus formation time (CITF) and the platelet hemostasis time (PHT). The effect of GP IIb/IIIa inhibitors was evaluated in a study using the CSA and platelet function was inhibited with prolongation of PHT and CITF (>30 minutes) independent of the agent. However, CSA lacked sensitivity to discriminate platelet function under conditions of profound inhibition by these agents [171].

Several antiplatelet regimens are used in patients undergoing percutaneous coronary intervention (PCI). Typically, the procedure is done under dual-antiplatelet coverage. GP IIb/IIIa inhibitors are commonly used as well. However, the most appropriate dosing, treatment duration, and choice of antiplatelet agents are still a subject of debate [172].

Limited data exists on platelet function monitoring in relation to neuroendovascular procedures. Using the VerifyNow assay, a study identified inadequate platelet inhibition in 13% of patients who took aspirin vs. 66% of patients who took clopidogrel (P <.0001) among patients who took aspirin or clopidogrel before their procedures. Inadequate platelet inhibition by POC testing was more common among patients who were administered 600 mg of clopidogrel within 6 hours of the procedure than in patients who had taken 300 mg within 24 hours or 75 mg daily for at least 7 days before the procedure

[173]. Another reported antiplatelet regimen included 300-mg loading dose of clopidogrel followed by 325 mg of aspirin and 75 mg of clopidogrel daily for five to ten days before their procedure. About 2% were found to be poor aspirin responders and 43% were poor clopidogrel responders with procedure-related thrombosis noted in patients with <20% platelet inhibition on testing [174].

Identifying variability in platelet inhibition between patients and ability to measure the degree of inhibition with POC testing may lead to the development of more effective strategies to reduce thromboembolic events.

Endovascular procedures and complications

Endovascular procedures are associated with a risk of immediate and delayed thromboembolic and ischemic complications. We reviewed the available clinical reports for selected endovascular procedures and used both clinical and laboratory data to establish recommendations for the prophylaxis and treatment of thromboembolic and ischemic complications associated with each procedure. We focused on the following procedures: (1) diagnostic cerebral angiography, (2) occlusion of intracranial aneurysms using coils, (3) occlusion of aneurysms using balloons, (4) parent vessel balloon occlusion for aneurysm treatment, (5) percutaneous transluminal angioplasty (PTA) of extracranial carotid artery stenosis, (6) percutaneous transluminal angioplasty and stenting (PTAS) of extracranial carotid artery stenosis, and (7) embolization of brain arteriovenous malformations (AVMs) using various agents (e.g., acrylic glue, particles, or coils).

Management of intracranial aneurysms may involve balloon occlusion during aneurysm coiling, and require thrombosis of the aneurysmal sac for successful results. Undesirable embolization must be prevented, without affecting the induced thrombosis in the aneurysmal sac. Angioplasty and stent placement involve deep arterial injury resulting from balloon inflation followed by the insertion of a potentially thrombogenic stent.

Diagnostic angiography

Diagnostic cerebral angiography, the initial step in endovascular procedures, is associated with a risk of ischemic events resulting from thromboembolic phenomena. Risk associated with diagnostic angiography

and the predisposing factors has been well researched and reported [19,20,32,100]. The overall periprocedural risk of thromboembolism-related complications occurring either during the procedure or within 24 hours thereafter ranged from 1.0 to 2.6%. Incidence of permanent neurological deficit is reported as 0.1 to 0.5% of the cases. The delayed risk between 24 and 72 hours after the procedure is noted as occurring in 1.8% of cases; one-third of the resultant deficits were permanent [19]. An interesting relationship between the indication for angiography and thromboembolic risk has been reported [20]. Patients with cerebrovascular disease carried a 4.2% risk (permanent deficits, 0.6%), followed by subarachnoid hemorrhage or aneurysm with a 3.8% risk (permanent deficits, 0%). Other factors conferring increased risk include age, procedural time, vascular anatomy of the case, operator experience, etc. Higher risk for neurological symptoms after cerebral angiography is reported in patients older than 60 years of age or with transient ischemic attacks (TIAs) or recent or evolving strokes [19,20,32,100]. A 4.5% risk for patients with TIAs and 7.7% for patients with evolving strokes is reported. There was no additional risk reported with history of previous strokes [100]. Longer procedure times (particularly longer than 60 minutes) and higher volumes of contrast material are associated with higher thromboembolic risks [19,32]. Catheter exchange was also suggested as an independent risk factor [19,20]. However, the reasons for catheter exchange, such as unexpected vessel tortuosity, the degree of atherosclerosis, or an inexperienced operator, may be responsible for this increase. Finally, elevated serum creatinine levels and the presence of diabetes were reported to present greater risks for thromboembolic events during diagnostic angiography [19,20].

Overall a relatively low risk of thromboembolic complications is reported with diagnostic angiography. Factors associated with increased risk with diagnostic angiography likely also influence the risk with other endovascular procedures.

Endovascular coil embolization of aneurysm

Complications associated with endovascular management of cerebral aneurysm are likely dependent on the treatment employed. Balloon occlusion and manipulation of the parent blood vessel causes stasis of distal flow potentially leading to intraluminal thrombosis. Progression of thrombus and distal embolization can produce neurological deficits. Additionally, during

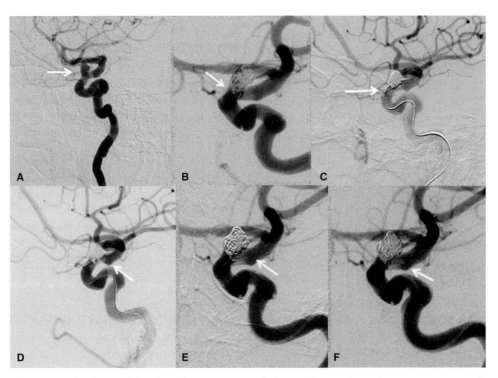

Figure 7.3 Coil prolapse and thrombosis during aneurysm embolization. (A) Internal carotid artery aneurysm protruding in anterior and superior direction (arrow). (B) Prolapse of coil loops into the parent artery (arrow). (C) A self-expanding nitinol stent 4.5 × 22 mm positioned across the aneurysm neck (arrow). (D) Filling defect (thrombus) in internal carotid artery in proximity to the stent and coil mass (arrow). (E) Partial resolution of filling defect (thrombus) in internal carotid artery in proximity to the stent and coil mass after administration of intra-arterial glycoprotein IIB/ IIIA inhibitor eptifibatide 5 mg (arrow). (F) Continued resolution of filling defect (thrombus) in internal carotid artery in proximity to the stent and coil mass after administration of intra-arterial glycoprotein IIB/ IIIA inhibitor eptifibatide 5 mg (arrow).

embolization of the aneurysmal sac with balloons or GDCs (Guglielmi Detachable Coils; Boston Scientific, Fremont, CA), embolism from a pre-existing aneurysmal thrombus is a possibility. Balloon or coil mass may slip or protrude into the vessel lumen and promote thrombus formation or become an embolus (Figure 7.3). Moreover, presence of a residual aneurysm postembolization may facilitate new thrombus formation. These possible thromboembolic mechanisms may occur either immediately after the procedure or could be delayed. For example, a thrombus already present within the aneurysm is likely to be dislodged and cause embolic complications during or shortly after the procedure. In contrast, a thrombus that develops during a procedure involving coil placement becomes symptomatic in the postprocedural period.

Several studies using GDCs for treatment of intracranial aneurysms of the anterior or posterior circulation were reviewed. We noted some studies focused on selected patient groups, such as patients with ruptured aneurysms [69,74,114] or vasospasm [128],

elderly patients [80], or patients with basilar tip [47,62,72,75] or anterior communicating artery [65] aneurysms. After exclusion of reports with overlapping patient samples [10,57,75], data on 1,547 patients remained for analysis. Various prophylactic regimens were used to prevent thromboembolic complications. Intraoperative intravenous heparin therapy is used in the majority of studies. In cases of acutely ruptured aneurysms, heparin therapy was initiated after the first coil was deployed. Heparin was used postoperatively in some studies [80,109,114]. The frequency of thromboembolic events (28 events among 472 patients, 5.9%) was lower than that in studies without postoperative heparin use (100 events among 1,075 patients, 9.3%). Only 1 of the 28 thromboembolic events reported in the studies using postoperative heparin therapy occurred postoperatively. Aspirin was used postoperatively in some studies [10,14,65,72,80]. The rate of thromboembolic events was lower among patients treated concurrently with aspirin (28 events among 435 patients, 6.4%), compared with patients not treated with aspirin in the perioperative period (99 events among 112 patients, 8.9%).

There are limited data on the demonstration of emboli or ischemia, during or after aneurysm coiling, using neuroimaging techniques. Lagalla *et al.* [52] observed minimal changes in the mean flow velocity in the middle cerebral artery, using intraoperative transcranial Doppler monitoring, in uncomplicated cases of aneurysm coiling. For patients who developed ischemic complications during the procedure, a 30% decrease in middle cerebral artery flow, which was unchanged 24 hours after the procedure, was observed. No observations were made regarding the detection of microemboli. Rowe *et al.* [79] observed 15 to 20% decreases in middle cerebral artery velocity during catheter placement in 20 patients undergoing GDC embolization of aneurysms. No episodes of embolization or changes in velocities were observed during GDC insertion.

Recently, a double-blinded, randomized trial of patients with ruptured or unruptured intracranial aneurysm was performed to evaluate the safety and clinical efficacy of the neuroprotective agent NA-1, an inhibitor of postsynaptic density-95 protein. The agent was administered after the endovascular treatment of aneurysms. Ninety-two of 185 randomized patients received the treatment with NA-1 and only two minor and no serious adverse events were associated with NA-1. Fewer ischemic infarcts in the NA-1 group compared to the placebo group based on diffusion-weighted MRI (adjusted incidence rate ratio 0·53, 95% CI 0·38–0·74) were noted. The study suggested a likely beneficial role of neuroprotection in ischemic stroke, calling for more research in this area [175].

Endovascular occlusion of intracranial aneurysms using balloons

Endovascular balloon therapy to occlude the aneurysmal sac or the parent vessel was previously evaluated. The overall risk of symptomatic thromboembolic complications with aneurysmal sac occlusion was reported as 11%. The overall risk of symptomatic complications associated with parent vessel occlusion was markedly higher (19%) [176]. The risks of ischemic complications for both detachable balloon techniques are higher than those associated with GDC treatment. However, balloon-based techniques are older than GDC occlusion and, considering the advancements

in endovascular technology in the past five to ten years, these complication rates may not be valid today.

Considering the complexity of the lesion and poor clinical condition of patients selected for endovascular intracranial aneurysm therapy, the risk of thromboembolic and ischemic complications is relatively low. Technical advances that may further reduce this risk in the future include stent placement and balloon protection. Inadvertent embolization of intra-aneurysmal thrombus may be prevented by placing a stent across the aneurysm neck before coil packing [63]. Thrombus formation promoted by coil prolapse into the parent vessel lumen may be minimized by placing an inflated balloon across the aneurysm neck while coils are being pushed into the aneurysm. The initial configuration of the coil as it is released from the tip of the catheter strongly influences the final shape assumed by the coil within the aneurysm. The balloon protection technique may preclude initial coil protrusion and later prolapse.

Percutaneous transluminal angioplasty (PTA) and PTA with stenting (PTAS)

During carotid PTA and PTAS, different mechanisms may produce thromboembolic events. Passing the lesion with the guide wire and angioplasty balloon catheter may dislodge plaque or thrombus. Inflation of the balloon may promote secondary thromboembolism by producing intimal cracks, flaps, or dissections, all of which act as thrombogenic surfaces. In addition, the usual risk associated with catheterization for routine angiography is increased with the use of larger caliber (7- or 8-French) sheaths [20].

A prior review of studies treating carotid stenosis with PTA revealed a risk of 5.9% for thromboembolic complications, of which 4 were asymptomatic, 9 were TIAs, and 14 were strokes [177]. Most complications occurred intraoperatively. PTAS was associated with more complications than PTA, with a risk of 8.8% for thromboembolic events of stroke or TIA. Unlike with PTA, the majority of thromboembolic events occurred postoperatively among patients who underwent PTAS. The stroke and death rate was also higher in patients with symptomatic carotid stenosis undergoing PTAS versus carotid endarterectomy (4.4% vs. 2.3%, hazard ratio: 1.90; 95% CI, 1.21 to 2.98) [178]. Studies utilizing MRI scans identified that three times more patients that underwent carotid stenting had new ischemic lesions on DWI post-treatment scans compared to those that underwent endarterectomy [179].

Several techniques have been introduced to limit thromboembolic complications in PTA and PTAS. Theron *et al.* [102] reported use of distal balloon protection to minimize inadvertent embolization in the cerebral circulation. A second balloon was inflated distal to the angioplasty balloon during lesion dilation, to keep emboli from flowing into the cerebral circulation. Initially, the second balloon was introduced through a contralateral femoral artery approach, which was later refined with use of a triple-lumen catheter. Temporary distal occlusion could theoretically lead to new thrombus formation, because stasis of blood flow is created. Other techniques that have been proposed to minimize inadvertent distal embolization include stent placement [50] and urokinase injection [31]. Before PTAS, urokinase is injected intra-arterially to dissolve loose emboli attached to the plaque.

With increased risk of stroke with PTAS compared to endarterectomy in patients with carotid stenosis [180–182] greater research focus was noted in identifying methods to lower the periprocedural stroke risk associated with stenting. Embolic protection during PTAS was proven effective in clinical trials [183,184]. A 30-day incidence of stroke was 3.9 (0.9 to 16.7) times higher in PTAS without compared to PTAS with cerebral protection [184]. Currently prevention of cerebral ischemic events is achieved using either the distal protection technique with different filters [185–187] or proximal occlusion with balloons [188,189] or in certain instances both [190]. While a randomized study found no difference in the incidence of cerebral ischemic events based on brain MR imaging, with a follow-up duration of one year [191], a recent meta-analysis revealed increased protection with use of a proximal balloon occlusion technique compared to a distal filter protection [192]. Additional evidence from a meta-analysis of carotid artery stenting (CAS) procedures performed with proximal occlusion devices demonstrated a very low incidence of adverse events at 30 days [193].

In a treatment comparison study of patients undergoing carotid stenting for primary atherosclerotic disease, ticlopidine 250 mg twice daily and aspirin 325 mg daily was found superior to IV heparin for 24 hours and aspirin 325 mg [194].

Similarly, a randomized controlled trial comparing aspirin and IV heparin with aspirin and clopidogrel for patients undergoing CAS, indicated benefit with dual antiplatelet regime without an additional increase in bleeding complications [195]. In a prospective, randomized, double-blind study comparing a loading dose of 300 mg of clopidogrel in combination with aspirin to clopidogrel dose of 600 mg was found equally effective in preventing periprocedural events in asymptomatic patients undergoing CAS [196].

Cilostazol as adjunctive treatment was found to reduce cerebral ischemic lesions more effectively in patients already on dual antiplatelet therapy (aspirin and clopidogrel) for carotid stenosis that underwent stenting. Benefit was noted in patients with clopidogrel resistance and recommendation [197]. Use of glycoprotein IIb/IIIa antagonists periprocedurally for CAS has revealed no significant benefit in lowering the risk of ischemic events. Analysis of 1,322 CAS cases revealed no difference in stroke or death (OR 1.81, 95% CI: 0.69–4.72) in patients that received abciximab, tirofiban, or eptifibatide compared to those that did not receive any glycoprotein IIb/IIa antagonists [198]. Similarly, administration of abciximab bolus injection did not reduce cerebral ischemic complications in elective CAS cases [199]. Additionally, increased frequency of intracranial hemorrhages was suggested with use of abciximab in a CAS study [200].

Embolization of AVMs

Different embolization techniques were used either alone or in combination with surgical excision or radiosurgery (for lesions considered incurable by endovascular methods alone). Embolic agents included n-butylcyanoacrylate [16,27,56,118,124], isobutylcyanoacrylate [7,22,23,40,56,64,113], polyvinyl alcohol particles of different sizes [67,86,113,118], ethanol [127], estrogen [40], polyfilament threads [7], and Gelfoam [96]. The most common complications were hemorrhage, vasogenic edema, and ischemic injury. Ischemic injury was predominantly caused by thromboembolism, the embolizing agent itself, or vasospasm.

In a review of embolization procedures in AVM management, 21% ischemic complications were noted. The overall risk per procedure of ischemic complications was 9.4%, on the basis of the total number of procedures performed (complications were observed for 21% of treated patients). The overall risk of transient neurological deficits (TIAs plus other deficits classified as "transient," without reports of exact recovery periods) was 2.6% for all procedures. The risk associated with acrylic glue (n-butylcyanoacrylate or isobutylcyanoacrylate) as an embolic agent was not different from the aggregate risk of all other materials. Specific agents other than glue could not be analyzed separately, because they were included in combination regimens.

Compared with the other endovascular techniques for treatment of cerebrovascular disease that are analyzed here, intracranial embolization of AVMs was associated with a higher risk (21%) of symptomatic thromboembolic complications. This high frequency was attributable to the multiple procedures required for each patient undergoing AVM embolization. The estimated risk per procedure performed was similar to that of other endovascular techniques. Most ischemic complications occur when flow through the AVM nidus is reduced and embolic material flows into normal blood vessels, either via reflux or through previously unrecognized vascular conduits. Less commonly, secondary thrombosis may occur proximal to occluded vascular channels, because of stasis, and may involve normal blood vessels by direct extension or embolization.

Catheter entrapment is a potential complication associated with Onyx embolization of AVMs and anecdotal reports have been published previously. This occurs when the microcatheter is encased within a cast of Onyx and retrieval of catheter after completion of Onyx injection is not possible [201,202]. Based on review of data in the medical device reports (MDRs) of the FDA, catheter entrapment is reportedly associated with ischemic stroke in <1% of all cases of Onyx embolization.

Mechanical thrombectomy

Arterial reocclusion and distal embolization is reported to occur in 16 to 18% of patients with stroke undergoing endovascular intervention, and arterial reocclusion was associated with poor long-term outcome [205]. With increasing utilization of mechanical thrombectomy for acute ischemic stroke, prospective studies evaluating the mechanism and risk factors associated with these phenomena will be critical to develop preventive strategies.

Intracranial angioplasty and stent placement

Intracranial angioplasty and stenting performed in the SAMMPRIS (Stenting vs. Aggressive Medical Management for Preventing Recurrent Stroke in Intracranial Stenosis) trial of patients with symptomatic intracranial stenosis revealed a significant 14% stroke and death rate in the stent-treated group [203]. However, the overall 30-day postprocedure stroke and death rate has been noted as lower (3.3%) in a similar patient population with more judicious use of primary angioplasty [204].

Summary

Preventive and therapeutic strategies for thromboembolic complications associated with endovascular procedures:

General principles

On the basis of pathophysiological features, procedures can be divided into the following two groups with respect to their thrombogenicity: (1) procedures in which deep arterial injury is involved (such as PTA or PTAS) or in which significant stasis of blood flow is observed (such as balloon occlusion of parent vessels; high ACT values (300–350 s) are recommended for such procedures because of the high thromboembolic risk; and (2) procedures in which the aforementioned thrombogenic components are absent (such as embolization of aneurysms or AVMs); moderate ACT elevation (250–300 s) is probably adequate for such procedures. Protamine reversal of heparin therapy after completion of the procedure should be considered for techniques such as AVM embolization, for which the risk is present primarily during the procedure. Removal of arterial sheaths after the procedure is another option. We think that early removal should be considered for all patients because of the high risk of clot formation within the sheath [49]. For patients receiving chronic warfarin treatment, Kearon and Hirsh [45] recommended the cessation of warfarin administration four days before the procedure, on the basis of a risk–benefit assessment.

Furthermore, recommended operator qualifications to perform neurointerventional procedures such as diagnostic cerebral angiography, intra-arterial thrombolysis, carotid angioplasty and stent placement, intracranial angioplasty and stent placement, and endovascular treatment of intracranial aneurysms and arteriovenous malformations has been previously proposed [205]. Adhering to these recommendations may likely result in better clinical outcomes of these procedures.

Diagnostic angiography

Given the low risk of thromboembolic events during cerebral angiography, the routine use of intravenously administered heparin or antiplatelet agents is not recommended. For patients who have experienced recent transient ischemic events, therapy with antiplatelet agents (aspirin in combination with either ticlopidine or clopidogrel) should be maintained or initiated three days before the procedure.

For patients with evolving strokes, heparin should be administered at least six hours before the procedure and then during the procedure, because of the high risk of thromboembolic complications [100]. Activated partial thromboplastin times (aPTTs) of 1.5 to 2.3 times the control values are considered adequate.

Coil embolization of aneurysms

As a majority of thromboembolic events associated with GDC treatment occur intraoperatively, emphasis is placed on intraoperative anticoagulation therapy. For patients with subarachnoid hemorrhage, heparin should be administered concurrently with microcatheter placement and deployment of the first coil and the dose should be titrated to maintained ACTs of 250 to 300 seconds. For patients with unruptured aneurysms, heparin should be administered early, before placement of the guide catheter. No clear benefit was observed with the postoperative use of aspirin or heparin, although a slightly lower rate of thromboembolic complications was observed with each regimen in the cumulative analysis. Given the risk of bleeding, we do not recommend the routine postoperative use of heparin. For selected patients, heparin administration may be continued for 24 hours postoperatively, to maintain aPTTs of 1.5 to 2.3 times the control values. Such patients include those with a protuberance of coils in the parent vessel, angiographic evidence of thrombus outside the aneurysm cavity, or ischemic symptoms in the intra- or postoperative period. The aPTT should be measured every six hours. A weight-based nomogram ensures safe and effective anticoagulation

[73]. After a 24-hour course of heparin, a combination of aspirin (325 mg, daily) and ticlopidine (250 mg, twice daily) may be used for four weeks, to ensure endothelialization of thrombogenic surfaces. For patients with a low risk of rupture, i.e., those with unruptured aneurysms or adequately coiled ruptured aneurysms, a combination of aspirin (325 mg, daily) and ticlopidine (250 mg, twice daily) may be used for four weeks, to ensure endothelialization of thrombogenic surfaces. As discussed previously, the risk of thromboembolic events is very low after the first four weeks.

Balloon occlusion of aneurysms or parent vessels harboring aneurysms

For parent vessel or aneurysm occlusion using a balloon, a regimen similar to that for endovascular coil embolization may be used. Because of the higher risk of thromboembolic events, higher ACTs (300–350 s) should be maintained during the procedure, and intravenous heparin administration should be continued for 24 hours postoperatively (aPTTs of 1.5–2.3 times the control values). The only exception to this approach is in patients with subarachnoid hemorrhage, where heparin administration should be discontinued after the procedure and aspirin and ticlopidine (or clopidogrel) therapy should be instituted. Heparin or antiplatelet treatment can be discontinued after 24 hours, to facilitate thrombosis of both the parent artery and the aneurysm.

PTA and PTAS

For PTA and PTAS, aspirin should be administered in conjunction with ticlopidine (or clopidogrel) for three days before the procedure, to allow ticlopidine to achieve full functional activity. The combination of the two drugs seems to have a synergistic effect. During the procedure, deep arterial injury associated with balloon angioplasty and the thrombogenicity of the stent result in a highly thrombogenic surface. Intramural thrombosis can be observed in more than 90% of the deeply injured arteries, even when elevation of the ACT to four to five times the control value has been achieved with intravenous heparin administration [53]. Animal studies suggest that heparin doses of more than 180 units/kg/hour are required to inhibit thrombosis during angioplasty [34,81]. These doses can be administered as two boluses 40 minutes apart, preferably before angioplasty, to maintain the ACT between 300 and 350 seconds. We recommend intravenous administration of an initial bolus of 100 units/kg heparin, hourly monitoring of ACTs, and administration of supplemental heparin to maintain the ACT between 300 and 350 seconds. Because most thromboembolic events occur postoperatively among patients who undergo PTAS, emphasis should be placed on postoperative prophylaxis and monitoring. Heparin administration may be discontinued after the procedure, but the administration of aspirin (325 mg, daily) and ticlopidine (250 mg, twice daily) or clopidogrel (75 mg, daily) should be continued for at least four weeks, until endothelialization of the stent is complete. Routine postprocedural intravenous administration of heparin cannot be recommended, because of the lack of evidence of definite benefits and the potential for increased bleeding complications, particularly at the site of sheath insertion. For patients who demonstrate angiographically visible dissections or mural thrombosis or progressive or new neurological symptoms, heparin may be administered to maintain aPTTs of 1.5 to 2.3 times the control values for a 24-hour period. Subcutaneous administration of enoxaparin (1 mg/kg, twice daily) is an alternative in such cases. Another approach that requires further evaluation is the use of abciximab for patients at high risk who undergo PTAS. On the basis of the coronary intervention literature, intravenous administration of an initial loading dose of 0.25 mg/kg abciximab, 10 to 60 minutes before the procedure, is recommended, followed by a 12-hour intravenous infusion at a rate of 10 µg/minute. Intravenous heparin therapy is used only during the procedure. An initial dose of 70 units/kg heparin is administered to maintain the ACT at approximately 200 seconds. The use of abciximab can be extended up to 24 hours for patients at high risk, such as those with arterial dissections, mural thrombosis, or ischemic symptoms during or after the procedure.

Embolization using glue, particles, or other materials

Because most thromboembolic complications associated with intracranial AVM embolization seem to occur in the early postoperative period, intraoperative heparin administration (70 units/kg) to achieve ACTs

between 250 and 300 seconds is recommended. Postprocedural heparin therapy is not required for most procedures, because most ischemic events occur during the procedure and are related to the passage of embolic materials into normal blood vessels. For uncomplicated procedures, protamine reversal of heparin therapy after completion of the procedure should be considered, to facilitate early safe sheath removal.

Intra-arterial thrombolysis

Vessel occlusion can occur during or shortly after endovascular procedures, as a result of local thrombosis or distal embolization. These occlusions are particularly amenable to selective intra-arterial administration of thrombolytic agents [14]. For early recognition of vessel occlusion, frequent control injections of contrast material or neurological examinations of non-anesthetized patients are recommended. Transcatheter thrombolysis treatments using recombinant tissue-type plasminogen activator (t-PA) or urokinase seem to be equally effective [25]. Most observations on the use of intra-arterially administered thrombolytic agents are based on studies of spontaneous thromboembolic events. Cronqvist *et al.* [14] reviewed 19 cases of thromboembolic events that occurred during endovascular treatment of aneurysms. Embolisms associated with the procedure were observed in the middle cerebral artery for 14 patients, the anterior cerebral artery for 3, and the basilar trunk for 2. Complete recanalization was observed for 10 of the 19 patients after intra-arterial administration of urokinase (mean dose, 975,000 IU; range, 450,000–1,300,000 IU; infusion rate, 20,000 IU/min). Partial recanalization was observed for nine patients. The authors observed that recanalization was best achieved when mechanical fragmentation of the thrombus and superselective drug infusion were possible.

Catheters previously placed for the primary endovascular procedure should be used for expeditious treatment of procedure-related complications [14]. A microcatheter should be navigated through the guide catheter into and across the thrombus [4]. Recombinant t-PA should be infused through the microcatheter in amounts of 5 to 40 mg. Slow infusion of the thrombolytic agent, at rates of 0.5 to 2.0 mg/min is preferred. Mechanical clot disruption or angioplasty can be effective if pharmacological recanalization alone is initially ineffective [4].

Heparinization during thrombolysis may enhance the thrombolytic efficacy of recombinant t-PA [46]. The intravenous administration of a heparin bolus (70 units/kg) before thrombolysis, to maintain the ACT between 250 and 300 seconds, may be considered.

Post-thrombolytic use of heparin to prevent reocclusion is recommended for patients with partial recanalization, arterial dissection, or persistent distal emboli not amenable to selective thrombolysis. Intravenous heparin administration should be titrated to maintain aPTTs of 1.5 to 2.3 times the control values. For thromboembolic complications that occur in the postoperative period, regimens similar to those used for the management of primary stroke may be considered. However, for prompt action, arterial access should be maintained for 12 to 24 hours for patients at high risk. In addition, patients should be closely monitored in a neurointensive care unit environment.

In a prior series, recanalization rates between 50 and 100% have been reported [68]; however, rates may be as low as 40% in cases of major stroke (initial National Institutes of Health Stroke Scale Score ≥24) [21,125]. Recanalization rates depend on the morphological features, site, and accessibility of the lesions. Clinical improvement is observed in 50 to 90% of cases [68] (20% for major strokes) [21]. Clinical outcomes clearly depend on the interval between symptom onset and treatment. Because this interval is expectedly shorter in cases with complications occurring during or shortly after endovascular interventions, the clinical outcomes in those cases may be better than those cited above.

Conclusions

In this chapter we report the high incidence of thromboembolic complications associated with endovascular procedures. Most of the existing prophylactic regimens either were derived empirically or are based on regimens reported in the coronary literature. Further research is required to develop both prophylactic and treatment strategies to reduce the rate of thromboembolic complications associated with neuroendovascular procedures and subsequently improve the overall success of such procedures.

In endovascular procedures, arterial injury and the use of catheters, contrast agents, and implanted devices with thrombogenic potential place patients at risk for thrombosis and embolization. Extensive research has been performed to elucidate the pathophysiological features underlying thrombosis associated with endovascular procedures. Recognition of the important role of platelet aggregation in arterial thrombosis has led to development and use of antiplatelet agents such as ticlopidine, clopidogrel, and antibodies to GP IIb/IIIa receptors. Administration of these agents should be initiated before the procedure for optimal antiplatelet effects. A combination of aspirin with ticlopidine or clopidogrel provides the best oral antiplatelet therapy. Treatment should be continued until endothelialization is complete (four to six weeks after the procedure). For patients at high risk, the use of antibodies to GP IIb/IIIa receptors during the period of maximal local prothrombotic activity (initial 24 hours) may be a reasonable alternative. The intraoperative use of heparin is well established; however, postprocedural use is restricted because of hemorrhagic complications and limited benefits. A better understanding of the limitations of standard treatments (such as aspirin and heparin) and the benefits of newer available agents will further the development of improved strategies for prophylaxis and treatment of thromboembolic complications associated with endovascular procedures.

References

1. Alberts M J, Brass L M, Perry A, Webb D, Dawson D V. Evaluation times for patients with in-hospital strokes. *Stroke*. 1993; 24:1817–22.

2. Emiru T, Adil M M, Suri M F, Qureshi A I. Thrombolytic treatment for in-hospital ischemic strokes in United States. *Journal of Vascular and Interventional Neurology*. 2014; 7:28–34.

3. Kelley R E, Kovacs A G. Mechanism of in-hospital cerebral ischemia. *Stroke*. 1986; 17:430–3.

4. Barnwell S L, Clark W M, Nguyen T T, *et al.* Safety and efficacy of delayed intraarterial urokinase therapy with mechanical clot disruption for thromboembolic stroke. *American Journal of Neuroradiology*. 1994; 15: 1817–22.

5. Bavinzski G, Killer M, Ferraz-Leite H, *et al.* Endovascular therapy of idiopathic cavernous aneurysms over 11 years. *American Journal of Neuroradiology*. 1998; 19:559–65.

6. Belan A, Vesela M, Vanek I, Weiss K, Peregrin J H. Percutaneous transluminal angioplasty of fibromuscular dysplasia of the internal carotid artery. *Cardiovascular and Interventional Radiology*. 1982; 5:79–81.

7. Benati A. Interventional neuroradiology for the treatment of inaccessible arterio-venous malformations. *Acta Neurochirurgica*. 1992; **118**: 76–9.

8. Brown M M, Butler P, Gibbs J, Swash M, Waterston J. Feasibility of percutaneous transluminal angioplasty for carotid artery stenosis. *Journal of Neurology, Neurosurgery, and Psychiatry*. 1990; **53**:238–43.

9. Casasco A E, Aymard A, Gobin Y P, *et al.* Selective endovascular treatment of 71 intracranial aneurysms with platinum coils. *Journal of Neurosurgery*. 1993; **79**:3–10.

10. Cognard C, Weill A, Castaings L, Rey A, Moret J. Intracranial berry aneurysms: Angiographic and clinical results after endovascular treatment. *Radiology*. 1998; **206**:499–510.

11. Crawley F, Clifton A, Buckenham T, *et al.* Comparison of hemodynamic cerebral ischemia and microembolic signals detected during carotid endarterectomy and carotid angioplasty. *Stroke*. 1997; **28**:2460–4.

12. Crawley F, Clifton A, Markus H, Brown M M. Delayed improvement in carotid artery diameter after carotid angioplasty. *Stroke*. 1997; **28**:574–9.

13. Criado F J, Wellons E, Clark N S. Evolving indications for and early results of carotid artery stenting. *American Journal of Surgery*. 1997; **174**:111–14.

14. Cronqvist M, Pierot L, Boulin A, *et al.* Local intraarterial fibrinolysis of thromboemboli occurring during endovascular treatment of intracerebral aneurysm: A comparison of anatomic results and clinical outcome. *American Journal of Neuroradiology*. 1998; **19**:157–65.

15. Debrun G, Vinuela F, Fox A, Drake C G. Embolization of cerebral arteriovenous malformations with bucrylate. *Journal of Neurosurgery*. 1982; **56**:615–27.

16. Debrun G M, Aletich V, Ausman J I, Charbel F, Dujovny M. Embolization of the nidus of brain arteriovenous malformations with n-butyl cyanoacrylate. *Neurosurgery*. 1997; **40**:112–20.

17. Debrun G M, Aletich V A, Kehrli P, *et al.* Selection of cerebral aneurysms for treatment using Guglielmi detachable coils: The preliminary University of Illinois at Chicago experience. *Neurosurgery*. 1998; **43**:1281–95.

18. Diethrich E B, Ndiaye M, Reid D B. Stenting in the carotid artery: Initial experience in 110 patients. *Journal of Endovascular Surgery*. 1996; **3**:42–62.

19. Dion J E, Gates P C, Fox A J, Barnett H J, Blom R J. Clinical events following neuroangiography: A prospective study. *Stroke*. 1987; **18**:997–1004.

20. Earnest F T, Forbes G, Sandok B A, *et al.* Complications of cerebral angiography: Prospective assessment of risk. *American Journal of Roentgenology*. 1984; **142**:247–53.

21. Endo S, Kuwayama N, Hirashima Y, *et al.* Results of urgent thrombolysis in patients with major stroke and atherothrombotic occlusion of the cervical internal carotid artery. *American Journal of Neuroradiology*. 1998; **19**:1169–75.

22. Fournier D, TerBrugge K G, Willinsky R, Lasjaunias P, Montanera W. Endovascular treatment of intracerebral arteriovenous malformations: Experience in 49 cases. *Journal of Neurosurgery*. 1991; **75**:228–33.

23. Fox A J, Pelz D M, Lee D H. Arteriovenous malformations of the brain: Recent results of endovascular therapy. *Radiology*. 1990; **177**:51–7.

24. Freitag G, Freitag J, Koch R D, Wagemann W. Percutaneous angioplasty of carotid artery stenoses. *Neuroradiology*. 1986; **28**:126–7.

25. Frey J L, Greene K A, Khayata M H, *et al.* Intrathrombus administration of tissue plasminogen activator in acute cerebrovascular occlusion. *Angiology*. 1995; **46**:649–56.

26. Gil-Peralta A, Mayol A, Marcos J R, *et al.* Percutaneous transluminal angioplasty of the symptomatic atherosclerotic carotid arteries. Results, complications, and follow-up. *Stroke*. 1996; **27**:2271–3.

27. Gobin Y P, Laurent A, Merienne L, *et al.* Treatment of brain arteriovenous malformations by embolization and radiosurgery. *Journal of Neurosurgery*. 1996; **85**:19–28.

28. Graves V B, Strother C M, Duff T A, Perl J 2nd. Early treatment of ruptured aneurysms with Guglielmi detachable coils: Effect on subsequent bleeding. *Neurosurgery*. 1995; **37**:640–7.

29. Guglielmi G, Vinuela F, Duckwiler G, *et al.* Endovascular treatment of posterior circulation aneurysms by electrothrombosis using electrically detachable coils. *Journal of Neurosurgery*. 1992; **77**:515–24.

30. Gurian J H, Martin N A, King W A, *et al.* Neurosurgical management of cerebral aneurysms following unsuccessful or incomplete endovascular embolization. *Journal of Neurosurgery*. 1995; **83**:843–53.

31. Guterman L R, Budny J L, Gibbons K J, Hopkins L N. Thrombolysis of the cervical internal carotid artery before balloon angioplasty and stent placement: Report of two cases. *Neurosurgery*. 1996; **38**:620–3.

32. Heiserman J E, Dean B L, Hodak J A, *et al.* Neurologic complications of cerebral angiography. *American Journal of Neuroradiology*. 1994; **15**:1401–7.

33. Henry M, Amor M, Masson I, *et al.* Angioplasty and stenting of the extracranial carotid arteries. *Journal of Endovascular Surgery*. 1998; **5**:293–304.

34. Heras M, Chesebro J H, Penny W J, *et al.* Importance of adequate heparin dosage in arterial angioplasty in a porcine model. *Circulation*. 1988; **78**:654–60.

35. Higashida R T, Halbach V V, Barnwell S L, *et al.* Treatment of intracranial aneurysms with preservation of the parent vessel: Results of percutaneous balloon embolization in 84 patients. *American Journal of Neuroradiology.* 1990; **11**:633–40.

36. Higashida R T, Halbach V V, Cahan L D, Hieshima G B, Konishi Y. Detachable balloon embolization therapy of posterior circulation intracranial aneurysms. *Journal of Neurosurgery.* 1989; **71**:512–19.

37. Higashida R T, Halbach V V, Dowd C, *et al.* Endovascular detachable balloon embolization therapy of cavernous carotid artery aneurysms: Results in 87 cases. *Journal of Neurosurgery.* 1990; **72**:857–63.

38. Higashida R T, Halbach V V, Dowd C F, Barnwell S L, Hieshima G B. Intracranial aneurysms: Interventional neurovascular treatment with detachable balloons – results in 215 cases. *Radiology.* 1991; **178**:663–70.

39. Hodes J E, Aymard A, Gobin Y P, *et al.* Endovascular occlusion of intracranial vessels for curative treatment of unclippable aneurysms: Report of 16 cases. *Journal of Neurosurgery.* 1991; **75**:694–701.

40. Huang Z, Dai Q, Suo J, *et al.* Percutaneous endovascular embolization of intracerebral arteriovenous malformations. Experience in 72 cases. *Chinese Medical Journal.* 1995; **108**:413–19.

41. Jordan W D, Jr., Schroeder P T, Fisher W S, McDowell H A. A comparison of angioplasty with stenting versus endarterectomy for the treatment of carotid artery stenosis. *Annals of Vascular Surgery.* 1997; **11**:2–8.

42. Jordan W D, Jr., Voellinger D C, Doblar D D, *et al.* Microemboli detected by transcranial Doppler monitoring in patients during carotid angioplasty versus carotid endarterectomy. *Cardiovascular Surgery.* 1999; **7**:33–8.

43. Kachel R, Basche S, Heerklotz I, Grossmann K, Endler S. Percutaneous transluminal angioplasty (PTA) of supra-aortic arteries especially the internal carotid artery. *Neuroradiology.* 1991; **33**:191–4.

44. Kachel R, Endert G, Basche S, Grossmann K, Glaser F H. Percutaneous transluminal angioplasty (dilatation) of carotid, vertebral, and innominate artery stenoses. *Cardiovascular and Interventional Radiology.* 1987; **10**:142–6.

45. Kearon C, Hirsh J. Management of anticoagulation before and after elective surgery. *New England Journal of Medicine.* 1997; **336**:1506–11.

46. Kesava P, Graves V, Salamat S, Rappe A. Intraarterial thrombolysis in a pig model: A preliminary note. *American Journal of Neuroradiology.* 1997; **18**:915–20.

47. Klein G E, Szolar D H, Leber K A, Karaic R, Hausegger K A. Basilar tip aneurysm: Endovascular treatment with Guglielmi detachable coils – midterm results. *Radiology.* 1997; **205**:191–6.

48. Klotzsch C, Nahser H C, Henkes H, Kuhne D, Berlit P. Detection of microemboli distal to cerebral aneurysms before and after therapeutic embolization. *American Journal of Neuroradiology.* 1998; **19**:1315–18.

49. Koenigsberg R A, Wysoki M, Weiss J, Faro S H, Tsai F Y. Risk of clot formation in femoral arterial sheaths maintained overnight for neuroangiographic procedures. *American Journal of Neuroradiology.* 1999; **20**:297–9.

50. Krupski W C, Bass A, Kelly A B, Hanson S R, Harker L A. Reduction in thrombus formation by placement of endovascular stents at endarterectomy sites in baboon carotid arteries. *Circulation.* 1991; **84**:1749–57.

51. Kuether T A, Nesbit G M, Barnwell S L. Clinical and angiographic outcomes, with treatment data, for patients with cerebral aneurysms treated with Guglielmi detachable coils: A single-center experience. *Neurosurgery.* 1998; **43**:1016–25.

52. Lagalla G, Ceravolo M G, Provinciali L, *et al.* Transcranial Doppler sonographic monitoring during cerebral aneurysm embolization: A preliminary report. *American Journal of Neuroradiology.* 1998; **19**:1549–53.

53. Lam J Y, Chesebro J H, Steele P M, *et al.* Deep arterial injury during experimental angioplasty: Relation to a positive indium-111-labeled platelet scintigram, quantitative platelet deposition and mural thrombosis. *Journal of the American College of Cardiology.* 1986; **8**:1380–6.

54. Larson J J, Tew J M, Jr., Tomsick T A, van Loveren H R. Treatment of aneurysms of the internal carotid artery by intravascular balloon occlusion: Long-term follow-up of 58 patients. *Neurosurgery.* 1995; **36**:26–30.

55. Lincoff A M, Tcheng J E, Califf R M, *et al.* Standard versus low-dose weight-adjusted heparin in patients treated with the platelet glycoprotein IIb/IIIa receptor antibody fragment abciximab (c7E3 Fab) during percutaneous coronary revascularization. PROLOG investigators. *American Journal of Cardiology.* 1997; **79**:286–91.

56. Lundqvist C, Wikholm G, Svendsen P. Embolization of cerebral arteriovenous malformations: Part II – aspects of complications and late outcome. *Neurosurgery.* 1996; **39**:460–7.

57. Malisch T W, Guglielmi G, Vinuela F, *et al.* Intracranial aneurysms treated with the Guglielmi detachable coil: Midterm clinical results in a consecutive series of 100 patients. *Journal of Neurosurgery.* 1997; **87**:176–83.

58. Markus H S, Clifton A, Buckenham T, Brown M M. Carotid angioplasty. Detection of embolic signals

during and after the procedure. *Stroke*. 1994; **25**: 2403–6.

59. Markus H S, Clifton A, Buckenham T, Taylor R, Brown M M. Improvement in cerebral hemodynamics after carotid angioplasty. *Stroke*. 1996; **27**:612–16.

60. Mathur A, Roubin G S, Gomez C R, *et al*. Elective carotid artery stenting in the presence of contralateral occlusion. *American Journal of Cardiology*. 1998; **81**: 1315–17.

61. Mathur A, Roubin G S, Iyer S S, *et al*. Predictors of stroke complicating carotid artery stenting. *Circulation*. 1998; **97**:1239–45.

62. McDougall C G, Halbach V V, Dowd C F, *et al*. Treatment of basilar tip aneurysms using electrolytically detachable coils. *Journal of Neurosurgery*. 1996; **84**:393–9.

63. Mericle R A, Lanzino G, Wakhloo A K, Guterman L R, Hopkins L N. Stenting and secondary coiling of intracranial internal carotid artery aneurysm: Technical case report. *Neurosurgery*. 1998; **43**: 1229–34.

64. Merland J J, Rufenacht D, Laurent A, Guimaraens L. Endovascular treatment with isobutyl cyano acrylate in patients with arteriovenous malformation of the brain. Indications, results and complications. *Acta Radiologica. Supplementum*. 1986; **369**:621–2.

65. Moret J, Pierot L, Boulin A, Castaings L, Rey A. Endovascular treatment of anterior communicating artery aneurysms using Guglielmi detachable coils. *Neuroradiology*. 1996; **38**:800–5.

66. Munari L M, Belloni G, Perretti A, *et al*. Carotid percutaneous angioplasty. *Neurological Research*. 1992; **14**:156–8.

67. Nakstad P H, Nornes H. Superselective angiography, embolisation and surgery in treatment of arteriovenous malformations of the brain. *Neuroradiology*. 1994; **36**:410–13.

68. Nesbit G M, Clark W M, O'Neill O R, Barnwell S L. Intracranial intraarterial thrombolysis facilitated by microcatheter navigation through an occluded cervical internal carotid artery. *Journal of Neurosurgery*. 1996; **84**:387–92.

69. Nichols D A, Brown R D, Jr., Thielen K R, *et al*. Endovascular treatment of ruptured posterior circulation aneurysms using electrolytically detachable coils. *Journal of Neurosurgery*. 1997; **87**:374–80.

70. Pasqualin A, Scienza R, Cioffi F, *et al*. Treatment of cerebral arteriovenous malformations with a combination of preoperative embolization and surgery. *Neurosurgery*. 1991; **29**:358–68.

71. Pelz D M, Lownie S P, Fox A J. Thromboembolic events associated with the treatment of cerebral aneurysms with Guglielmi detachable coils. *American Journal of Neuroradiology*. 1998; **19**:1541–7.

72. Pierot L, Boulin A, Castaings L, Rey A, Moret J. Selective occlusion of basilar artery aneurysms using controlled detachable coils: Report of 35 cases. *Neurosurgery*. 1996; **38**:948–53.

73. Raschke R A, Reilly B M, Guidry J R, Fontana J R, Srinivas S. The weight-based heparin dosing nomogram compared with a "standard care" nomogram. A randomized controlled trial. *Annals of Internal Medicine*. 1993; **119**:874–81.

74. Raymond J, Roy D. Safety and efficacy of endovascular treatment of acutely ruptured aneurysms. *Neurosurgery*. 1997; **41**:1235–45.

75. Raymond J, Roy D, Bojanowski M, Moumdjian R, L'Esperance G. Endovascular treatment of acutely ruptured and unruptured aneurysms of the basilar bifurcation. *Journal of Neurosurgery*. 1997; **86**:211–19.

76. Raymond J, Theron J. Intracavernous aneurysms: Treatment by proximal balloon occlusion of the internal carotid artery. *American Journal of Neuroradiology*. 1986; **7**:1087–92.

77. Rich L F, Weimar V L, Squires E L, Haraguchi K H. Stimulation of corneal wound healing with mesodermal growth factor. *Archives of Ophthalmology*. 1979; **97**:1326–30.

78. Roubin G S, Yadav S, Iyer S S, Vitek J. Carotid stent-supported angioplasty: A neurovascular intervention to prevent stroke. *American Journal of Cardiology*. 1996; **78**:8–12.

79. Rowe J G, Byrne J V, Molyneux A, Rajagopalan B. Haemodynamic consequences of embolizing aneurysms: A transcranial Doppler study. *British Journal of Neurosurgery*. 1995; **9**:749–57.

80. Rowe J G, Molyneux A J, Byrne J V, Renowden S, Aziz T Z. Endovascular treatment of intracranial aneurysms: A minimally invasive approach with advantages for elderly patients. *Age and Ageing*. 1996; **25**:372–6.

81. Sawyer P N, Stanczewski B, Pomerance A, Stoner G, Srinivasan S. Utility of anticoagulant drugs in vascular thrombosis: Electron microscopic and biophysical study. *Surgery*. 1973; **74**:263–75.

82. Scarborough R M, Rose J W, Hsu M A, *et al*. Barbourin. A GPIIB-IIIa-specific integrin antagonist from the venom of *Sistrurus m.* barbouri. *Journal of Biological Chemistry*. 1991; **266**:9359–62.

83. Schatz R A, Baim D S, Leon M, *et al*. Clinical experience with the Palmaz-Schatz coronary stent. Initial results of a multicenter study. *Circulation*. 1991; **83**:148–61.

84. Schlossman D. Thrombogenic properties of vascular catheter materials in vivo. The differences between materials. *Acta Radiologica: Diagnosis*. 1973; **14**:186–92.

85. Schomig A, Neumann F J, Kastrati A, *al*. A randomized comparison of antiplatelet and anticoagulant therapy

after the placement of coronary-artery stents. *New England Journal of Medicine.* 1996; **334**:1084–9.

86. Schumacher M, Horton J A. Treatment of cerebral arteriovenous malformations with PVA. Results and analysis of complications. *Neuroradiology.* 1991; **33**: 101–5.

87. Segi E, Sugimoto Y, Yamasaki A, *et al.* Patent ductus arteriosus and neonatal death in prostaglandin receptor EP4-deficient mice. *Biochemical and Biophysical Research Communications.* 1998; **246**:7–12.

88. Serbinenko F A. Balloon catheterization and occlusion of major cerebral vessels. *Journal of Neurosurgery.* 1974; **41**:125–45.

89. Serruys P W, de Jaegere P, Kiemeneij F, *et al.* A comparison of balloon-expandable-stent implantation with balloon angioplasty in patients with coronary artery disease. Benestent study group. *New England Journal of Medicine.* 1994; **331**:489–95.

90. Sharis P J, Cannon C P, Loscalzo J. The antiplatelet effects of ticlopidine and clopidogrel. *Annals of Internal Medicine.* 1998; **129**:394–405.

91. Smedema J P, Saaiman A. Carotid stent-assisted angioplasty. *South African Medical Journal.* 1997; **87** Suppl 1:C9–14.

92. Smith D C, Smith L L, Hasso A N. Fibromuscular dysplasia of the internal carotid artery treated by operative transluminal balloon angioplasty. *Radiology.* 1985; **155**:645–8.

93. Smyth S S, Joneckis C C, Parise L V. Regulation of vascular integrins. *Blood.* 1993; **81**:2827–43.

94. Sobel M, McNeill P M, Carlson P L, *et al.* Heparin inhibition of von Willebrand factor-dependent platelet function in vitro and in vivo. *Journal of Clinical Investigation.* 1991; **87**:1787–93.

95. Speidel C M, Eisenberg P R, Ruf W, Edgington T S, Abendschein D R. Tissue factor mediates prolonged procoagulant activity on the luminal surface of balloon-injured aortas in rabbits. *Circulation.* 1995; **92**: 3323–30.

96. Spetzler R F, Martin N A, Carter L P, *et al.* Surgical management of large AVM's by staged embolization and operative excision. *Journal of Neurosurgery.* 1987; **67**:17–28.

97. Stormorken H. Effects of contrast media on the hemostatic and thrombotic mechanisms. *Investigative Radiology.* 1988; **23** Suppl 2:S318–25.

98. Taki W, Nishi S, Yamashita K, *et al.* Selection and combination of various endovascular techniques in the treatment of giant aneurysms. *Journal of Neurosurgery.* 1992; **77**:37–42.

99. Teitelbaum G P, Lefkowitz M A, Giannotta S L. Carotid angioplasty and stenting in high-risk patients. *Surgical Neurology.* 1998; **50**:300–11.

100. Theodotou B C, Whaley R, Mahaley M S. Complications following transfemoral cerebral angiography for cerebral ischemia. Report of 159 angiograms and correlation with surgical risk. *Surgical Neurology.* 1987; **28**:90–2.

101. Theron J, Courtheoux P, Alachkar F, Bouvard G, Maiza D. New triple coaxial catheter system for carotid angioplasty with cerebral protection. *American Journal of Neuroradiology.* 1990; **11**:869–74.

102. Theron J G, Payelle G G, Coskun O, Huet H F, Guimaraens L. Carotid artery stenosis: Treatment with protected balloon angioplasty and stent placement. *Radiology.* 1996; **201**:627–36.

103. Theroux P. Antiplatelet therapy: Do the new platelet inhibitors add significantly to the clinical benefits of aspirin? *American Heart Journal.* 1997; **134**:S62–70.

104. Theroux P, Waters D, Lam J, Juneau M, McCans J. Reactivation of unstable angina after the discontinuation of heparin. *New England Journal of Medicine.* 1992; **327**:141–5.

105. Thielen K R, Nichols D A, Fulgham J R, Piepgras D G. Endovascular treatment of cerebral aneurysms following incomplete clipping. *Journal of Neurosurgery.* 1997; **87**:184–9.

106. Topol E J. Ultrathrombolysis. *Journal of the American College of Cardiology.* 1990; **15**:922–4.

107. Topol E J, Bonan R, Jewitt D, *et al.* Use of a direct antithrombin, hirulog, in place of heparin during coronary angioplasty. *Circulation.* 1993; **87**:1622–9.

108. Touho H. Percutaneous transluminal angioplasty in the treatment of atherosclerotic disease of the anterior cerebral circulation and hemodynamic evaluation. *Journal of Neurosurgery.* 1995; **82**:953–60.

109. Tournade A, Courtheoux P, Sengel C, Ozgulle S, Tajahmady T. Saccular intracranial aneurysms: Endovascular treatment with mechanical detachable spiral coils. *Radiology.* 1997; **202**:481–6.

110. Tsai F Y, Matovich V, Hieshima G, *et al.* Percutaneous transluminal angioplasty of the carotid artery. *American Journal of Neuroradiology.* 1986; **7**: 349–58.

111. Turpie A G. Successors to heparin: New antithrombotic agents. *American Heart Journal.* 1997; **134**:S71–77.

112. Van Belle E, Tio F O, Chen D, *et al.* Passivation of metallic stents after arterial gene transfer of phVEGF165 inhibits thrombus formation and intimal thickening. *Journal of the American College of Cardiology.* 1997; **29**:1371–9.

113. Vinuela F, Dion J E, Duckwiler G, *et al.* Combined endovascular embolization and surgery in the management of cerebral arteriovenous malformations: Experience with 101 cases. *Journal of Neurosurgery.* 1991; **75**:856–64.

114. Vinuela F, Duckwiler G, Mawad M. Guglielmi detachable coil embolization of acute intracranial aneurysm: Perioperative anatomical and clinical outcome in 403 patients. *Journal of Neurosurgery.* 1997; **86**:475–82.

115. Vorchheimer D A, Badimon JJ, Fuster V. Platelet glycoprotein IIb/IIIa receptor antagonists in cardiovascular disease. *JAMA.* 1999; **281**:1407–14.

116. Vozzi C R, Rodriguez A O, Paolantonio D, Smith J A, Wholey M H. Extracranial carotid angioplasty and stenting. Initial results and short-term follow-up. *Texas Heart Institute Journal.* 1997; **24**:167–72.

117. Waigand J, Gross C M, Uhlich F, *et al.* Elective stenting of carotid artery stenosis in patients with severe coronary artery disease. *European Heart Journal.* 1998; **19**:1365–70.

118. Wallace R C, Flom R A, Khayata M H, *et al.* The safety and effectiveness of brain arteriovenous malformation embolization using acrylic and particles: The experiences of a single institution. *Neurosurgery.* 1995; **37**:606–15.

119. Wardlaw J M, Warlow C P, Counsell C. Systematic review of evidence on thrombolytic therapy for acute ischaemic stroke. *Lancet.* 1997; **350**:607–14.

120. Warkentin T E, Levine M N, Hirsh J, *et al.* Heparin-induced thrombocytopenia in patients treated with low-molecular-weight heparin or unfractionated heparin. *New England Journal of Medicine.* 1995; **332**: 1330–5.

121. Weitz J I. Low-molecular-weight heparins. *New England Journal of Medicine.* 1997; **337**:688–98.

122. Weitz J I, Hudoba M, Massel D, Maraganore J, Hirsh J. Clot-bound thrombin is protected from inhibition by heparin-antithrombin III but is susceptible to inactivation by antithrombin III-independent inhibitors. *Journal of Clinical Investigation.* 1990; **86**:385–91.

123. Wholey M H, Wholey M H, Jarmolowski C R, *et al.* Endovascular stents for carotid artery occlusive disease. *Journal of Endovascular Surgery.* 1997; **4**: 326–38.

124. Wikholm G, Lundqvist C, Svendsen P. Embolization of cerebral arteriovenous malformations: Part I – technique, morphology, and complications. *Neurosurgery.* 1996; **39**:448–57.

125. Wityk R J, Pessin M S, Kaplan R F, Caplan L R. Serial assessment of acute stroke using the NIH stroke scale. *Stroke.* 1994; **25**:362–5.

126. Yadav J S, Roubin G S, King P, Iyer S, Vitek J. Angioplasty and stenting for restenosis after carotid endarterectomy. Initial experience. *Stroke.* 1996; **27**: 2075–9.

127. Yakes W F, Krauth L, Ecklund J, *et al.* Ethanol endovascular management of brain arteriovenous malformations: Initial results. *Neurosurgery.* 1997; **40**: 1145–52.

128. Yalamanchili K, Rosenwasser R H, Thomas J E, *et al.* Frequency of cerebral vasospasm in patients treated with endovascular occlusion of intracranial aneurysms. *American Journal of Neuroradiology.* 1998; **19**:553–8.

129. CAPRIE Steering Committee. A randomised, blinded, trial of clopidogrel versus aspirin in patients at risk of ischaemic events (CAPRIE). *Lancet.* 1996; **348**:1329–39.

130. Ansara A J, Shiltz D L, Slavens J B. Use of cilostazol for secondary stroke prevention: An old dog with new tricks? *Annals of Pharmacotherapy.* 2012; **46**:394–402.

131. Gotoh F, Tohgi H, Hirai S, *et al.* Cilostazol stroke prevention study: A placebo-controlled double-blind trial for secondary prevention of cerebral infarction. *Journal of Stroke and Cerebrovascular Diseases.* 2000; **9**:147–57.

132. Dinicolantonio J J, Lavie C J, Fares H, *et al.* Meta-analysis of cilostazol versus aspirin for the secondary prevention of stroke. *American Journal of Cardiology.* 2013; **112**:1230–4.

133. Kamal A K, Naqvi I, Husain M R, Khealani B A. Cilostazol versus aspirin for secondary prevention of vascular events after stroke of arterial origin. *Cochrane Database of Systematic Reviews.* 2011; CD008076.

134. Ikeda Y. Antiplatelet therapy using cilostazol, a specific PPE3 inhibitor. *Thrombosis and Haemostasis.* 1999; **82**:435–8.

135. Jeng J S, Sun Y, Lee J T, *et al.* The efficacy and safety of cilostazol in ischemic stroke patients with peripheral arterial disease (SPAD): Protocol of a randomized, double-blind, placebo-controlled multicenter trial. *International Journal of Stroke.* 2015; **10**:123–7.

136. Lefkovits J, Plow E F, Topol E J. Platelet glycoprotein IIb/IIIa receptors in cardiovascular medicine. *New England Journal of Medicine.* 1995; **332**:1553–9.

137. PRISM-PLUS study investigators. Inhibition of the platelet glycoprotein IIb/IIIa receptor with tirofiban in unstable angina and non-Q-wave myocardial infarction. Platelet receptor inhibition in ischemic syndrome management in patients limited by unstable signs and symptoms (PRISM-PLUS). *New England Journal of Medicine.* 1998; **338**:1488–97.

138. Ciccone A, Motto C, Abraha I, Cozzolino F, Santilli I. Glycoprotein IIb-IIIa inhibitors for acute ischaemic stroke. *Cochrane Database of Systematic Reviews.* 2014; 3:CD005208.

139. Adams H P, Jr., Effron M B, Torner J, *et al.* Emergency administration of abciximab for treatment of patients with acute ischemic stroke: Results of an international

phase III trial: Abciximab in emergency treatment of stroke trial (ABESTT-II). *Stroke*. 2008; **39**:87–99.

140. Velat G J, Burry M V, Eskioglu E, *et al.* The use of abciximab in the treatment of acute cerebral thromboembolic events during neuroendovascular procedures. *Surgical Neurology*. 2006; **65**:352–8.

141. Siebler M, Hennerici M G, Schneider D, *et al.* Safety of tirofiban in acute ischemic stroke: The SATIS trial. *Stroke*. 2011; **42**:2388–92.

142. Kellert L, Hametner C, Rohde S, *et al.* Endovascular stroke therapy: Tirofiban is associated with risk of fatal intracerebral hemorrhage and poor outcome. *Stroke*. 2013; **44**:1453–5.

143. Cannon C P. Oral platelet glycoprotein IIb/IIIa receptor inhibitors – part I. *Clinical Cardiology*. 2003; **26**:358–64.

144. Second S I. Randomized trial of aspirin, sibrafiban, or both for secondary prevention after acute coronary syndromes. *Circulation*. 2001; **103**:1727–33.

145. Cannon C P, McCabe C H, Wilcox R G, *et al.* Oral glycoprotein IIb/IIIa inhibition with orbofiban in patients with unstable coronary syndromes (OPUS-TIMI 16) trial. *Circulation*. 2000; **102**:149–56.

146. O'Neill W W, Serruys P, Knudtson M, *et al.* Long-term treatment with a platelet glycoprotein-receptor antagonist after percutaneous coronary revascularization. EXCITE trial investigators. Evaluation of oral xemilofiban in controlling thrombotic events. *New England Journal of Medicine*. 2000; **342**:1316–24.

147. Mousa S A, Khurana S, Forsythe M S. Comparative in vitro efficacy of different platelet glycoprotein IIb/IIIa antagonists on platelet-mediated clot strength induced by tissue factor with use of thromboelastography: Differentiation among glycoprotein IIb/IIIa antagonists. *Arteriosclerosis, Thrombosis, and Vascular Biology*. 2000; **20**:1162–7.

148. The SYMPHONY investigators. Comparison of sibrafiban with aspirin for prevention of cardiovascular events after acute coronary syndromes: A randomised trial. Sibrafiban versus aspirin to yield maximum protection from ischemic heart events post-acute coronary syndromes. *Lancet*. 2000; **355**:337–45.

149. Chew D P, Bhatt D L, Sapp S, Topol E J. Increased mortality with oral platelet glycoprotein IIb/IIIa antagonists: A meta-analysis of phase III multicenter randomized trials. *Circulation*. 2001; **103**:201–6.

150. Saw J, Bajzer C, Casserly I P, *et al.* Evaluating the optimal activated clotting time during carotid artery stenting. *American Journal of Cardiology*. 2006; **97**:1657–60.

151. Batchelor W B, Mahaffey K W, Berger P B, *et al.* A randomized, placebo-controlled trial of enoxaparin after high-risk coronary stenting: The ATLAST trial. *Journal of the American College of Cardiology*. 2001; **38**:1608–13.

152. Hassan A E, Memon M Z, Georgiadis A L, *et al.* Safety and tolerability of high-intensity anticoagulation with bivalirudin during neuroendovascular procedures. *Neurocritical Care*. 2011; **15**:96–100.

153. Zidar J P. Rationale for low-molecular weight heparin in coronary stenting. *American Heart Journal*. 1997; **134**:S81–87.

154. McDougall C G, Johnston S C, Gholkar A, *et al.* Bioactive versus bare platinum coils in the treatment of intracranial aneurysms: The MAPS (matrix and platinum science) trial. *American Journal of Neuroradiology*. 2014; **35**:935–42.

155. Molyneux A J, Clarke A, Sneade M, *et al.* Cerecyte coil trial: Angiographic outcomes of a prospective randomized trial comparing endovascular coiling of cerebral aneurysms with either cerecyte or bare platinum coils. *Stroke*. 2012; **43**:2544–50.

156. Coley S, Sneade M, Clarke A, *et al.* Cerecyte coil trial: Procedural safety and clinical outcomes in patients with ruptured and unruptured intracranial aneurysms. *American Journal of Neuroradiology*. 2012; **33**:474–80.

157. Butteriss D, Gholkar A, Mitra D, Birchall D, Jayakrishnan V. Single-center experience of cerecyte coils in the treatment of intracranial aneurysms: Initial experience and early follow-up results. *American Journal of Neuroradiology*. 2008; **29**:53–5.

158. Kallmes D F, Ding Y H, Dai D, *et al.* A new endoluminal, flow-disrupting device for treatment of saccular aneurysms. *Stroke*. 2007; **38**:2346–52.

159. Nelson P K, Lylyk P, Szikora I, *et al.* The pipeline embolization device for the intracranial treatment of aneurysms trial. *American Journal of Neuroradiology*. 2011; **32**:34–40.

160. De Vries J, Boogaarts J, Van Norden A, Wakhloo A K. New generation of flow diverter (surpass) for unruptured intracranial aneurysms: A prospective single-center study in 37 patients. *Stroke*. 2013; **44**:1567–77.

161. Darsaut T E, Bing F, Makoyeva A, *et al.* Flow diversion to treat aneurysms: The free segment of stent. *Journal of Neurointerventional Surgery*. 2013; **5**:452–7.

162. Augsburger L, Farhat M, Reymond P, *et al.* Effect of flow diverter porosity on intraaneurysmal blood flow. *Klinische Neuroradiologie*. 2009; **19**:204–14.

163. Walcott B P, Pisapia J M, Nahed B V, Kahle K T, Ogilvy C S. Early experience with flow diverting endoluminal stents for the treatment of intracranial aneurysms. *Journal of Clinical Neuroscience*. 2011; **18**:891–4.

164. McAuliffe W, Wycoco V, Rice H, *et al.* Immediate and midterm results following treatment of unruptured intracranial aneurysms with the pipeline embolization device. *American Journal of Neuroradiology.* 2012; **33**:164–70.

165. Stabile E, Salemme L, Sorropago G, *et al.* Proximal endovascular occlusion for carotid artery stenting: Results from a prospective registry of 1,300 patients. *Journal of the American College of Cardiology.* 2010; **55**:1661–7.

166. Ang L, Mahmud E. Monitoring oral antiplatelet therapy: Is it justified? *Therapeutic Advances in Cardiovascular Disease.* 2008; **2**:485–96.

167. Smith J W, Steinhubl S R, Lincoff A M, *et al.* Rapid platelet-function assay: An automated and quantitative cartridge-based method. *Circulation.* 1999; **99**:620–5.

168. Antman E M, Wiviott S D, Murphy S A, *et al.* Early and late benefits of prasugrel in patients with acute coronary syndromes undergoing percutaneous coronary intervention: A triton-timi 38 (trial to assess improvement in therapeutic outcomes by optimizing platelet inhibition with prasugrel-thrombolysis in myocardial infarction) analysis. *Journal of the American College of Cardiology.* 2008; **51**:2028–33.

169. Steinhubl S R, Talley J D, Braden G A, *et al.* Point-of-care measured platelet inhibition correlates with a reduced risk of an adverse cardiac event after percutaneous coronary intervention: Results of the GOLD (AU-Assessing Ultegra) multicenter study. *Circulation.* 2001; **103**:2572–8.

170. Helena Laboratories. 2015

171. Simon D I, Liu C B, Ganz P, *et al.* A comparative study of light transmission aggregometry and automated bedside platelet function assays in patients undergoing percutaneous coronary intervention and receiving abciximab, eptifibatide, or tirofiban. *Catheterization and Cardiovascular Interventions.* 2001; **52**:425–32.

172. Mukherjee D, Chew D P, Robbins M, *et al.* Clinical application of procedural platelet monitoring during percutaneous coronary intervention among patients at increased bleeding risk. *Journal of Thrombosis and Thrombolysis.* 2001; **11**:151–4.

173. Pandya D J, Fitzsimmons B F, Wolfe T J, *et al.* Measurement of antiplatelet inhibition during neurointerventional procedures: The effect of antithrombotic duration and loading dose. *Journal of Neuroimaging.* 2010; **20**:64–9.

174. Lee D H, Arat A, Morsi H, *et al.* Dual antiplatelet therapy monitoring for neurointerventional procedures using a point-of-care platelet function test: A single-center experience. *American Journal of Neuroradiology.* 2008; **29**:1389–94.

175. Hill M D, Martin R H, Mikulis D, *et al.* Safety and efficacy of NA-1 in patients with iatrogenic stroke after endovascular aneurysm repair (ENACT): A phase 2, randomised, double-blind, placebo-controlled trial. *Lancet. Neurology.* 2012; **11**:942–50.

176. Qureshi A I, Luft A R, Sharma M, *et al.* Prevention and treatment of thromboembolic and ischemic complications associated with endovascular procedures: Part II – clinical aspects and recommendations. *Neurosurgery.* 2000; **46**:1360–75.

177. Qureshi A I, Janardhan V, Memon M Z, *et al.* Initial experience in establishing an academic neuroendovascular service: Program building, procedural types, and outcomes. *Journal of Neuroimaging.* 2009; **19**:72–9.

178. Silver F L, Mackey A, Clark W M, *et al.* Safety of stenting and endarterectomy by symptomatic status in the carotid revascularization endarterectomy versus stenting trial (CREST). *Stroke.* 2011; **42**:675–80.

179. Bonati L H, Jongen L M, Haller S, *et al.* New ischaemic brain lesions on MRI after stenting or endarterectomy for symptomatic carotid stenosis: A substudy of the International Carotid Stenting Study (ICSS). *Lancet. Neurology.* 2010; **9**:353–62.

180. Economopoulos K P, Sergentanis T N, Tsivgoulis G, Mariolis A D, Stefanadis C. Carotid artery stenting versus carotid endarterectomy: A comprehensive meta-analysis of short-term and long-term outcomes. *Stroke.* 2011; **42**:687–92.

181. Halliday A, Mansfield A, Marro J, *et al.* Prevention of disabling and fatal strokes by successful carotid endarterectomy in patients without recent neurological symptoms: Randomised controlled trial. *Lancet.* 2004; **363**:1491–502.

182. Rothwell P M, Eliasziw M, Gutnikov S A, *et al.* Analysis of pooled data from the randomised controlled trials of endarterectomy for symptomatic carotid stenosis. *Lancet.* 2003; **361**:107–16.

183. Yadav J S, Wholey M H, Kuntz R E, *et al.* Protected carotid-artery stenting versus endarterectomy in high-risk patients. *New England Journal of Medicine.* 2004; **351**:1493–501.

184. Mas J L, Chatellier G, Beyssen B, EVA-3S Investigators. Carotid angioplasty and stenting with and without cerebral protection: Clinical alert from the Endarterectomy Versus Angioplasty in Patients with Symptomatic Severe Carotid Stenosis (EVA-3S) Trial. *Stroke.* 2004; **35**:e18–20.

185. Matsumura J S, Gray W, Chaturvedi S, *et al.* Results of carotid artery stenting with distal embolic protection with improved systems: Protected Carotid Artery Stenting in Patients at High Risk for Carotid Endarterectomy (PROTECT) Trial. *Journal of Vascular Surgery.* 2012; **55**:968–76.

186. Myla S, Bacharach J M, Ansel G M, *et al.* Carotid artery stenting in high surgical risk patients using the fibernet embolic protection system: The EPIC trial results. *Catheterization and Cardiovascular Interventions.* 2010; **75**:817–22.

187. Higashida R T, Popma J J, Apruzzese P, Zimetbaum P; MAVErIC I and II Investigators. Evaluation of the Medtronic exponent self-expanding carotid stent system with the Medtronic guardwire temporary occlusion and aspiration system in the treatment of carotid stenosis: Combined from the MAVErIC (Medtronic AVE self-expanding carotid stent system with distal protection in the treatment of carotid stenosis) I and MAVErIC II trials. *Stroke.* 2010; **41**:e102–9.

188. Ansel G M, Hopkins L N, Jaff M R, *et al.* Safety and effectiveness of the INVATEC MO.MA proximal cerebral protection device during carotid artery stenting: Results from the ARMOUR pivotal trial. *Catheterization and Cardiovascular Interventions.* 2010; **76**:1–8.

189. Ohki T, Parodi J, Veith F J, *et al.* Efficacy of a proximal occlusion catheter with reversal of flow in the prevention of embolic events during carotid artery stenting: An experimental analysis. *Journal of Vascular Surgery.* 2001; **33**:504–9.

190. Harada K, Kakumoto K, Morioka J, Saito T, Fukuyama K. Combination of flow reversal and distal filter for cerebral protection during carotid artery stenting. *Annals of Vascular Surgery.* 2014; **28**:651–8.

191. Cano M N, Kambara A M, de Cano S J, *et al.* Randomized comparison of distal and proximal cerebral protection during carotid artery stenting. *Cardiovascular Interventions.* 2013; **6**:1203–9.

192. Stabile E, Sannino A, Schiattarella G G, *et al.* Cerebral embolic lesions detected with diffusion-weighted magnetic resonance imaging following carotid artery stenting: A meta-analysis of 8 studies comparing filter cerebral protection and proximal balloon occlusion. *Cardiovascular Interventions.* 2014; **7**:1177–83.

193. Bersin R M, Stabile E, Ansel G M, *et al.* A meta-analysis of proximal occlusion device outcomes in carotid artery stenting. *Catheterization and Cardiovascular Interventions.* 2012; **80**:1072–8.

194. Dalainas I, Nano G, Bianchi P, *et al.* Dual antiplatelet regime versus acetyl-acetic acid for carotid artery stenting. *Cardiovascular and Interventional Radiology.* 2006; **29**:519–21.

195. McKevitt F M, Randall M S, Cleveland T J, *et al.* The benefits of combined anti-platelet treatment in carotid artery stenting. *European Journal of Vascular and Endovascular Surgery.* 2005; **29**:522–7.

196. Van Der Heyden J, Van Werkum J, Hackeng C M, *et al.* High versus standard clopidogrel loading in patients undergoing carotid artery stenting prior to cardiac surgery to assess the number of microemboli detected with transcranial Doppler: Results of the randomized IMPACT trial. *Journal of Cardiovascular Surgery.* 2013; **54**:337–47.

197. Nakagawa I, Wada T, Park H S, *et al.* Platelet inhibition by adjunctive cilostazol suppresses the frequency of cerebral ischemic lesions after carotid artery stenting in patients with carotid artery stenosis. *Journal of Vascular Surgery.* 2014; **59**:761–7.

198. Zahn R, Ischinger T, Hochadel M, *et al.* Glycoprotein IIb/IIIa antagonists during carotid artery stenting: Results from the Carotid Artery Stenting (CAS) registry of the Arbeitsgemeinschaft Leitende Kardiologische Krankenhausarzte (ALKK). *Clinical Research in Cardiology.* 2007; **96**:730–7.

199. Hofmann R, Kerschner K, Steinwender C, *et al.* Abciximab bolus injection does not reduce cerebral ischemic complications of elective carotid artery stenting: A randomized study. *Stroke.* 2002; **33**: 725–7.

200. Qureshi A I, Suri M F, Ali Z, *et al.* Carotid angioplasty and stent placement: A prospective analysis of perioperative complications and impact of intravenously administered abciximab. *Neurosurgery.* 2002; **50**:466–73.

201. Walcott B P, Gerrard J L, Nogueira R G, *et al.* Microsurgical retrieval of an endovascular microcatheter trapped during onyx embolization of a cerebral arteriovenous malformation. *Journal of Neurointerventional Surgery.* 2011; **3**:77–9.

202. Huk W, Becker H. [Complication after embolization of an AVM with onyx]. *Klinische Neuroradiologie.* 2009; **19**:145–52.

203. Chimowitz M I, Lynn M J, Derdeyn C P, *et al.* Stenting versus aggressive medical therapy for intracranial arterial stenosis. *New England Journal of Medicine.* 2011; **365**:993–1003.

204. Siddiq F, Chaudhry S A, Khatri R, *et al.* Rate of postprocedural stroke and death in SAMMPRIS trial-eligible patients treated with intracranial angioplasty and/or stent placement in practice. *Neurosurgery.* 2012; **71**:68–73.

205. Qureshi A I, Abou-Chebl A, Jovin T G. Qualification requirements for performing neurointerventional procedures: A report of the Practice Guidelines Committee of the American Society of Neuroimaging and the Society of Vascular and Interventional Neurology. *Journal of Neuroimaging.* 2008; **18**:433–47.

Chapter 8

Stroke after diagnostic endovascular procedures

Anastasios Mpotsaris and Tommy Andersson

Introduction

Since its advent in 1927 [1] diagnostic intra-arterial cerebral angiography has for decades been essential in the diagnosis and evaluation of diseases of the central nervous system (CNS). It has contributed to the understanding of vascular lesions such as aneurysms, arteriovenous malformations, and fistulas, as well as CNS vasculitis, and atherosclerotic disease. It remains, however, an invasive procedure, requiring the placement of catheters in arteries that supply the brain. These arteries are naturally not only important, but also sometimes sensitive and iatrogenic harm can lead to a devastating impact on the patient's life. In the light of current advances in non-invasive imaging of the craniocervical vasculature, the role of conventional intra-arterial diagnostic cerebral angiography has to be evaluated by the physician on the basis of the individual patient's risk–benefit ratio [2]. A close cooperation between all involved clinical subspecialties is of paramount importance, especially in cases where interventional neuroangiographic procedures might be necessary. From a technical point of view, conventional intra-arterial cerebral angiography is still unmatched in terms of spatial and time resolution as well as selectivity of the depicted vessel; these factors can translate into clinically meaningful – and for any interventional treatment crucial – advantages in accuracy [2,3]. Consequently, an understanding of the complications that may arise and the means to reduce the inherent risk of this procedure is the basis of any responsible decision-making process.

Complications of intra-arterial cerebral angiography

Definition and prerequisites

With the exemption of two major clinical studies [4,5] most authors have defined a 24 hour interval after the procedure as a sensible timeframe for relating a change in the patient's status to the angiography. In order to avoid bias due to subjective judgment on behalf of the physician, seemingly a consensus has evolved in the literature, that any change in the patient's condition, whether subjective or objective, has to be recorded as a complication of the angiography if it occurs during the procedure or within 24 hours [6–10].

It has to be taken into account, though, that this definition is not uncontroversial; Baum *et al.* reported on 1,600 consecutive cardiovascular and peripheral catheter-based angiographies, assessing all causes for cancellation within 48 hours of scheduled exams as complications of "no arteriography" if they were complications of the primary disease. Interestingly, the rate of serious or fatal complications among subjects with performed arteriographies was as high as the corresponding rate for subjects with "no arteriography" (0.9%) [11]. A clinical worsening can thus happen due to a progress of the primary disease, independently from any invasive examination, presumably even during the procedure.

Non-neurological complications

Local and systemic complications of catheter-based cerebral angiography have been evaluated repeatedly

Treatment-Related Stroke, ed. Alexander Tsiskaridze, Arne Lindgren and Adnan Qureshi. Published by Cambridge University Press. © Cambridge University Press 2016.

in large retrospective or prospective clinical studies [4–9,12–16]. The observed results have been consistent through the decades. Methodically inherent complications independent from the targeted organ, such as puncture site related complications, are comparable to the experiences in other disciplines, e.g., interventional cardiology [17].

The most common complication of diagnostic cerebral angiography is a local hematoma in the groin [4,7,8]. It has been reported in 4.2 to 10.7% of patients; besides technical aspects such as sheath size, age seems to be an important risk factor that can increase the complication rate to 18% in patients older than 70 years [4]. It is rare, though, that groin hematomas lead to more serious complications, necessitating invasive countermeasures such as surgery for evacuation (0.03% of cases) [7].

Nausea, vomiting, headaches, and transient hypotension are the most common systemic adverse effects, ranging between 0.2 and 1.2% of cases [4,7,15,16]. We felt from our personal experience at the Karolinska University Hospital that migraine-like symptoms occur in a number of younger patients after the initial application of contrast or within hours after the examination. This observation is not reflected in the literature, though; severe headaches were described in less than 1.0% of patients [7]. Anaphylactic conditions and circulatory collapse were uncommon (0.03%) in the largest published series with nearly 20,000 cerebral angiography procedures; death occurred in 0.06% of examined patients and was mostly attributable to severe neurological complications [7].

Clinically detectable neurological complications

Since the 1970s a substantial number of studies have reported in detail on clinically evident neurological complications of cerebral angiography; Table 8.1 provides an overview.

Overall, the combined rate of transient (resolving within 24 hours) and reversible (resolving within 10 days) neurologic deficits attributable to cerebral angiography has been reported to be as low as 0.06% and as high as 3.3% in a selected cohort of patients examined explicitly for cerebrovascular disease. Furthermore, the reported transient and reversible rate of stroke ranged between 0 and 1.2% for the studies where a more detailed description of symptoms was available

(see Table 8.1). Interestingly, most of these ischemic complications were exacerbations of the underlying primary disease, which was especially true for patients with atheromatous cerebrovascular disease. A meta-analysis conducted by Cloft et al. has shown that the combined risk of permanent and transient neurological complications was significantly lower in patients with aneurysm and AVM (with and without subarachnoid hemorrhage) compared to patients with TIA or stroke [18].

The reported permanent neurologic complication rate varies between 0 and 0.52% (Table 8.1). A closer analysis of the described permanent complications attributed to intra-arterial cerebral angiography shows that almost all of the permanent deficits are based on ischemia and a consecutive stroke. Consequently, stroke is the leading etiology for severe and disabling neurologic complications after diagnostic cerebral angiography in all patients, not only those with cerebrovascular disease. The reported risk can be as high as 0.52% [5] in patients with atheromatous cerebrovascular disease but can also approach zero in a dedicated neurointerventional department with a homogenous distribution of underlying etiologies, where atheromatous disease represents a fraction of patients [9]. Stroke-related mortality was as low as 0 and as high as 0.05% in the largest examined cohort, featuring nearly 20,000 cerebral angiographies in a university department between 1981 and 2003 [7]. The authors were also able to show that the overall risk for a neurologic complication decreased significantly over the course of time, reaching its nadir between 1997 and 2003. Willinsky et al. reported a similar effect; the rate of neurologic complications decreased in the last quartile of their study [10].

Risk factors associated with clinically detectable neurological complications

The following risk factors for clinically evident neurological complications in the first 24 hours after diagnostic cerebral angiography were identified by multiple studies:

> age – the risk increases with patient age [6,10,13,19]
>
> (concomitant) atheromatous cardiovascular or cerebrovascular disease [7,10,19]
>
> subarachnoid hemorrhage and intracerebral hemorrhage [7,12]

Table 8.1 Clinically evident neurological complication rates in major studies (1977–2010).

Study/year	Type of analysis	No. of cases	Transient neurological deficit (<10 d)	Transient stroke (<10 d)	Persistent neurological deficit	Persistent stroke (mortality)	Time interval for definition as complication	Significant risk factors for neurologic complications
Olivecrona [8]/1977	Pro	5,531	2.9%	0.13%	0.11%	0.11% (0.02%)	24 h	1. No significance of operator experience 2. No significance of procedure length
Mani et al. [15]/1978[a]	Retro	5,000	0.86%	0.76%	0.04%	0.04% (0.02%)	24 h	1. Operator experience 2. Duration >80 min 3. Age >40 years
Earnest et al. [6]/1984	Pro	1,517	2.3%	0.13%	0.33%	0.33% (0%)	24 h	1. Patient age 2. Serum creatinine↑ 3. Utilization of more than one catheter
Dion et al. [4]/1987	Pro	1,002	1.2%	1.2%	0.1%	0.1% (0%)	24 h	1. Duration >60 min 2. Systolic hypertension
Waugh et al. [16]/1992	Pro	939	0.9%	n.a.	0.3%	n.a.	24 h	n.a.
Warnock et al. [5]/1993[b]	Retro	395	3.3%	n.a.	0.52%	0.52% (0%)	48 h	No increased risk for patients with cerebrovascular disease
Heiserman et al. [19]/1994	Pro	1,000	0.5%	0.5%	0.5%	0.5% (0%)	24 h	1. Age 2. Duration >60 min 3. Stenosis >70% in injected vessel
Willinsky et al. [10]/2003	Pro	2,899	0.86%	n.a.	0.5%	0.25% (0%)	24 h	1. Age >55 years 2. Cardiovascular disease 3. Fluoroscopy >10 min

Table 8.1 (cont.)

Study/year	Type of analysis	No. of cases	Transient neurological deficit (<10 d)	Transient stroke (<10 d)	Persistent neurological deficit	Persistent stroke (mortality)	Time interval for definition as complication	Significant risk factors for neurologic complications
Dawkins et al. [12]/2007[c]	Pro	2,924	0.34%	0.17%	0%	0% (0%)	6 h	1. ICH and SAH 2. Emergency setting
Kaufmann et al. [7]/2007[d]	Retro	19,826	2.45%	n.a.	0.14%	0.14% (0.05%)	24 h	1. Cerebrovascular disease 2. SAH 3. History of TIA
Thiex et al. [9]/2010	Retro	1,715	0.06%	0%	0%	0% (0%)	24 h	n.a.
Summary		**42,748**	**0.06–3.3%**	**0–1.2%**	**0–0.52%**	**0–0.52% (0–0.05%)**		

Olivecrona (1977) calculated the risks based on the total number of patients examined and not on the total number of angiographies in the studied period. In order to ensure comparability with following authors who calculated the risks based on the total number of angiographies in the studied period, the risks given in the table were recalculated based on the original publication in relation to the total number of angiographies.

Pro: prospective study; Retro: retrospective study.

[a] Neurologic event within 24 h counted as a complication if the examiner classified it as an angiographic complication (investigator-related bias).

[b] All patients underwent angiography exclusively due to clinical suspicion of cerebrovascular disease (preselected cohort); for two thirds of patients this diagnosis was confirmed angiographically

[c] Ten dissections of cervical vessels were classified as "asymptomatic technical complications"; none necessitated emergent stent placement.

[d] Largest study to date, featuring all consecutive cerebral angiographies in a single center from 1981 to 2003.

The given mortality rate in brackets is the stroke-related mortality rate in cerebral angiographies.

prolonged examinations (overall duration >60 min or fluoroscopy >10 min) [4,10,13].

Factors that may also play a role but were only reported in single larger series are:

systolic hypertension [4]

elevated serum creatinine [6]

examination conducted as emergency [12]

operator experience [15].

Pathophysiology of stroke-related complications

Several mechanisms have been proposed to account for the stroke-related complications in diagnostic cerebral angiography. From a technical point of view, the most obvious cause is thromboembolism from the catheters or guide wires. These thrombi develop inside the dead space of the catheter while manipulating with the guide wire [10]. Especially stagnant blood in this dead space is prone to clot formation. Thus it should be common practice to keep guide-wire manipulations at a minimum. A roadmap technique for a quick and precise overview of any underlying vessel anatomy in conjunction with continuous flushing of the catheter with heparinized saline may be helpful to reduce the rate of thromboembolic events [4,9].

Disruptions of pre-existing atherosclerotic plaques are rare but have been described; they seem to lead to more severe ischemic events, provoking proximal occlusions of cerebral arteries and sometimes even leading to stroke-related mortality [6,8]. Other potential causes include arterial wall dissections related to catheter or wire manipulations. However, the rate of dissection-related thromboembolism leading to clinically evident ischemic events seems to be lower than expected. Dawkins *et al.* reported ten intraprocedural dissections of the selectively catheterized vertebral or internal carotid artery in a series of 2,924 diagnostic cerebral angiograms. There was no clinically apparent stroke and furthermore eight out of the ten patients had a subsequent MRI examination showing no abnormalities on diffusion-weighted imaging (DWI) indicative of embolism or stroke. All patients were treated medically; there were no emergency stentings [12].

Diffusion-weighted imaging abnormalities after diagnostic cerebral angiography

Aside from clinically evident neurological deficits, the phenomenon of microemboli and microbubbles in cerebral angiography has given rise to concern in recent times. This phenomenon, taking place after injection of contrast or saline in catheterized vessels, had been studied earlier by transcranial Doppler, but its clinical impact remained largely unknown [20,21]. The advent of MRI in routine clinical practice was followed by initial reports of T2 abnormalities in patients after diagnostic cerebral angiography with no clinically evident ischemic event [22,23]. This led to more robustly designed clinical studies, alluding to the conclusion that clinically obvious strokes may only be the tip of the iceberg. The frequency of so-called "silent" microembolizations is reported in the range of 15 to 26% [24–28]. The indication for conventional intra-arterial angiography plays a role, as patients with vasculopathies (atheromatous disease, vasculitis) showed an increased risk for silent emboli [24,28,29]. A prolonged examination also increases the risk for silent emboli, a finding that is concomitant with previous observations and a known risk factor for clinically apparent ischemic events [4,13,24].

The clinical significance of silent DWI abnormalities has been debated. The body of evidence that speaks in favor of DWI lesions being an adequate surrogate marker for structural brain damage has increased [25,30]. The presentation characteristics on MRI do not differ between clinically evident and clinically silent lesions. It is the anatomical location of the lesion that constitutes the extent of clinically observable neurological deficits and even small emboli in eloquent areas can cause substantial neurological deficits [30]. Such deficits have not been described in patients without DWI lesions.

In all mentioned major clinical studies (Table 8.1) the definition of a clinically apparent deficit was based on common, routine clinical neurological examinations before and after angiography. This clinical examination looks systematically for focal abnormalities such as paresis, ataxia, hypesthesia, visual defects, and oculomotor syndromes. The screening for neuropsychological deficits is often restricted to aphasia, apraxia, and dyscalculia. Global dysfunctions of the brain, e.g., cognitive decline, memory loss, mood disturbances, and personality changes may be missed. In this setting, the available data on the role of postangiographic DWI abnormalities is controversial, which can be partially attributed to small patient samples. The cumulative burden of ischemic brain injury, though, might be responsible for neuropsychological deficits and/or aggravation of vascular dementia [31–35].

It has been demonstrated that the burden of microemboli can be significantly reduced by appropriate technical means such as continuous flush in closed systems, the use of air filters, and heparin administration during the procedure [29]. Interestingly, Brockmann *et al.* were recently not able to show a significant reduction of microemboli through the intraprocedural administration of abciximab (IIb/IIIa receptor inhibition in platelets) in a randomized placebo-controlled trial [36]. Patients in both groups, though, received heparin, which is known to reduce the rate of thromboembolism during angiography significantly [29]. The conclusion might then be that abciximab does not further reduce the rate of thromboembolism compared to heparin alone.

Diagnostic cerebral angiography in children

Cerebral angiography conducted in children has substantial technical and procedural differences compared to adults. The majority of examinations are conducted under general anesthesia. The underlying pathologies are different, being dominated by intracranial shunts and arteriovenous malformations, with and without concomitant intracranial hemorrhage [37]. The presence of atheromatous disease is far less important compared to adults and stands behind e.g., moyamoya disease or cerebral vasculitis [37,38]. In recent studies, the rate of intraprocedural complications in children was very low, reported to be 0% for thromboembolic events and iatrogenic dissections as well as for systemic or local complications at the access site [37,38]. Burger *et al.* observed a single postangiographic rebleeding of a complex dural arteriovenous fistula after three hours in a cohort of 205 consecutive patients with 241 diagnostic angiograms [38]. Regarding infants and very young children up to the age of 36 months, Hoffman *et al.* analyzed 309 consecutive cerebral angiograms obtained in 87 children from 2004 to 2010 at a single institution [39]. Their rate of neurological complications was 0.0%, the rate of non-neurological complications was 2.9%. The rate of radiographic complications was as low as 1.3% and there were no delayed complications during a mean follow-up of 16.6 months. No association was found between complications and age, duration of anesthesia, number of vessels catheterized, size of the sheath, or diagnostic vs. interventional procedures. Overall, their rate of complications was comparable to reported rates for older children and lower than for adults.

In comparison with studies conducted in adults, studies in children have smaller sample sizes and conclusions are more difficult to draw. Thus, in view of limited data, the exact incidence of stroke as a procedural complication in pediatric cerebral angiography is unknown.

Conclusions

Diagnostic intra-arterial cerebral angiography remains technically the gold standard in the evaluation of cerebrovascular disease. As an invasive procedure, though, it has a persistent inherent risk for a permanent deficit, which can be as high as 0.5%. This rate has not substantially decreased in recent times compared to the 1970s and 1980s in spite of significant technical improvements in hardware and contrast agents. The reason for this might be an overall decrease of conducted examinations and the increased age and comorbidity of examined patients. Consequently, from a practical point of view, alternative diagnostic methods should be considered in patients who are investigated for diseases that are known to increase the risk of diagnostic cerebral angiography. However, this should not lead to an exclusion of patients from a technically superior, high-quality diagnostic intra-arterial cerebral angiogram, which does provide critical information in patients with potentially life-threatening neurovascular conditions and forms the basis of any decision-making process in case of an interventional endovascular procedure. Those patients must still accept these risks in order to gain potentially life-saving information otherwise unobtainable.

References

1. Moniz E. L'encéphalographie artérielle, son importance dans la localisation des tumeurs cérébrales. *Revue Neurologique.* 1927; **2**:63.

2. Kaufmann T J, Kallmes D F. Diagnostic cerebral angiography: Archaic and complication-prone or here to stay for another 80 years? *American Journal of Roentgenology.* 2008; **190**:1435–7.

3. Kallmes D F, Layton K, Marx W F, Tong F. Death by nondiagnosis: why emergent CT angiography should not be done for patients with subarachnoid hemorrhage. *American Journal of Neuroradiology.* 2007; **28**:1837–8.

4. Dion J E, Gates P C, Fox A J, Barnett H J, Blom R J. Clinical events following neuroangiography: a prospective study. *Stroke.* 1987; **18**:997–1004.

5. Warnock N G, Gandhi M R, Bergvall U, Powell T. Complications of intraarterial digital subtraction

angiography in patients investigated for cerebral vascular disease. *British Journal of Radiology.* 1993; **66**: 855–8.

6. Earnest F T, Forbes G, Sandok B A, *et al.* Complications of cerebral angiography: prospective assessment of risk. *American Journal of Roentgenology.* 1984; **142**:247–53.

7. Kaufmann T J, Huston J, 3rd, Mandrekar J N, *et al.* of diagnostic cerebral angiography: evaluation of 19,826 consecutive patients. *Radiology.* 2007; **243**:812–19.

8. Olivecrona H. Complications of cerebral angiography. *Neuroradiology.* 1977; **14**:175–81.

9. Thiex R, Norbash A M, Frerichs K U. *et al.* The safety of dedicated-team catheter-based diagnostic cerebral angiography in the era of advanced noninvasive imaging. *American Journal of Neuroradiology.* 2010; **31**: 230–4.

10. Willinsky R A, Taylor S M, TerBrugge K, et al. Neurologic complications of cerebral angiography: prospective analysis of 2,899 procedures and review of the literature. *Radiology.* 2003; **227**:522–8.

11. Baum S, Stein G N, Kuroda K K. Complications of "no arteriography". *Radiology.* 1966; **86**:835–8.

12. Dawkins A A, Evans A L, Wattam J, *et al.* Complications of cerebral angiography: a prospective analysis of 2,924 consecutive procedures. *Neuroradiology.* 2007; **49**:753–9.

13. Mani R L, Eisenberg R L. Complications of catheter cerebral arteriography: analysis of 5,000 procedures. III. Assessment of arteries injected, contrast medium used, duration of procedure, and age of patient. *American Journal of Roentgenology.* 1978; **131**:871–4.

14. Mani R L, Eisenberg R L. Complications of catheter cerebral arteriography: analysis of 5,000 procedures. II. Relation of complication rates to clinical and arteriographic diagnoses. *American Journal of Roentgenology.* 1978; **131**:867–9.

15. Mani R L, Eisenberg R L, McDonald E J, Jr., Pollock J A, Mani J R. Complications of catheter cerebral arteriography: analysis of 5,000 procedures. I. Criteria and incidence. *American Journal of Roentgenology.* 1978; **131**:861–5.

16. Waugh J R, Sacharias N. Arteriographic complications in the DSA era. *Radiology.* 1992; **182**:243–6.

17. Pohler E, Gunther H, Diekmann M, Eggeling T. Outpatient coronary angiography–safety and feasibility. *Cardiology.* 1994; **84**:305–9.

18. Cloft H J, Joseph G J, Dion J E. Risk of cerebral angiography in patients with subarachnoid hemorrhage, cerebral aneurysm, and arteriovenous malformation: a meta-analysis. *Stroke.* 1999; **30**:317–20.

19. Heiserman J E, Dean B L, Hodak J A, *et al.* Neurologic complications of cerebral angiography. *American Journal of Neuroradiology.* 1994; **15**:1401–7.

20. Dagirmanjian A, Davis D A, Rothfus W E, Deeb Z L, Goldberg A L. Silent cerebral microemboli occurring during carotid angiography: frequency as determined with Doppler sonography. *American Journal of Roentgenology.* 1993; **161**:1037–40.

21. Markus H, Loh A, Israel D, *et al.* Microscopic air embolism during cerebral angiography and strategies for its avoidance. *Lancet.* 1993; **341**:784–7.

22. Gerraty R P, Bowser D N, Infeld B, Mitchell P J, Davis S M. Microemboli during carotid angiography. Association with stroke risk factors or subsequent magnetic resonance imaging changes? *Stroke.* 1996; **27**: 1543–7.

23. Mamourian A, Drayer B P. Clinically silent infarcts shown by MR after cerebral angiography. *American Journal of Neuroradiology.* 1990; **11**:1084.

24. Bendszus M, Koltzenburg M, Burger R, *et al.* Silent embolism in diagnostic cerebral angiography and neurointerventional procedures: a prospective study. *Lancet.* 1999; **354**:1594–7.

25. Chuah K C, Stuckey S L, Berman I G. Silent embolism in diagnostic cerebral angiography: detection with diffusion-weighted imaging. *Australasian Radiology.* 2004; **48**:133–8.

26. Hahnel S, Bender J, Jansen O, et al. [Clinically silent cerebral embolisms after cerebral catheter angiography]. *Fortschritte auf dem Gebiete der Rontgenstrahlen und der Nuklearmedizin.* 2001; **173**: 300–5.

27. Kato K, Tomura N, Takahashi S, Sakuma I, Watarai J. Ischemic lesions related to cerebral angiography: Evaluation by diffusion weighted MR imaging. *Neuroradiology.* 2003; **45**:39–43.

28. Krings T, Willmes K, Becker R, *et al.* Silent microemboli related to diagnostic cerebral angiography: a matter of operator's experience and patient's disease. *Neuroradiology.* 2006; **48**:387–93.

29. Bendszus M, Koltzenburg M, Bartsch A J, *et al.* Heparin and air filters reduce embolic events caused by intra-arterial cerebral angiography: a prospective, randomized trial. *Circulation.* 2004; **110**:2210–15.

30. Bendszus M, Stoll G. Silent cerebral ischaemia: hidden fingerprints of invasive medical procedures. *Lancet Neurology.* 2006; **5**:364–72.

31. Bendszus M, Reents W, Franke D, *et al.* Brain damage after coronary artery bypass grafting. *Archives of Neurology.* 2002; **59**:1090–5.

32. Knipp S C, Matatko N, Wilhelm H, *et al.* Evaluation of brain injury after coronary artery bypass grafting. A prospective study using neuropsychological assessment and diffusion-weighted magnetic resonance imaging. *European Journal of Cardio-Thoracic Surgery.* 2004; **25**:791–800.

33. Lund C, Nes R B, Ugelstad T P, *et al.* Cerebral emboli during left heart catheterization may cause acute brain injury. *European Heart Journal.* 2005; **26:** 1269–75.

34. Lund C, Sundet K, Tennoe B, *et al.* Cerebral ischemic injury and cognitive impairment after off-pump and on-pump coronary artery bypass grafting surgery. *Annals of Thoracic Surgery.* 2005; **80:** 2126–31.

35. Restrepo L, Wityk R J, Grega M A, *et al.* Diffusion- and perfusion-weighted magnetic resonance imaging of the brain before and after coronary artery bypass grafting surgery. *Stroke.* 2002; **33:** 2909–15.

36. Brockmann C, Hoefer T, Diepers M, *et al.* Abciximab does not prevent ischemic lesions related to cerebral angiography: a randomized placebo-controlled trial. *Cerebrovascular Disease.* 2011; **31:**353–7.

37. Wolfe T J, Hussain S I, Lynch J R, Fitzsimmons B F, Zaidat O O. Pediatric cerebral angiography: analysis of utilization and findings. *Pediatric Neurology.* 2009; **40:**98–101.

38. Burger I M, Murphy K J, Jordan L C, Tamargo R J, Gailloud P. Safety of cerebral digital subtraction angiography in children: complication rate analysis in 241 consecutive diagnostic angiograms. *Stroke.* 2006; 37:2535–9.

39. Hoffman C E, Santillan A, Rotman L, Gobin Y P, Souweidane M M. Complications of cerebral angiography in children younger than 3 years of age: clinical article. *Journal of Neurosurgery Pediatrics.* 2014; **13:**414–19.

Stroke after endovascular cardiac procedures and cardiothoracic surgery

Christian Weimar and Stephan C. Knipp

Introduction

The interactions between heart disease and stroke are close and well known. Advances in therapeutics are leading to the development of a broad gamut of cardiac interventions, including medical, surgical, and endovascular procedures that are aimed at improving outcomes in persons with severe heart disease. Unfortunately, these procedures may be accompanied by neurologic complications that result in considerable morbidity or even death. Stroke and neuropsychologic impairments are well-recognized complications of cardiovascular operations, with stroke being one of the most devastating potential complications [1].

Stroke and endovascular cardiac procedures

Coronary intervention-related stroke

Stroke is one of the most feared complications of percutaneous coronary intervention (PCI). Use of guiding catheters and mechanical devices to provide circulatory support during PCI can cause fragmentation of atherosclerotic debris from the aorta and cerebral embolization leading to ischemic stroke [2,3]. Other potential mechanisms of PCI-related ischemic stroke include embolization of air, arterial dissection from catheter or guide wire manipulation, thrombus formation through warming of the tip or other parts of catheter, thrombocyte activation through endothelial lesions, and hemodynamic hypoperfusion due to systemic hypotension [4]. In addition, use of adjunctive antithrombotic medications during PCI may increase the risk of intracranial hemorrhage, which constitutes about 10% of PCI-related strokes [5].

In support of the hypothesis of plaque dislodgement during catheterization, transcranial Doppler signals have shown to increase during the passage of catheters around the aortic arch, suggestive of microembolization [6]. Analysis of 1,000 consecutive guiding catheters removed after PCI showed macroscopic aortic debris within the guide lumen in more than 50% [7]. While PCI-related mortality has declined over the last two decades [8], the rate of stroke remains unchanged at approximately 0.3 to 0.4% [9–11], which may be due to the fact that PCI is increasingly performed in high-risk patients. Representative data comes from the National Cardiovascular Data Registry sponsored by the American College of Cardiology, which included 706,782 patients undergoing PCI between January 2004 and March 2007 [10]. Periprocedural stroke (defined as a central neurological deficit persisting >72 h with onset at starting time in the catheterization laboratory until the time of hospital discharge) was documented in 1,540 patients (0.22%). Patients with periprocedural stroke were more likely to present with an acute coronary syndrome, had a greater percentage of high-risk coronary lesions, and worse PCI results. In a multivariate analysis, known cerebrovascular disease, older age, admission with an acute coronary syndrome, and use of an intra-aortic balloon pump were independently associated with stroke. In-hospital mortality was 30-fold higher in patients who developed a stroke compared with those who did not (30% vs. 1%), and length of hospital stay after PCI was considerably longer (10.9 vs. 3.1 days). In this registry, however, classification of the stroke events as ischemic or hemorrhagic was not available and there was no routine neurological follow-up or an independent adjudication of stroke events. Previously reported higher incidences for PCI-related stroke mentioned above

Treatment-Related Stroke, ed. Alexander Tsiskaridze, Arne Lindgren and Adnan Qureshi. Published by Cambridge University Press. © Cambridge University Press 2016.

are most likely due to a different definition of stroke as a neurological deficit lasting >24 h instead of >72 h [5,9,10]. Even in these studies, however, stroke symptoms may have been overlooked because no routine neurological follow-up was available.

While age, sex, multivessel coronary disease, and previous stroke or TIA cannot be modified, several procedural-related risk factors of stroke have been identified. In a large retrospective single center study, stroke during PCI involved the use of more catheters, greater contrast volumes, and larger guide caliber. PCI-stroke patients were also more likely to have undergone rotational arterectomy (10% vs. 3%) [8]. Presence of atheromatous plaque in the aortic arch poses the main risk of spontaneous embolism and the aforementioned procedural risk factors increase the chance of dislodging atherosclerotic debris from the aorta by physical abrasion. While imaging of aortic plaque distribution in high-risk patients could influence the choice of access site, several studies have suggested that the likelihood of displacing debris is greater in large vs. small caliber catheters, which therefore should be given preference in high-risk patients [11]. Because multiple catheter exchanges were independently associated with an increased risk of stroke, use of a single diagnostic or guiding catheter designed to intubate both coronary arteries may additionally lower the risk of stroke.

Catheter ablation of atrial fibrillation

Atrial fibrillation (AF) is the most common arrhythmia and constitutes a major risk factor for ischemic stroke. Catheter ablation is increasingly being utilized for treating both paroxysmal and persistent AF. The procedure is aimed at elimination or isolation of arrhythmogenic tissue by either heating (radiofrequency) or cooling (cryothermia). Another technology, laser treatment, is currently undergoing clinical trials. Most AF ablation procedures aim at electrical isolation of the pulmonary veins, which are electrically active structures with a sleeve of syncytial myocardium that extends from the left atrium. Electric separation by placing lesions in the left atrium around the ostia of the pulmonary veins disconnects the pulmonary veins from the rest of the atria. Various studies at different time periods have reported a stroke incidence in the range of 0.28 to 1.09% [12,13]. Studies looking for silent infarctions on post-interventional 1.5T MRI have reported stroke rates

between 8 and 18%, which went up to 40% when using 3T MRI [14,15]. Stroke and TIA may result from either dislodgement of pre-existing thrombus, or other material (including air) during ablation in the left atrium. A potential disadvantage is that RF ablation has been shown to reduce the left atrial transport function up to 30%, which may predispose to thrombus formation even during sinus rhythm [16]. Atrial endothelium has intrinsic anticoagulant properties, but when denuded, during e.g., RF ablation, this may promote the formation of a procoagulant state and ultimately the formation of thrombus [17].

Anticoagulation with warfarin appears to reduce the risk of stroke compared to stopping warfarin for the ablation procedure and bridging with low molecular weight heparin [18]. Intravenous heparin must be given during the ablation procedure to reduce the risk of thromboembolism, even when procedures are performed on therapeutic warfarin treatment. Hematological studies show that left atrial spontaneous echo contrast on transesophageal echocardiography arises from an interaction between red blood cells and plasma proteins such as fibrinogen. This finding has been described as a major predisposing factor for thrombus formation and may also predict the risk of embolism [19,20]. Patients with presence of left-atrial spontaneous echo contrast can therefore perhaps be managed with a more aggressive anticoagulation regimen. A study on 511 patients concluded that the detection of spontaneous echo contrast can be utilized to identify patients at increased risk of development of left atrial thrombus and that increased intensity of heparin anticoagulation (Activated Clotting Time >300 s) during left atrial ablation may prevent thrombus formation in these high-risk patients [21]. Because of a high rate of recurrent atrial fibrillation even after left atrial ablation, these patients remain at long-term risk for ischemic stroke and therefore should be considered for long-term anticoagulation treatment.

Percutaneous closure of patent foramen ovale

The foramen ovale is a congenital connection between the right and left atrium, which remains patent in about 20 to 25% of the general population. In several case-control studies and systematic reviews thereof, a patent foramen ovale (PFO) was associated with cryptogenic stroke [22]. Catheter-based closure of

PFO was introduced in 1992 to reduce the rate of recurrent stroke in patients with cryptogenic cerebrovascular events. However, no randomized study so far could show any clear benefit of PFO closure in patients with cryptogenic stroke [23–25] and no clear evidence exists for PFO closure benefit in patients with migraine [26]. Notwithstanding, PFO closure is still widely performed by cardiologic interventionalists. According to a review by Khairy *et al.* atrial arrhythmias, device thrombosis, and systemic embolism are both periprocedural and long-term potential complications after PFO closure, which may lead to (recurrent) stroke events [27]. In randomized trials, stroke was a rare periprocedural complication and occurred in between 0 and 0.75% of patients undergoing PFO closure. In addition, patients with PFO closure are at increased risk of paroxysmal atrial fibrillation, which in turn can cause ischemic stroke up to several weeks later [23].

The use of clopidogrel or aspirin is believed to reduce the incidence of thrombus formation and thromboembolism on the surface of the PFO closing devices. Furthermore, device-related complications are reported less frequently using newer devices. In this case, like for any other procedure, the experience of the interventionalist is probably more important than a specific device or technique. Given the lack of evidence for a secondary preventive effect of PFO closure, the best prevention of procedure-related complications, however, is to refrain from the intervention unless strongly indicated or within a randomized controlled study. Patients should receive aspirin and/or clopidogrel during and after the intervention and be monitored for paroxysmal atrial fibrillation following the intervention.

Stroke after cardiac surgery

Coronary artery bypass graft (CABG) surgery

The incidence of stroke in cardiac surgical patients has been studied by many investigators, yielding estimates being as high as 5% in patients undergoing coronary artery bypass graft (CABG) surgery, increasing to almost 9% in CABG patients ≥75 years of age and nearly 16% in patients undergoing valve surgery or those with pre-existing cerebrovascular disease [28–31]. Stroke significantly affects survival and quality of life. Moreover, adverse neurologic events have important economic consequences, with estimated

costs that exceed $2 to $4 billion annually worldwide for patients with stroke after CABG [29].

Despite the increasing prevalence of atherosclerotic disease in patients undergoing coronary revascularization, the incidence of stroke after CABG has declined over the past decade, with a recent study reporting an overall rate of stroke of 1.6% (95% confidence interval, 1.4 to 1.7%) after isolated CABG surgery [32]. Stroke rates vary, depending on the underlying risks of the patient population as well as on the definition of stroke. Estimated frequencies are increased by a factor of ten, when radiographic cerebral infarction is included in the definition of stroke, and the use of magnetic resonance imaging (MRI) rather than computed tomography results in higher rates of radiographic cerebral infarct. These radiographic infarcts are not always accompanied by clinical deficits. In addition, more subtle deficits from stroke are frequently not diagnosed in the perioperative period, since patients are often experiencing pain, are receiving medications including sedatives, or have other symptoms that can mask subtle neurologic signs [33]. Some patients develop stroke intraoperatively, with neurologic deficit apparent immediately after awakening from anesthesia, others develop it postoperatively, after initially awakening without neurologic deficit. Among 45,432 patients who underwent isolated primary or reoperative CABG surgery at a single US academic medical center from 1982 through 2009, the occurrence of stroke declined despite an increasing patient risk profile [32]. More than half of strokes (60 to 65%) occurred postoperatively and 40% intraoperatively [30,32]. Postoperative stroke peaked at 40 hours.

Pathogenetic causes of stroke related to cardiac surgery include the traditionally invoked mechanisms of brain infarction, such as macroembolization or microembolization. More recent data suggest, however, that hypoperfusion and systemic inflammatory response may also be presumed sources of neurologic injury, possibly in conjunction with embolization [34]. Persons with chronic hypertension may be exposed to relative intraoperative arterial hypotension in the brain if their blood pressure is maintained at a normal or slightly low level during surgery, thus placing them at risk for a borderzone cerebral infarction [35]. Caplan and Hennerici have proposed that the combination of hypoperfusion and microembolization increases the risk of neurologic injury owing to decreased washout of emboli [36]. Because of the likely multifactorial mechanisms underlying stroke after CABG, preventive strategies may need to be designed not only to avoid excessive release of emboli, but also to avoid relative hypotension or a systemic inflammatory response.

Several risk factors have been identified as predictors of stroke. Risk factors common to both intraoperative and postoperative stroke were older age, previous stroke, preoperative atrial fibrillation, variables representing atherosclerotic burden (hypertension, diabetes, carotid artery stenosis, peripheral artery disease), on-pump CABG with hypothermic circulatory arrest, and smaller body surface area [32]. The mechanisms of these factors are probably related to the health of the blood vessels, both those surrounding the heart and those in the neck and brain. Persons with chronic hyperlipidemia and diabetes mellitus may have plaques in the aorta, increasing the risk of perioperative embolism to the brain. New onset postoperative atrial fibrillation has also been found to be a major macroembolic cause of stroke in some studies [30,32,37]. Moreover, anemia is strongly associated with the risk of adverse perioperative neurological outcomes including stroke [38,39]. The above factors may not only affect risk of stroke occurring during the intraoperative period but also lead to stroke with an onset in the postoperative period, which accounts for up to two thirds of all perioperative strokes. With the increasing availability of MRI, evidence of pre-existing cerebrovascular disease has been shown to predict postoperative neurological complications. In a study involving patients who underwent brain MRI before CABG, those with small (often subclinical) infarctions had increased rates of clinical stroke of 5.6% compared to 1.4% among patients with normal preoperative MRI scans [40]. The development of strategies to reduce the incidence of postoperative neurologic events has been hampered by the lack of a clear understanding of the pathophysiology of such outcomes [41].

Several strategies have been suggested to lower the risk of stroke in cardiac surgery. Owing partly to the assumption that adverse neurologic events were specifically related to the use of extracorporeal circulation with cardiopulmonary bypass (CPB), techniques were developed for performing CABG without the use of CPB. However, recent large, prospective, randomized studies comparing the rate of adverse neurologic outcomes after conventional on-pump surgery with the rate after off-pump surgery have not shown a significant risk reduction associated with the use of off-pump surgery [42,43]. In other, non-randomized studies, off-pump bypass surgery was associated with lower rates of early strokes (i.e., immediately after surgery) but with similar rates of delayed stroke (i.e., after an initially uneventful neurologic recovery from surgery) [44]. Consequently, efforts to reduce the incidence of postoperative neurologic injury have begun to focus on patient-related factors such as the degree of atherosclerosis of the aorta, the carotid arteries, and the cerebral arteries, rather than procedure-related variables. Hyperlipidemia is such a potential atherosclerotic risk factor, and although the effect of statins for decreasing the risk of postoperative stroke and adverse cognitive outcomes is limited to observational studies, the combination of a preoperative statin and beta-blockers may reduce the risk of postoperative stroke [45]. Aspirin is also frequently used by patients undergoing CABG, and when used during the first 48 hours after surgery, it is associated with a reduced risk of postoperative stroke [46].

Transcatheter aortic valve implantation (TAVI)

Stroke is a potential complication of treating patients with aortic stenosis via surgical valve replacement (AVR), transcatheter aortic valve implantation (TAVI), and balloon aortic valvuloplasty (BAV). Based on recent randomized data from the PARTNER (Placement of Aortic Transcatheter Valves) trial, TAVI has emerged as the preferred therapy for inoperable patients and as an alternative to surgical AVR in high-risk patients [47, 48].

Reported stroke outcomes with the balloon-expandable Edwards SAPIEN transcatheter heart valve (Edwards Lifesciences, Irvine, California, USA) using a transfemoral approach ranged from 2.4 to 6% [47–49]. Two feasibility trials evaluating only the transapical approach using the Edwards SAPIEN valve reported strokes in 2% and 5% of patients [50,51]. Four registries reported stroke-related clinical outcomes with the self-expanding CoreValve Revalving system (Medtronic, Minneapolis, Minnesota, USA). In these registries, 30-day strokes ranged between 1.9 and 4.5% with the TF approach with the 18-F device [52]. There are limited data on the subclavian approach with the CoreValve and the largest cohort of subclavian patients reported a 1.9% in-hospital stroke rate [53].

In a multidevice series of 697 patients treated with TAVI, the overall rate of in-hospital stroke was 2.8%; a TF approach was used in most patients (92.4%) and most (84.4%) were treated with the CoreValve prosthesis [54].

In addition to the clinically apparent neurologic events, several cerebral diffusion-weighted magnetic resonance imaging (DW-MRI) studies have shown a very high incidence (58 to 91%) of new ischemic lesions after TAVI, regardless of the transcatheter valve type and approach [55,56]. These small, usually asymptomatic, DWI lesions are most probably caused by microembolic particles arising during the valve implantation procedure, specifically during the positioning and expansion of the prosthesis [57,58]. Although the consequences of silent ischemic brain lesions are still uncertain, in some studies they have been associated with cognitive decline and an increased risk of dementia and depression [59]. The typically silent aspect of the majority of TAVI-related DWI lesions might be explained by their location in the brain and their size.

With the emergence of TAVI, there has been a resurgence in BAV. In recent studies of BAV, the observed stroke rates were found to be approximately 1 to 2% [60].

Open valve replacement (AVR)

The overall risk of stroke for isolated AVR in the general US population is approximately 1.5% based on the Society of Thoracic Surgeons database [61]. Several studies have specifically examined the outcomes of high-risk elderly patients undergoing heart surgery. In these multiple small series, the stroke frequency in high-risk patients undergoing AVR was increased, and important predictors were age (>80 years) and mean logistic EuroSCORE (European System for Cardiac Operative Risk Evaluation) [62]. In the largest single-center study including 249 octogenarians (STS score 10.5%) who underwent AVR, there was a 3% perioperative mortality, but 4% of patients had strokes [63].

In much of the current AVR literature, stroke is poorly defined and usually is not independently adjudicated. Definitions have varied from crude determinations of a new neurologic deficit to more sensitive discriminations of stroke severity [64]. In contrast, most TAVI studies have 30-day and often one-year follow-up and attempt to apply a more consistent definition of stroke, but with varying ascertainment and adjudication. It is likely that without prospective assessment and follow-up, dedicated neurologic evaluations to adjudicate events, and confirmatory neuroimaging studies, strokes were systematically underreported in many registries. Another barrier to the interpretation of available data relates to discrepancies in the treated population across studies (e.g., important comorbidity) and the type of surgery performed (e.g., AVR alone, AVR + CABG). These limitations render cross-study comparisons of published observational data problematic [65]. In the PARTNER randomized trial comparing TAVI and surgical AVR in high-risk patients (n = 348 TAVI [TA and TF]; n = 351 AVR), the AVR group had a two-fold lower event rate for strokes and transient ischemic attacks at both 30-days and one year (30 days: 2.4% AVR vs. 5.5% TAVI, p = 0.04; and one year: 4.3% AVR vs. 8.3% TAVI, p = 0.04) [48].

Pathophysiology

Although strokes during either AVR or TAVI are undoubtedly multifactorial, the dominant etiology is likely intraprocedural embolic events. A transcranial Doppler study during TAVI demonstrated that the majority of procedural embolic events occurred during balloon valvuloplasty, manipulation of catheters across the aortic valve, and valve implantation [66]. During AVR, evidence of emboli from transcranial Doppler imaging was mainly seen during insertion of the cannula at the start of cardiopulmonary bypass and after removing the clamp from the aorta with the heart beating while empty [67]. Late embolic events post-AVR are presumably caused by debris from the prosthesis [68].

Risk factors for stroke after valve procedures

A number of variables have been identified as independent risk factors for stroke after cardiac valve operations. A multivariable analysis in patients undergoing valve surgery revealed four baseline characteristics and two procedural events that were associated with early postprocedure stroke: female sex, EF <30%, diabetes, age older than 70 years, duration of extracorporeal circulation >120 min, and atherosclerosis of the ascending aorta. Of note, atrial fibrillation was not included in this model [69]. Among patients with an EF <40% in another study, additional multivariate predictors of stroke were peripheral vascular disease and history of stroke or cerebrovascular disease [70].

Late embolic stroke after surgical AVR is also a concern. Follow-up of 2,317 patients with AVR revealed an annual rate of stroke of 1.3% for bio-prostheses and 1.4% for mechanical valves [71]. In the PARTNER randomized trial of AVR vs. TAVI, independent predictors of early stroke were assignment to TAVI and a smaller aortic valve area [48,64].

Combined cardiac interventions

The addition of coronary bypass surgery or other procedures to AVR appears to significantly increase the risk of neurologic events. In two studies on octogenarians receiving AVR combined with other procedures, the observed incidence of stroke was 4% (67% had AVR + CABG, 11.3% had concomitant mitral valve replacement or repair) [72] and 4.9% (AVR + CABG) [73]. Significant carotid artery stenosis is present in approximately 6 to 8% of all patients undergoing CABG and is associated with an increased risk of stroke during and after surgery [74,75]. Treatment of these patients is handled controversially. Staged or synchronous carotid endarterectomy (CEA) has been advocated by many cardiovascular surgeons to reduce the increased perioperative and long-term risk of stroke associated with polyvascular disease. During the synchronous operation, CEA is usually performed before CABG. Pooled data from single-center observational studies and a nationwide US registry of 26,197 patients treated between 2000 and 2004 with synchronous CEA + CABG revealed a perioperative stroke rate of approximately 4% [76,77]. In the absence of any randomized controlled trials, however, no systematic evidence exists that staged or synchronous operations (CEA + CABG) confer any benefit over CABG without CEA. Conversely, it remains questionable whether the observed risk of the synchronous procedure is justified in any asymptomatic patient with high-grade carotid stenosis. On the other hand, evidence for isolated CABG, the least invasive and least expensive strategy, is limited to self-reported, uncontrolled, mostly retrospective case series. Very soon, the Coronary Artery Bypass graft surgery in patients with Asymptomatic Carotid Stenosis (CABACS) randomized clinical trial will report its results to finally settle this open question by comparing safety and efficacy of isolated CABG with combined synchronous CABG and CEA in patients with asymptomatic atherosclerotic carotid artery stenosis [78].

Conclusion

While stroke is rather rare after endovascular cardiac procedures, it becomes a more frequent complication in cardiac surgery. Because focal neurological deficits tend to be overlooked by surgeons, postoperative strokes may often remain undetected and therefore untreated. While routine cerebral MRI for stroke detection is clearly not feasible, a routine neurological evaluation before discharge would certainly improve detection and awareness to further lower the risk of this important complication.

References

1. Gottesman R F, McKhann G, Hogue C V. Neurological complications of cardiac surgery. *Semin Neurol.* 2008; 703–15.

2. Karalis D G, Quinn V, Victor M F, *et al.* Risk of catheter-related emboli in patients with atherosclerotic debris in the thoracic aorta. *Am Heart J.* 1996; **131**(6): 1149–55.

3. Eggebrecht H, Oldenburg O, Dirsch O *et al.* Potential embolization by atherosclerotic debris dislodged from aortic wall during cardiac catheterization: histological and clinical findings in 7,621 patients. *Catheter Cardiovasc Interv.* 2000; **49**(4):389–94.

4. Qureshi A I, Luft A R, Sharma M, Guterman L R, Hopkins L N. Prevention and treatment of thromboembolic and ischemic complications associated with endovascular procedures: Part I – Pathophysiological and pharmacological features. *Neurosurgery.* 2000; **46**(6):1344–59.

5. Hoffman S J, Holmes D R Jr, Rabinstein A A, *et al.* Trends, predictors, and outcomes of cerebrovascular events related to percutaneous coronary intervention: A 16-year single-center experience. *JACC Cardiovasc Interv.* 2011; **4**(4):415–22.

6. Lund C, Nes R B, Ugelstad T P, *et al.* Cerebral emboli during left heart catheterization may cause acute brain injury. *Eur Heart J.* 2005; **26**(13):1269–75.

7. Keeley E C, Grines C L. Scraping of aortic debris by coronary guiding catheters: A prospective evaluation of 1,000 cases. *J Am Coll Cardiol.* 1998; **32**(7): 1861–5.

8. Hilliard A A, From A M, Lennon R J, *et al.* Percutaneous revascularization for stable coronary artery disease temporal trends and impact of drug-eluting stents. *JACC Cardiovasc Interv.* 2010; **3**(2):172–9.

9. Dukkipati S, O'Neill W W, Harjai K J, *et al.* Characteristics of cerebrovascular accidents after percutaneous coronary interventions. *J Am Coll Cardiol.* 2004; **43**(7):1161–7.

10. Aggarwal A, Dai D, Rumsfeld, J S, Klein L W, Roe M T. Incidence and predictors of stroke associated with percutaneous coronary intervention. *Am J Cardiol.* 2009; **104**(3):349–53.

11. Hoffman S J, Routledge H C, Lennon R J, *et al.* Procedural factors associated with percutaneous coronary intervention-related ischemic stroke. *JACC Cardiovasc Interv.* 2012; **5**(2):200–6.

12. Cappato R, Calkins H, Chen S A, *et al.* Updated worldwide survey on the methods, efficacy, and safety of catheter ablation for human atrial fibrillation. *Circ Arrhythm Electrophysiol.* 2010; **3**(1):32–8.

13. Maan A, Shaikh A Y, Mansour M, Ruskin J N, Heist E K. Complications from catheter ablation of atrial fibrillation: a systematic review. *Crit Pathw Cardiol.* 2011; **10**(2):76–83.

14. Haeusler K G, Kirchhof P, Endres M. Left atrial catheter ablation and ischemic stroke. *Stroke.* 2012; **43**(1):265–70.

15. Haeusler K G, Koch L, Herm J, *et al.* 3 Tesla MRI-detected brain lesions after pulmonary vein isolation for atrial fibrillation: results of the MACPAF study. *J Cardiovasc Electrophysiol.* 2013; **24**(1):14–21.

16. Oral H, Chugh A, Ozaydin M, *et al.* Risk of thromboembolic events after percutaneous left atrial radiofrequency ablation of atrial fibrillation. *Circulation.* 2006; **114**(8):759–65.

17. Lemola K, Desjardins B, Sneider M, *et al.* Effect of left atrial circumferential ablation for atrial fibrillation on left atrial transport function. *Heart Rhythm.* 2005; **2**(9):923–8.

18. Di Biase L, Burkhardt J D, Mohanty P, *et al.* Periprocedural stroke and management of major bleeding complications in patients undergoing catheter ablation of atrial fibrillation: the impact of periprocedural therapeutic international normalized ratio. *Circulation.* 2010; **121**(23):2550–6.

19. Rastegar R, Harnick D J, Weidemann P, *et al.* Spontaneous echo contrast videodensity is flow-related and is dependent on the relative concentrations of fibrinogen and red blood cells. *J Am Coll Cardiol.* 2003; **41**(4):603–10.

20. Ren J F, Marchlinski F E, Callans D J. Left atrial thrombus associated with ablation for atrial fibrillation: identification with intracardiac echocardiography. *J Am Coll Cardiol.* 2004; **43**(10):1861–7.

21. Ren J F, Marchlinski F E, Callans D J, *et al.* Increased intensity of anticoagulation may reduce risk of thrombus during atrial fibrillation ablation procedures in patients with spontaneous echo contrast. *J Cardiovasc Electrophysiol.* 2005; **16**(5):474–7.

22. Handke M, Harloff A, Olschewski M, Hetzel A, Geibel A. Patent foramen ovale and cryptogenic stroke in older patients. *N Engl J Med.* 2007; **357**(22):2262–8.

23. Furlan A J, Reisman M, Massaro J, *et al.* Closure or medical therapy for cryptogenic stroke with patent foramen ovale. *N Engl J Med.* 2012; **366**(11):991–9.

24. Carroll J D, Saver J L, Thaler D E, *et al.* Closure of patent foramen ovale versus medical therapy after cryptogenic stroke. *N Engl J Med.* 2013; **368**(12): 1092–100.

25. Meier B, Kalesan B, Mattle H P, *et al.* Percutaneous closure of patent foramen ovale in cryptogenic embolism. *N Engl J Med.* 2013; **368**(12):1083–91.

26. Dowson A, Mullen M J, Peatfield R, *et al.* Migraine Intervention with STARFlex Technology (MIST) trial: a prospective, multicenter, double-blind, sham-controlled trial to evaluate the effectiveness of patent foramen ovale closure with STARFlex septal repair implant to resolve refractory migraine headache. *Circulation.* 2008; **117**(11):1397–404.

27. Khairy P, O'Donnell C P, Landzberg M J. Transcatheter closure versus medical therapy of patent foramen ovale and presumed paradoxical thromboemboli: A systematic review. *Ann Intern Med.* 2003; **139**(9):753–60.

28. Ricotta J J, Faggioli G L, Castilone A, Hassett J M. Risk factors for stroke after cardiac surgery. *J Vasc Surg.* 1995; **21**:359–64.

29. Roach G W, Kanchuger M, Mora-Mangano C, *et al.* Adverse cerebral outcomes after coronary bypass surgery. *N Engl J Med.* 1996; **335**:1857–63.

30. Hogue C W, Murphy S F, Schechtman K B, Davilla-Roman V G. Risk factors for early or delayed stroke after cardiac surgery. *Circulation.* 1999; **100**:642–7.

31. Almassi G H, Sommers T, Moritz T E, *et al.* Stroke in cardiac surgical patients: determinants and outcome. *Ann Thorac Surg.* 1999; **68**:391–8.

32. Tarakji K G, Sabik JF III, Bhudia S K, Batzy L H, Blackstone E H. Temporal onset, risk factors, and outcomes associated with stroke after coronary artery bypass grafting. *JAMA.* 2011; **305**:381–90.

33. Selnes O A, Gottesman R F, Grega M A, *et al.* Cognitive and neurologic outcomes after coronary-artery bypass surgery. *N Engl J Med.* 2012; **366**:250–7.

34. Raja S G, Berg G A. Impact of off-pump coronary artery bypass surgery on systemic inflammation: Current best available evidence. *J Card Surg.* 2007; **22**:445–55.

35. Gottesman R F, Sherman P M, Grega M A *et al.* Watershed strokes after cardiac surgery: diagnosis, etiology and outcome. *Stroke.* 2006; **37**:2306–11.

36. Caplan L R, Hennerici M. Impaired clearance of emboli (washout) is an important link between hypoperfusion, embolism, and ischemic stroke. *Arch Neurol.* 1998; **55**:1475–82.

37. Hedberg M, Boivie P, Engström K G. Early and late stroke after coronary surgery: An analysis of risk

factors and the impact of short-term and long-term survival. *Eur J Cardiothorac Surg.* 2011; **40**:379–87.

38. McKhann G M, Grega M A, Borowicz L M Jr, Baumgartner W A, Selnes O A. Stroke and encephalopathy after cardiac surgery. An update. *Stroke.* 2006; **37**:562–71.

39. Karkouti K, Djalani G, Borger M A, *et al.* Low hematocrit during cardiopulmonary bypass is associated with increased risk of perioperative stroke in cardiac surgery. *Ann Thorac Surg.* 2005; **80**:1381–7.

40. Goto T, Baba T, Honma K, *et al.* Magnetic resonance imaging findings and postoperative neurologic dysfunction in elderly patients undergoing coronary artery bypass grafting. *Ann Thorac Surg.* 2001; **72**: 137–42.

41. Selnes O A, Gottesman R F, Grega M A, *et al.* Cognitive and neurologic outcomes after coronary-artery bypass surgery. *N Engl J Med.* 2012; **366**:250–7.

42. Shroyer A L, Grower F L, Hattler B, *et al.* On-pump vs. off-pump coronary-artery bypass surgery. *N Engl J Med.* 2009; **361**:1827–37.

43. Møller C H, Perko M J, Lund J T, *et al.* No major differences in 30-day outcomes in high-risk patients randomized to off-pump vs. on-pump coronary bypass surgery. The Best Bypass Surgery Trial. *Circulation.* 2010; **121**:498–504.

44. Nishijama K, Horiguchi M, Shizuta S, *et al.* Temporal pattern of strokes after on-pump and off-pump coronary artery bypass graft surgery. *Ann Thorac Surg.* 2009; **87**:1839–44.

45. Bouchard D, Carrier M, Demers P, *et al.* Statins in combination with beta-blocker therapy reduces postoperative stroke after coronary artery bypass graft surgery. *Ann Thorac Surg.* 2011; **91**:654–9.

46. Mangano D T. Aspirin and mortality from coronary bypass surgery. *N Engl J Med.* 2002; **347**:1309–17.

47. Leon M B, Smith C R, Mack M, *et al.* Transcatheter aortic valve implantation for aortic stenosis in patients who cannot undergo surgery. *N Engl J Med.* 2010; **363**: 1597–607.

48. Smith C R, Leon M B, Mack M J, *et al.* Transcatheter versus surgical aortic valve replacement in high-risk patients. *N Engl J Med.* 2011; **364**:2187–98.

49. Thomas M, Schymik G, Walther T, *et al.* Thirty-day results of the SAPIEN aortic Bioprosthesis European Outcome (SOURCE) registry: A European registry of transcatheter aortic valve implantation using the Edwards SAPIEN valve. *Circulation.* 2010; **122**:62–9.

50. Walther T, Kasimir M T, Doss M, *et al.* One-year interim follow-up of the TRAVERSE trial: the initial feasibility study for transapical aortic valve implantation. *Eur J Cardiothorac Surg.* 2010; **39**:532–7.

51. Svenson L G, Dewey T, Kapadia S, *et al.* United States feasibility study of transcatheter insertion of a stented aortic valve by the left ventricular apex. *Ann Thorac Surg.* 2008; **86**:46–55.

52. Piazza N, Grube E, Gerckens U, *et al.* Procedural and 30-day outcomes following transcatheter aortic valve implantation using the third generation (18 Fr) CoreValve revalving system: results from the multicentre, expanded evaluation registry 1-year following CE mark approval. *EuroIntervention.* 2008; **4**:242–9.

53. Petronio A S, De Carlo M, Bedogni F, *et al.* Safety and efficacy of the subclavian approach for transcatheter aortic valve implantation with the CoreValve Revalving system. *Circ Cardiovasc Interv.* 2010; **3**: 359–66.

54. Zahn R, Gerckens U, Grube E, *et al.* Transcatheter aortic valve implantation: first results from a multi-centre real-world registry. *Eur Heart J.* 2011; **32**:198–204.

55. Arnold M, Schulz-Heise S, Achenbach S, *et al.* Embolic cerebral insults after transapical aortic valve implantation detected by magnetic resonance imaging. *JACC Cardiovasc Int.* 2010; **3**:1126–32.

56. Rodes-Cabau J, Dumont E, Boone R H, *et al.* Cerebral embolism following transcatheter aortic valve implantation: comparison of transfemoral and transapical approaches. *J Am Coll Cardiol.* 2011; **57**:18–28.

57. Kahlert P, Al-Rashid F, Döttger P, *et al.* Cerebral embolization during transcatheter aortic valve implantation: a transcranial Doppler study. *Circulation.* 2012; **126**:1245–55.

58. Reinsfelt B, Wetsrelind A, Ioanes D, *et al.* Transcranial Doppler microembolic signals and serum evidence of brain injury during transcatheter aortic valve implantation. *Acta Anaesthesiol Scand.* 2012; **56**:240–7.

59. Vermeer S E, Prins N D, den Heijer T, *et al.* Silent brain infarcts and the risk of dementia and cognitive decline. *N Engl J Med.* 2003; **348**:1215–22.

60. Ben-Dor I, Pichard A D, Satler L F, *et al.* Complications and outcome of balloon aortic valvuloplasty in high-risk or inoperable patients. *J Am Coll Cardiol Intv.* 2010; **3**:1150–6.

61. O'Brien S M, Shahain D M, Filardo G, *et al.* The Society of Thoracic Surgeons 2008 cardiac surgery risk models: Part 2-isolated valve surgery. *Ann Thorac Surg.* 2009; **88**-S23-42.

62. Ferrari E, Tozzi P, Hurni M, *et al.* Primary isolated aortic valve surgery in octogenarians. *Eur J Cardiothorac Surg.* 2010; **38**:128–33.

63. Elbardissi A W, Shekar P, Couper G S, Cohn L H. Minimally invasive aortic valve replacement in octogenarian, high-risk, transcatheter aortic valve

implantation candidates. *J Thorac Cardiovasc Surg.* 2010; **141**:328–35.

64. Leon M B, Piazza N, Nikolsky E, *et al.* Standardized endpoint definitions for transcatheter aortic valve implantation clinical trials. A consensus report from the valve academic research consortium. *J Am Coll Cardiol.* 2011; **57**:253–69.

65. Daneault B, Kirtane A J, Kodali S K, *et al.* Stroke associated with surgical and transcatheter treatment of aortic stenosis. *J Am Coll Cardiol.* 2011; **58**:2143–50.

66. Drews T, Pasic M, Bus S, *et al.* Transcranial Doppler sound detection of cerebral microembolism during transapical aortic valve implantation. *Thorac Cardiovasc Surg.* 2011; **59**:237–42.

67. van der Linden J, Casimir-Ahn H. When do cerebral emboli appear during open heart operation? A Transcranial Doppler study. *Ann Thorac Surg.* 1991; **51**:237–41.

68. Guerrieri Wolf L, Choudhary B P, Abu-Omar Y, Taggert D P. Solid and gaseous cerebral microembolization after biologic and mechanical aortic valve replacement: investigation with multirange and multifrequency transcranial Doppler ultrasound. *J Thorac Cardiovasc Surg.* 2008; **135**:512–20.

69. Filsoufi F, Rahmanian P B, Castillo J G, Bronster D, Adams D H. Incidence, imaging analysis, and early and late outcomes of stroke after cardiac valve operation. *Am J Cardiol.* 2008; **101**:1472–8.

70. Sharony R, Grossi E A, Saunders P C, *et al.* Aortic valve replacement in patients with impaired ventricular function. *Ann Thorac Surg.* 2003; **75**:1808–14.

71. Ruel M, Masters R G, Rubens F D, *et al.* Late incidence and determinants of stroke after aortic and mitral valve replacement. *Ann Thorac Surg.* 2004; **78**:77–84.

72. Sundt T M, Bailey M S, Moon M R, *et al.* Quality of life after aortic valve replacement at the age of >80 years. *Circulation.* 2000; **102**:III70–4.

73. Alexander K P, Anstrom K J, Muhlbaier L H, *et al.* Outcomes of cardiac surgery in patients > or = 80 years: Results from the National Cardiovascular Network. *J Am Coll Cardiol.* 2000; **35**:731–8.

74. Naylor A R, Mehta Z, Rothwell P M, Bell P R. Carotid artery disease and stroke during coronary artery bypass: a critical review of the literature. *Eur J Vasc Endovasc Surg.* 2002; **23**:283–94.

75. Li Y, Walicki D, Mathiesen C, Jenny D, *et al.* Strokes after cardiac surgery and relationship to carotid stenosis. *Arch Neurol.* 2009; **66**:1091–6.

76. Naylor A R. Does the risk of post-CABG stroke merit staged or synchronous reconstruction in patients with symptomatic or asymptomatic carotid disease? *J Cardiovasc Surg.* 2009; **50**:71–81.

77. Timaran C H, Rosero E B, Smith S T, *et al.* Trends and outcomes of concurrent carotid revascularization and coronary bypass. *J Vasc Surg.* 2008; **48**:355–61.

78. Knipp S C, Scherag A, Beyersdorf F, *et al.* for the CABACS study group. Randomized comparison of synchronous CABG and carotid endarterectomy vs. isolated CABG in patients with asymptomatic carotid stenosis: The CABACS trial. *Int J Stroke.* 2012; **7**:354–60.

Stroke after carotid revascularization procedure

Andrei V. Alexandrov, Kristian Barlinn and Robert Mikulik

Introduction

Carotid revascularization procedures include carotid endarterectomy and stenting for atheromatous disease, and thrombectomy for acute thromboembolic lesions. This chapter will describe stroke types that can occur during and shortly after these procedures. Although the clinical discovery of a new neurological deficit could be delayed by anesthesia, diagnostic tools are available for clinicians to detect neuronal dysfunction early with electroencephalography (EEG), cerebral perfusion changes in real time with transcranial Doppler (TCD), and to ascertain tissue damage and cerebral blood flow changes with multimodal magnetic resonance imaging (MRI) and advance computed tomography (CT) tests. Even though these adverse events are rare in the hands of experienced operators, perioperative stroke rates are far from zero and even the most advanced surgeons and interventionalists should utilize monitoring and clinicians should know how to suspect a potential perioperative stroke and rapidly determine its mechanism. This in turn provides critical information to make quick management decisions and avert many of these strokes.

Carotid endarterectomy

Carotid endarterectomy (CEA) was introduced by Eastcott [1] and its efficacy and durability were established in two large randomized trials for symptomatic patients with carotid stenosis [2,3]. The number needed to treat to prevent one stroke is 8:1 for symptomatic patients with ≥70% carotid stenosis, and 15:1 for those with 50 to 69% stenosis [4]. In asymptomatic patients, the overall risk of stroke is 2% per year, and CEA offers a small protection by reducing it to 1% per year if the complication rate from angiography and surgery is kept at or below 2% [5]. Perioperative complications from

CEA in symptomatic patients amount to 6.5% in the NASCET trial [6] and are even higher in general practice [7].

In general, there are four mechanisms that can lead to perioperative stroke [8,9]:

1. Embolism
2. Thrombosis
3. Hypoperfusion
4. Hyperperfusion.

Non-invasive monitoring of CEA can identify patients developing ischemia during surgery. Intraoperative cerebral blood flow measurements [10,11] are of historic interest since these helped us to understand critical levels of cerebral blood flow in the development and tolerance of cerebral ischemia. More widely used methods include EEG [11–16], evoked potentials [17–18], cerebral oximetry [19,20], and direct stump pressure measurements [21,22]. Electrodiagnostic tools are very sensitive to the neuronal malfunction but non-specific to the mechanism of damage. Direct stump pressure measurements are helpful in assessment of competency of the circle of Willis but are limited as to when these can be performed. Finally, if CEA is performed under local anesthesia, the patient can also be assessed with repeat clinical examinations [23]. The above-mentioned tests help suspect perioperative stroke but provide limited clues to the mechanism of cerebral ischemia.

Real-time ultrasound monitoring [8,24–28] can be used for the purpose of detection of thromboembolism and perfusion changes that can lead to cerebral ischemia as well as to identify the pathogenic mechanism of this potentially hazardous event. This information is complementary to other monitoring modalities. Ultrasound has sensitivity equal to EEG in predicting

Treatment-Related Stroke, ed. Alexander Tsiskaridze, Arne Lindgren and Adnan Qureshi. Published by Cambridge University Press. © Cambridge University Press 2016.

Table 10.1 Common mechanisms and findings on imaging modalities in patients with perioperative strokes with carotid revascularization.

Event	Ultrasound	CT or MRI
Embolism	TCD: unilateral or bilateral microembolic signals (transient increases in intensity on spectral Doppler or motion-mode); appearance of an abnormal waveform in the middle cerebral artery (MCA) indicating acute occlusion.	Wedge-shaped cortical stroke or a large subcortical lesion or scattered small cortical or subcortical strokes.
Thrombosis	Carotid duplex: direct evidence of a thrombus at the surgical site on brightness mode (B-mode), OR TCD: evidence for a proximal hemodynamically significant obstruction or artery-to-artery embolism.	Wedge-shaped cortical stroke or a large subcortical lesion or scattered small cortical or subcortical strokes, OR Strokes located in border-zone territories, i.e., between the MCA and anterior (ACA) or posterior (PCA) cerebral arteries.
Hypoperfusion	TCD: evidence of unilateral or bilateral reduction in the mean flow velocities to less than 50% of preclamp or prior to the observed reduction values.	Strokes located in border-zone territories, i.e., between the MCA and anterior (ACA) or posterior (PCA) cerebral arteries.
Hyperperfusion	TCD: evidence of a unilateral increase of the MCA mean flow velocities to 1.5 times preclamp value or by ≥50% compared to the contralateral side and pulsatility index reduction by 30% or more compared to the contralateral side.	No new changes or the presence of gyral enhancement with blood or blood products or hemorrhagic transformation on the side unilateral to revascularization.

cerebral ischemia and can be superior to EEG, particularly in cases under general anesthesia [29].

Although multicenter randomized trials of monitoring techniques targeted to reduce perioperative stroke or TIA are lacking, several prospective studies showed very low complication rates with monitoring compared to historic controls [30–33], and a single-center randomized trial investigated reduction of microemboli after CEA as a surrogate marker for the risk of perioperative stroke [34,35].

The following criteria can be helpful in prompt detection of perioperative strokes with ultrasound (Table 10.1). Table 10.1 also lists subsequent findings on CT and MRI (Figure 10.1) confirming clinical and ultrasound suspicions. Of note, patients developing embolic, thrombotic, and hemodynamic strokes may present with similar focal neurological deficits that could be blood pressure (BP) and head of bed (HOB) elevation sensitive, i.e., one can observe transient improvement with manipulations of BP and HOB. The last one (hyperperfusion) may lead to a specific syndrome that manifests in headache and possible seizure and can occur at blood pressures just exceeding 140/80 mm Hg.

Carotid artery stenting

Carotid artery stenting (CAS) has become an alternative to CEA in selected patients. Strokes related to CAS usually occur in between 2 to 10% of cases [9,36]. In addition to symptomatic thromboembolic events, brain embolism can be detected by TCD in almost every case even if flow-diversion techniques are deployed to protect the brain. The finding of microembolic signals on TCD is linked to the introduction of air-containing dye during diagnostic runs and inability of the distal protection devices to capture all small particulate and gaseous emboli. Even though largely regarded as clinically silent events, these microembolic signals may reflect a greater likelihood of cerebral embolization that can produce subtle or subclinical changes. Recently, a prospective study of neurocognitive functions after CEA and CAS was performed in patients who have MRI evidence of periprocedural embolic events [37]. Though preliminary, this study underscores the importance of optimization of carotid revascularization procedures not only to reduce the risk of frank thromboembolic events but

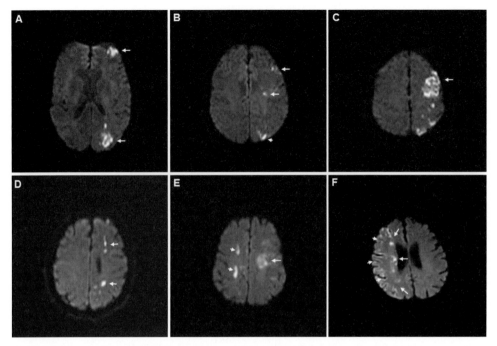

Figure 10.1 Axial diffusion-weighted magnetic resonance imaging showing typical cerebral infarct patterns in patients with high-grade internal carotid artery (ICA) stenosis. (A) Cortical watershed or external borderzone infarcts between the left middle (MCA) and anterior and the left MCA and posterior cerebral artery territories (arrows). (B) Scattered embolic infarcts in the left MCA territory (arrows) and hemodynamic infarct in left posterior borderzone (arrow head). (C) Embolic infarct in the left middle cerebral artery territory (arrow). (D) Hemodynamic infarcts in the left internal border zone (arrows). (E) Embolic infarcts in the left MCA territory (arrow) and hemodynamic infarcts in the right internal border zone (arrow heads) in a patient with bilateral high-grade ICA stenosis. (F) Multiple hemodynamic (internal and external border zone, arrows) and cortical embolic infarcts (arrow heads) in the right MCA territory in a patient who underwent carotid artery stenting for a high-grade ICA stenosis.

also microscopic embolization with air or particulate materials that could not be captured effectively with current distal protection devices.

Hypoperfusion and especially thromboembolism are the major complications of CAS and TCD detects numerous microembolic signals, most being associated with wire manipulations particularly along the aortic arch and during dye injections [38]. However, it is unclear how these signals (likely most being air microbubbles) affect the intracranial circulation and if they contribute to cerebral ischemia or cognitive dysfunction. Hypoperfusion is commonly seen during CAS with lesion crossing with a wire and balloon expansions/occlusions [38]. Transcranial Doppler demonstrates a significant velocity drop and flattening of the waveform that in turn may worsen the washout of embolic material from the border zone and small vessels in the brain. The most promising technique to reduce embolism to the brain during CAS is to reverse the carotid artery flow, which results in far fewer microembolic signals detected by TCD [39]. Depending on the exact flow-reversal technique,

flow reversal is commonly seen in the ACA and terminal ICA on periprocedural TCD monitoring [39]. A recent analysis of microembolic counts by TCD showed that flow-reversal techniques are associated with fewer emboli than CAS but still higher counts than during CEA [40].

Although TCD is able to detect hyperperfusion syndrome that can complicate both CEA and CAS, the criteria and most experiences were described for CEA, much fewer for CAS [41]. A recent review advocates for more studies of TCD applications to monitor the occurrence of cerebral hyperperfusion syndrome that can occur in up to 3% of CAS as well as CEA cases [40]. Although the criteria listed in Table 10.1 indicate mean flow velocity increase up to 1.5 times preclamp value (i.e., 50% increase), some use 100% increase in velocity values (or double the velocity) [41]. The lower velocity increase cut-off is more sensitive and probably should be deployed during or shortly after revascularization procedures when this syndrome is just developing (Figure 10.2). The persistence of velocity elevation over time serves as an additional

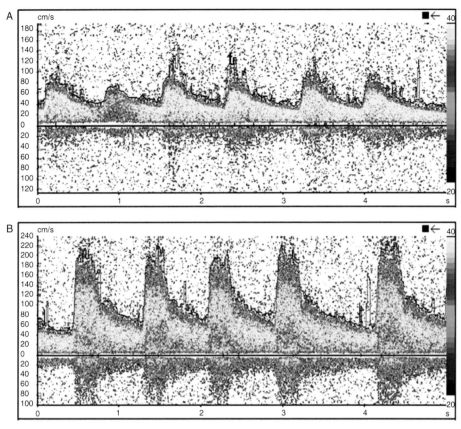

Figure 10.2 Transcranial Doppler shows right (A) and left (B) proximal middle cerebral artery waveforms in a patient who underwent carotid artery angioplasty and stenting for left high-grade internal carotid artery stenosis. (A) Normal MCA mean flow velocity (45 cm/s) at 62 mm depth in the RMCA. (B) An increased mean flow velocity of 80 cm/s at 63 mm depth suggestive of early post-revascularization hyperemia in the left MCA.

criterion. A more robust and specific 100% velocity increase will more likely correlate with hyperperfusion at delayed assessments. Regardless, both criteria require a comparison vessel and ideally should be compared with baseline velocities measured for the same vessel at a steady angle of insonation. In the absence of such baseline data, comparison to the contralateral vessel should be made.

Head CT or MRI can further show signs of hyperperfusion such as excessive presence of blood in the cortical areas on the side of revascularization. This extravasation of blood or the increase of blood pool in the cortical vessels is due to maximal vasodilation and inability of autoregulation to control the incoming blood flow volume. Prompt blood pressure lowering to normotension is paramount to avoid frank hemorrhagic transformation (Figure 10.3) when hyperperfusion syndrome evolves from headache and seizures to focal neurological deficits.

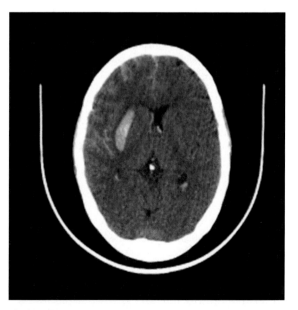

Figure 10.3 A non-contrast CT scan showing hemorrhagic transformation with subarachnoid and intraparenchymal hemorrhage.

109

References

1. Eastcott H H G, Pickering G W, Rob C G. Reconstruction of internal carotid artery in a patient with intermittent attacks of hemiplegia. *Lancet.* 1954; **ii**:954.

2. North American Symptomatic Carotid Endarterectomy Trial Collaborators. Beneficial effect of carotid endarterectomy in symptomatic patients with high-grade carotid stenosis. *N Engl J Med.* 1991; **325**:445–53.

3. European Carotid Surgery Trialists' Collaborative Group. Randomised trial of endarterectomy for recently symptomatic carotid stenosis: final results of the MRC European Carotid Surgery Trial (ECST). *Lancet.* 1998; **351**:1379–87.

4. Barnett H J, Taylor D W, Eliasziw M, *et al.* Benefit of carotid endarterectomy in patients with symptomatic moderate or severe stenosis. North American Symptomatic Carotid Endarterectomy Trial Collaborators. *N Engl J Med.* 1998; **339**:1415–25.

5. Executive Committee of the Asymptomatic Carotid Atherosclerosis Study. Endarterectomy for asymptomatic carotid artery stenosis. *JAMA.* 1995; **273**:1421–8.

6. Ferguson G G, Eliasziw M, Barr H W, *et al.* The North American Symptomatic Carotid Endarterectomy Trial: surgical results in 1415 patients. *Stroke.* 1999; **30**:1751–8.

7. Chaturvedi S, Aggarwal R, Murugappan A. Results of carotid endarterectomy with prospective neurologist follow-up. *Neurology.* 2000; **26**:55:769–72.

8. Spencer M P. Transcranial Doppler monitoring and causes of stroke from carotid endarterectomy. *Stroke.* 1997; **28**:685–91.

9. Huibers A, Calvet D, Kennedy F, *et al.* Mechanism of procedural stroke following carotid endarterectomy or carotid artery stenting within the International Carotid Stenting Study (ICSS) randomised trial. *Eur J Vasc Endovasc Surg.* 2015; doi:10.1016/j.ejvs.2015.05.017. [Epub ahead of print].

10. Sundt T M. The ischemic tolerance of neural tissue and the need for monitoring and selective shunting during carotid endarterectomy. *Stroke.* 1983; **14**:93–8.

11. Sharbrough F M, Messik J M, Sundt T M. Correlation of continuous electroencephalograms with cerebral blood flow measurements during carotid endarterectomy. *Stroke.* 1973; **4**:674–83.

12. Blackshear W M, Di Carlo V, Seifert K B, Connar R G. Advantages of continuous electroencephalographic monitoring during carotid surgery. *J Cardiovasc Surg.* 1986; **27**:146–53.

13. Cho I, Smullens S N, Streletz L J, Fariello R G. The value of intraoperative EEG monitoring during carotid endarterectomy. *Ann Neurol.* 1986; **20**:508–12.

14. Blume W T, Ferguson G G, McNeil D K. Significance of EEG changes at carotid endarterectomy. *Stroke.* 1986; **17**:891–97.

15. McCarthy W J, Park A E, Koushanpour E, *et al.* Carotid endarterectomy. Lessons from intraoprative monitoring – a decade of experience. *Ann Surg.* 1996; **224**:291–307.

16. Balotta E, Daigau G, Saladini M, *et al.* Results of electroencephalographic monitoring during 369 consecutive carotid artery revascularizations. *Eur Neurol.* 1997; **37**:43–7.

17. Kearse L A, Brown E N, McPeck K. Somatosensory evoked potential sensitivity relative to electroencephalography for cerebral ischemia during carotid endarterectomy. *Stroke.* 1992; **23**:498–505.

18. Haupt W F, Horsch S. Evoked potential monitoring in carotid surgery: A review of 994 cases. *Neurology.* 1992; **42**:835–8.

19. Duncan L A, Ruckley C V, Wildsmith J A W. Cerebral oximetry: a useful monitor during carotid artery surgery. *Anesthesiology.* 1995; **50**:1041–5.

20. Samra S K, Dorje P, Zelenock G B, Stanley J C. Cerebral oximetry in patients undergoing carotid endarterectomy under regional anesthesia. *Stroke.* 1996; **27**:49–55.

21. Cherry K J, Roland C F, Hallett J W, *et al.* Stump pressure, the contralateral carotid artery, and electroencephalographic changes. *Am J Surg.* 1991; **162**:185–9.

22. Harada R N, Comerota A J, Good G M, *et al.* Stump pressure, electroencephalographic changes, and the contralateral carotid artery: another look at selective shunting. *Am J Surg.* 1995; **170**:148–53.

23. Benjamin M E, Silva M B, Watt C, *et al.* Awake patient monitoring to determine the need for shunting during carotid endarterectomy. *Surgery.* 1993; **114**:673–81.

24. Padayachee T S, Bishop C C R, Gosling R G, *et al.* Monitoring middle cerebral artery blood flow velocity during carotid endarterectomy. *Br J Surg.* 1986; **73**:98–100.

25. Steiger H J, Schaffler L, Boll J, Liechti S. Results of microsurgical carotid endarterectomy: a prospective study with transcranial Doppler and EEG monitoring, and selective shunting. *Acta Neurochir.* 1989; **100**:31–8.

26. Spencer M P, Thomas G I, Nicholls S C, Sauvage L R. Detection of middle cerebral artery emboli during carotid endarterectomy using transcranial Doppler ultrasonography. *Stroke.* 1990; **21**:415–23.

27. Ackerstaff R G A, Janes C, Moll F L, *et al.* The significance of emboli detection by means of transcranial Doppler ultrasonography monitoring in carotid endarterectomy. *J Vasc Surg.* 1995; **21**:415–23.

28. Canthelmo N L, Babikian V L, Samaraweera R N, *et al.* Cerebral microembolism and ischemic changes associated with carotid endarterectomy. *J Vasc Surg.* 1998; **27**:1024–31.

29. Arnold M, Sturzenegger M, Schaffler L, Seiler R. Continuous intraoperative monitoring of middle cerebral artery flow velocities and electroencephalography during carotid endarterectomy. *Stroke.* 1997; **28**:1345–50.

30. Spencer M P. Transcranial Doppler monitoring and causes of stroke from carotid endarterectomy. *Stroke.* 1997; **28**:685–91.

31. Jansen C, Ramos L M, van Heesewijk J P, *et al.* Impact of microembolism and hemodynamic changes in the brain during carotid endarterectomy. *Stroke.* 1994; **25**: 992–7.

32. Ackerstaff R G, Moons K G, van de Vlasakker C J, *et al.* Association of intraoperative transcranial Doppler monitoring variables with stroke from carotid endarterectomy. *Stroke.* 2000; **31**:1817–23.

33. Babikian V L, Canthelmo N L. Cerebrovascular monitoring during carotid endarterectomy. *Stroke.* 2000; **31**:1799–801.

34. Levy C R, O'Malley H M, Fell G, *et al.* Transcranial Doppler detected cerebral microembolism following carotid endarterectomy. High intensity signal loads predict postoperative cerebral ischemia. *Brain.* 1997; **120**:621–9.

35. Kaposzta Z, Baskerville P A, Madge D, *et al.* L-arginine and S-nitrosoglutathione reduce embolization in humans. *Circulation.* 2001; **103**:2371–5.

36. Chen C I, Iguchi Y, Garami Z, *et al.* Analysis of emboli during carotid stenting with distal protection device. *Cerebrovasc Dis.* 2006; **21**(4):223–8.

37. Zhou W, Hitchner E, Gillis K, *et al.* Prospective neurocognitive evaluation of patients undergoing carotid interventions. *J Vasc Surg.* 2012; **56**:1571–8.

38. Garami Z, Lumsden A B. Intra-operative and peri-procedural TCD monitoring. In Alexandrov A V (ed). *Cerebrovascular Ultrasound in Stroke Prevention and Treatment* (2nd edn). Oxford: Wiley-Blackwell Publishers. 2011.

39. Garami Z, Charlton-Ouw K M, Broadbent K C, Lumsden A B. A practical guide to transcranial Doppler monitoring during carotid interventions. Part 1: basics and blood flow changes. *Vascular Ultrasound Today.* 2008; **13**(1).

40. Gupta N, Corriere M A, Dodson T F, *et al.* Incidence of microemboli to the brain is less with endarterectomy than with percutaneous revascularization with distal filters or flow reversal. *J Vasc Surg.* 2011; **53**:316–22.

41. Pennekamp C W, Moll F L, De Borst G J. Role of transcranial Doppler in cerebral hyperperfusion syndrome. *J Cardiovasc Surg.* 2012; **53**:765–71.

Radiation therapy and stroke

Jelle Demeestere and Vincent Thijs

Introduction

Radiation therapy is commonly used for treatment of malignancies occurring in the brain or in the head and neck region. As more and more patients survive their malignancy, late effects of radiation therapy are increasingly encountered. Stroke is one of the most devastating long-term complications that can occur in patients who have been otherwise successfully treated for their malignancy. Traditionally, the side effects of radiation therapy are classified into those occurring in the acute phase, the early delayed (within six months) phase, and the late delayed phase occurring after six months. It is in the latter phase that two complications arise, which are of most importance to the stroke neurologist: white matter changes; and stroke occurring as a result of indirect damage to the intracerebral vasculature or the precerebral vessels. Changes induced by radiation include moyamoya-like patterns, cavernous angiomas, aneurysms, progressive stenosis, and occlusion of small, medium, and large precerebral and intracranial arteries. There is typically a long latency between radiotherapy (RT) and the development of these complications. A new entity, stroke-like migraine attacks after radiation therapy (SMART) syndrome, has received increased attention recently. Determining a causal relationship between radiation therapy and stroke is difficult, because this therapy is often given to patients at high risk of vascular complications; other oncological treatments and the presence of a malignancy itself may also increase the stroke risk. Moreover, there is a dearth of prospective, controlled studies with long-term follow up in cancer survivors to estimate the magnitude of this problem and factors that influence the occurrence of stroke.

Epidemiology

Radiation therapy is a common and effective treatment for cancer. In the United States it is estimated that about one million people undergo radiation therapy annually. About 60% of patients with cancer will receive radiation from high-energy sources at some stage during their disease course. There is a tendency for an increase in the indications for radiation [1].

Radiation is used to treat common cancers such as breast cancer, nasopharyngeal carcinoma, larynx carcinoma, or hematological malignancies. Prophylactic whole-brain radiation therapy is used in many patients with small cell lung cancer [2]. Malignant brain tumor patients often undergo radiotherapy both in childhood and adulthood.

There are few epidemiological data estimating the global risk of stroke in patients who undergo radiation therapy per se due to the heterogeneity of cancers, use of concomitant therapies, and the relative scarcity of events [3]. High-quality estimates of the frequency of stroke occurring in patients surviving tumors are lacking.

One controlled study found a 29-fold increase in the risk of self-reported stroke in patients who underwent brain irradiation [4]. A recent long-term follow-up study compared the incidence of neurovascular events in patients receiving irradiation because of brain tumors in childhood with patients who did not undergo brain irradiation or where no direct irradiation of the circle of Willis had occurred [5]. Again, a remarkable increase in risk of stroke and TIA was observed after a median of 4.9 years. The highest risk occurred in patients who underwent direct radiation to the circle of Willis, with a risk in absolute numbers of 6 per 1,000 patient years. Of note, patients who had concomitant chemotherapy seemed to be at a particularly high risk.

Table 11.1 Causes of stroke in cancer patients [6].

Tumor related

Intravascular lymphoma

Direct invasion of blood vessels by tumor

Hematological malignancies with hyperviscosity

Embolism or aneurysm from atrial myxoma

Therapy related

Radiation therapy

L-asparaginase

Cisplatinum

Intrathecal methotrexate

Hormonal therapy

Surgery

Immune-suppression related

Opportunistic vasculotropic fungal infection
(Aspergillus)

Coagulation related

Non-bacterial thrombotic endocarditis

Diffuse intravascular coagulation

Thrombotic microangiopathy

Traditional causes

Heart disease including atrial fibrillation

Large vessel disease due to atherosclerosis

Small vessel disease including lacunar stroke related to
hypertension

Other traditional causes

Before radiation therapy is considered to be related to stroke, other reasons for stroke in cancer patients have to be taken into account (see Table 11.1) [6]. Several types of vascular abnormalities can develop after radiotherapy. It has to be kept in mind that traditional causes can also be the reason for stroke in patients treated with radiotherapy and that it is possible that irradiation may accelerate the process of e.g., arterial atherosclerotic changes.

Cavernomas

Cavernous angiomas, also called cavernous malformations (CMs) – consisting of small berry-like lesions with disorganized and enlarged capillaries – are common cerebral vascular malformations found in 0.5% of patients undergoing MRI scans or autopsy. They typically have a popcorn aspect on T2/FLAIR imaging. Cavernous malformations are easily visualized on GRE or SWI sequences but are not identifiable with MRA or intra-arterial digital subtraction angiography (IADSA). However, they may be associated with a venous malformation that can be found on vascular imaging or as a flow void on standard MRI. They are typically found in the CNS but may also occur in the spinal cord. Cavernous malformations are typically sporadic occurring lesions; however, genetic autosomal-dominant forms have been found [7]. Lesions are dynamic with new lesions arising during lifetime in genetic forms. A genetic form should be suspected when multiple lesions are seen on imaging, although this can also be found in patients who underwent radiation therapy. Mutations in *CCM2, KRIT1,* and *PDCD10* have been identified [8–10].

Cavernous malformations may be entirely asymptomatic, but often present as seizures, focal neurologic deficits, or as a brain hemorrhage. Cavernous malformations in the brain and spinal cord can be found in patients treated with RT. Lesions are mostly found in patients that underwent RT as children, or in adults that received very high RT doses. The delay between RT and detection of the CM is quite variable. It is unclear whether early development is related to a higher RT dosage.

In one review of patients who underwent RT more than half of the lesions were incidental findings [11]. In another series of 59 patients with medulloblastoma who underwent craniospinal irradiation, CMs developed in 18 (31%) over a mean follow up of 7.2 years. Here almost all of the lesions were clinically silent [12].

It is unclear why CM lesions occur after radiation. Vessel wall necrosis and changes to the vessel wall induced by radiation may predispose to CM formation. Others have suggested that radiation uncovers radiographically occult lesions.

The management of CMs is not based on randomized clinical trials. The bleeding risk is considered to be quite low, but this depends on how the lesions are uncovered, for example, if incidental or if patients present with seizures, the risk of bleeding is considered to be low. In a recent population-based study the five-year risk of hemorrhage was about 2.5% [13]. On the contrary, patients who had a history of intracerebral hemorrhage (ICH) or presented with ICH had a risk of up to 29.5%. Patients with brainstem cavernomas and female patients seem to be at higher risk of brain hemorrhage [13].

Treatment of cavernous malformations

If patients present with seizures, antiepileptic medication may be quite effective. Surgery may be considered if lesions are accessible [14]. The high risk of recurrent bleeding may favor an initial surgical approach in patients who present with ICH. Paradoxically, CMs can sometimes be treated with stereotactic radiosurgery, although this treatment approach is controversial and severe complications can occur [15]. However, it is important to note that these prognostic data and treatment approaches have not been evaluated in patients with a history of RT. No firm recommendations can therefore be made and case-by-case decisions have to be made.

When confronted with a brain hemorrhage or epilepsy in a patient who underwent RT, the neurologist should consider the presence of a CM. For the neuro-oncologist or radiotherapy specialist, the identification of CMs and consultation with a vascular neurologist would be advised regarding the right course of action. As incidental CMs are now more frequently uncovered with advanced brain imaging, the question arises whether these patients can safely receive antithrombotic agents in case of coronary artery disease, TIA, or atrial fibrillation. Pilot data suggest this may be the case, although larger studies are obviously warranted [16].

Stenosis of the extracranial carotid arteries or vertebral arteries

Stenosis of the large precerebral vessels is a frequent condition in the general population. In a meta-analysis of four population-based studies, the prevalence of severe carotid stenosis was 3.1% in male octogenarians and about 1% in female octogenarians [17]. The prevalence of VA stenosis in the general population is not known, but ultrasound studies found a prevalence of 7.5% of ostial stenosis in patients with established vascular disease [18,19]. In clinical situations, VA stenosis is less commonly assessed because the most frequently used non-invasive technique, duplex ultrasound, is more reliable for carotid stenosis and only a portion of the VA can be probed. Also, the benefit of surgical or interventional treatment has mostly been evaluated in

trials that focused on internal carotid artery stenosis. Stenosis or occlusion of the internal carotid arteries and vertebral arteries can be incidental or found in TIA or stroke in patients undergoing neck or vessel imaging. Most stenoses are due to carotid atherosclerosis, with other vasculopathies of the arteries such as fibromuscular dysplasia or dissection, being much less common. These rarer vasculopathies tend to present with particular imaging patterns, whereas internal carotid artery atherosclerosis is usually confined to the bifurcation. Extracranial atherosclerosis affecting the vertebral artery is mostly found at the ostium of the VA. Intracranial atherosclerosis is much less common in Caucasians, but is thought to be quite common in Asians, who may have lesions in the middle cerebral artery, or in the distal vertebral arteries [20]. Stenosis or occlusion of intracranial vessels may also be due to embolism from a proximal source, such as an embolus resulting from atrial fibrillation and originating in the left atrial appendix. This makes a definite diagnosis of intracranial stenosis sometimes difficult. In practice, the absence of a proximal source together with worsening or persistent stenosis with serial imaging argues strongly for intracranial artery atherosclerosis, rather than embolic remnants producing a pseudo-stenotic aspect.

Patients who underwent RT for head and neck cancer are at risk for development of large-vessel stenosis and for resulting embolic stroke or TIA [21,22]. Table 11.2 provides an overview of the larger studies reported to date. Mantle irradiation and irradiation of the neck for squamous cell carcinoma, parotid tumors, lymphomas, and Hodgkin's disease result in an increased risk for stroke. There are several limitations to these studies, but despite these limitations the conclusions remain quite similar. There may be a delay of up to 20 years between RT and development of the stenosis. The delay is often shorter when RT was done at a younger age, presumably because of the smaller diameter of the artery at that age. There is apparently no increase in risk with breast cancer irradiation where the carotid artery is only minimally exposed, although some studies find a slightly higher risk, which cannot be clearly attributed to radiation per se [23–26].

Imaging studies with ultrasound show increased risk of stenosis in mostly cross-sectional studies of patients undergoing head and neck cancer therapy. A recent study compared angiographic patterns of

Table 11.2 Epidemiological studies assessing risk of extracranial carotid stenosis in cancer survivors who underwent RT.

Type of treatment (sample size)	Risk	Control group	Type of disease	Delay	Comment	Reference
Head and neck RT (n = 6,862)	RR 1.5 (95% CI 1.7–4.4)	Indirect comparison to population-based incidence rates	Squamous cell carcinoma	9 years	No distinction between ischemic or hemorrhagic stroke	[79]
Head and neck RT (n = 413)	RR 2.09 (95% CI 1.28–3.22)	Indirect comparison to population-based incidence rates	Squamous cell carcinoma	4.6 years	No dose effect	[80]
Head and neck RT (n = 367)	RR 5.6 (95% CI 3.1–9.4)	Indirect comparison to population-based incidence rates	Various	10.9 years	Only patients under 60 years	[81]
Head and neck RT (n = 910)	Increased but not significantly	Age, sex-matched controls	Various	9 years		[82]
Neck irradiation (n = 2,201)	RR 2.5 (95% CI 1.1–5.6)	General population	Hodgkin lymphoma survivors	17 years	Radiation dose lacking Self-reported stroke	[83]
Neck irradiation (n = 1,926)	5.6 RR (95% CI 2.6–12)	Siblings	Hodgkin lymphoma	17.5 years	Self-reported stroke	[4]
Neck irradiation (n = 476)	2.3 RR (if more than 40 Gray)	Matched control population and no RT	Non-Hodgkin lymphoma	3.7 years	No stroke subclassification	[84]

RT: radiotherapy; RR: relative risk.

TIA or stroke patients who had undergone RT with a control group of TIA or stroke patients with atherosclerotic disease [27]. Radiotherapy-associated lesions were more diffusely distributed over the common and internal carotid arteries, more frequently bilateral or tandem, and more often also associated with external carotid artery and vertebral artery involvement. Plaque ulcers and dissections were more frequently found. Collateral development was more extensive. In this population of patients, irradiated for head and neck cancer, no aneurysm or moyamoya syndrome patterns were found.

There is discussion whether RT induces acceleration of atherosclerosis or induces a separate fibrotic vasculopathy due to damage to the vasa vasorum. In histopathological examinations of human specimens, adventitial fibrosis, scarring, and atherosclerosis is found [28,29].

One should keep in mind that many patients with head and neck cancer have risk factors for atherosclerosis, as smoking is both a risk factor for many of these cancers and for atherosclerosis development. However, it is quite clear that in patients who underwent RT, stenoses are often located within the radiation field outside the bifurcation. This is a strong argument indicating that RT is linked to medium- to large-vessel stenosis.

Surgeons often prefer to treat carotid artery stenosis induced by radiotherapy with stenting rather than with carotid endarterectomy. Skin and vessel fibrosis is often a feature of these lesions, which makes endarterectomy more difficult to perform. Also, the atypical locations of the stenosis favor stenting. Moreover, wound healing may be impeded in areas that were previously irradiated. However, reports suggest a high restenosis rate in patients who underwent stenting for radiation-induced arteriopathy [30]. The evidence base regarding treatment of irradiated carotid arteries is based on mostly small case series, in highly selected centers [31,30].

There are no randomized trials to guide treatment decisions in this population. Often a similar stance is adopted as in atherosclerotic disease, with surgical intervention or stenting being recommended in symptomatic high-grade internal carotid artery stenosis and aggressive medical management with antiplatelet therapy, antihypertensive medication, and statins, along with smoking cessation and exercise recommended for all patients – symptomatic or asymptomatic.

An extraordinary complication, rupture of the carotid artery, often in combination with skin necrosis and wound infection, has been reported in the first few weeks after RT at very high doses, especially in the context of re-irradiation after head and neck cancer [32]. Blowout of the carotid artery occurs more frequently in previously irradiated arteries and anecdotal evidence suggests this often-fatal complication can be treated with endovascular therapy [33].

Large- and medium-vessel intracranial disease

Intracranial occlusive disease affecting the intracranial carotid artery and medium-sized vessels such as the middle cerebral artery or basilar artery can result from RT. That RT of the brain at childhood increases the risk of stroke is well established. Incidences of non-perioperative stroke of 4 per 1,000 years have been described. In one cohort 5% of all patients developed stroke attributable to stenosis of irradiated cerebral vessels [34,35].

A direct link between RT and stroke remains controversial when RT is not used for the treatment of brain cancer. For instance, whether radiation for pituitary adenoma is a risk factor for stroke is not as clearly established and studies have contradicted each other [36–39]. The lack of a direct link of RT and intracranial vessel stenosis, except for small case series and case reports, may be due to the relative lack of well-designed studies with appropriate imaging techniques of the intracranial vasculature.

Small-vessel disease, white matter tissue changes, and microbleeds

Small infarcts located within the deep, non-cortical areas of the brain, including the basal ganglia, thalamus, and brain stem, occur as a result of occlusion of small penetrating brain arteries [32]. The pathology is diverse

and includes lipohyalinosis and microatheromatosis [40]. In animal models, microemboli can also theoretically occlude these small arteries, but this is considered a more infrequent event in humans [41–43]. These small infarcts can remain entirely silent but also manifest as minor and occasionally as major strokes or as progressive cognitive changes or as a gait disturbance [44]. From an imaging standpoint, acute lacunar infarcts are diagnosed as small hyperintense lesions on diffusion-weighted imaging (DWI) and subacute or chronic lacunes as T2/FLAIR hyperintense lesions or a small hypodensity on CT [45]. They should be differentiated from enlarged perivascular spaces (Virchow–Robin spaces), which often occur in specific locations, are well circumscribed, and can include a central punctiform hyperintensity, corresponding to a vessel that is cut transversally [46]. Often lacunar infarcts are found in conjunction with white matter hyperintensities on FLAIR imaging or leukoaraiosis on CT, and can also be seen in patients with evidence of prior intracerebral bleeding, so-called microbleeds on gradient echo or susceptibility weighted imaging.

White matter hyperintensities (WMH) on FLAIR or T2-based imaging reflect increased water content in the brain and signal a change in the permeability of the blood–brain barrier of small cerebral vessels. Pathologically, white matter rarefaction and axonal loss are found in regions of white matter hyperintensity [47].

White matter hyperintensities can evolve from initial punctiform changes to large confluent areas of hyperintensity. Risk factors include a genetic predisposition, hypertension, and diabetes. There seems to be a strong genetic background with a high concordance between monozygotic twins compared to dizygotic twins, and a strong heritability [48,49].

Patients with white matter changes on imaging are at risk for development of cognitive disorders and stroke, especially small lacunar infarcts [50]. There is a frequent co-occurrence of WMH with lacunar infarcts on imaging and clinical lacunar stroke.

White matter changes can also result from RT [51]. The distinction between sporadically occurring white matter changes and RT-induced leukoencephalopathy or radiation necrosis is not easy. Radiotherapy in itself may accelerate the development of white matter disease. Consequences may be devastating with development of recurrent strokes or dementia [52].

117

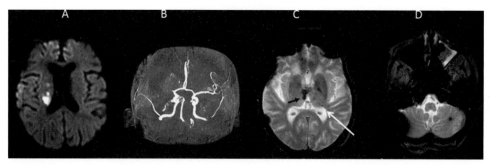

Figure 11.1 Magnetic resonance imaging scan of a female patient treated with radiotherapy for a right-sided thalamic astrocytoma grade II at age 15. She suffered an acute ischemic stroke 19 years later with left-sided weakness. (A) An acute ischemic lesion in the periventricular white matter was demonstrated on diffusion-weighted imaging. (B) Time-of-flight magnetic resonance angiography shows occlusion of the proximal middle cerebral artery. (C) Gradient echo imaging shows a right-sided thalamic hypointensity at the location of the primary tumor (black arrow). Note multiple hypointensities, corresponding to microbleeds or small cavernous angiomas in the thalamus bilaterally (white arrow). (D) Left ring-like cerebellar hypointensity corresponding to cavernous angioma on T2-weighted imaging.

Microbleeds are small deposits of blood products located within the cerebral arterioles and capillaries [53]. Typically, the iron deposits are found within macrophages, but their presence in pericytes has also been described. On a macroscopic level, if visible, they correspond to microhemorrhages or hemorrhagic lacunar holes [54–56]. Some of these microbleeds can be detected using T2*-weighted imaging or even better with susceptibility-weighted magnetic resonance imaging (MRI) [57].They appear as oval or round hypointensities with a size ranging up to 10 mm. The exact sensitivity and specificity with which microbleeds can be detected using MRI when compared to pathology is not exactly defined. Microbleeds on MRI are found in more than 50% of patients with ICH or vascular dementia, and to a lesser extent in patients with ischemic stroke. Population studies have found microbleeds in about 5% of the general population [58,59]. No studies have systematically evaluated the presence of microbleeds in RT patients. Anecdotal evidence suggests that there may be a relationship (Figure 11.1).

Secondary prevention after small-vessel stroke includes blood pressure control, smoking cessation, statin treatment, and antiplatelet therapy. Combination therapy of aspirin and clopidogrel is harmful for patients with SVD [60]. However, none of these preventive strategies have been specifically tested in patients who underwent RT.

Aneurysms

Cerebral aneurysms are most commonly found in or near vessels of the circle of Willis [61]. Rarely, aneurysms can form as a result of embolization from atrial myxoma. Other causes of more distally located aneurysms can be the result of mycotic aneurysms in the course of infectious endocarditis. Some aneurysms are found in conjunction with arteriovenous malformations. The clinical manifestations of aneurysms are diverse. They can remain asymptomatic, but also induce life-threatening subarachnoid bleedings [62]. Large aneurysms can compress cranial nerves or brain structures. Rarely, aneurysms can be a source of distal embolization and produce ischemic stroke. The frequency of aneurysms is relatively high in the general population [63]. Cerebral aneurysms are a complex disease where multiple factors interplay. These include genetic risk factors, familial predisposition, and environmental risk factors such as smoking [64]. The risk of bleeding is thought to be related to size, location, smoking, and the presence of familial disease [65]. A few case reports have described the development of cerebral aneurysms in the context of RT [66,67]. This is considered an exceptional development. However, these aneurysms had a very high rate of subsequent bleeding making this a condition that should be detected as soon as possible and preventive treatment should be strongly considered.

Moyamoya phenomenon development

The moyamoya phenomenon refers to the development of a progressive intracranial stenosis or occlusion of vessels within the circle of Willis with concomitant development of very fine collateral vessels within the lenticulostriate arteries, described on angiography as moyamoya-type vessels [68]. Other collaterals also develop over time to compensate for the reduction in blood flow. Moyamoya-type vessels can occur in the context of RT, neurofibromatosis type 1, polycystic kidney disease, or even atherosclerosis. Clinical manifestations include ischemic or hemorrhagic strokes, TIA, and recurrent movement disorder with dystonia and seizures. Some patients have few or no symptoms. Moyamoya disease is a distinct entity, which is more frequent in Asian populations, where the vasculopathy does not occur in relation to other diseases. Sometimes it is associated with stenosis of renal arteries and with cerebral aneurysms. Recently, two genes have been found that are very strongly associated with development of moyamoya disease, mainly in Asians [69,70].

Moyamoya-type vasculopathy has been described as a direct result of RT to the base of the brain, most often in the context of RT for optic glioma, brainstem glioma, or craniopharyngioma [71,72]. Most strikingly, in a series of 69 patients with optic glioma treated with RT, 19% of patients developed moyamoya over a median follow up of three years [35].

The therapeutic strategy for moyamoya-type vessels is complex and should take into account several factors such as the age of the patient, the cerebrovascular reserve, the presence or absence of symptoms, and the nature of the symptoms. Several surgical approaches have been described; however, no controlled studies are available. These surgical techniques include direct revascularization techniques such as superficial temporal artery to middle cerebral artery (STA-MCA) bypass [73]. Indirect revascularization such as pial synangiosis is favored where the cortical recipient artery is not available. Regression of moyamoya vessels can be seen after these types of surgery. It is not clear whether the approach should be different for moyamoya patients who underwent RT.

Stroke mimics

An infrequent delayed complication of brain irradiation sometimes confused with stroke, the stroke-like migraine attacks after radiation therapy (SMART) syndrome was first described in 1995 [74]. The syndrome is characterized by single or recurrent attacks of subacute severe headache and stroke-like focal neurological deficits several years after RT [75]. Seizures are a frequent symptom, often evolving to focal status epilepticus. Consciousness can be

markedly reduced [76]. There is a male preponderance and the syndrome occurs more often in patients irradiated at a younger age [77]. The prognosis is good, with symptoms usually resolving completely after a period of several weeks to months. A recent case series, however, described residual neurological cognitive or language-related symptoms in up to 45% of patients [75]. MRI usually shows a unilateral increased cortical T2 hyperintensity with contrast enhancement and gyral swelling not restricted to a specific vascular territory. The findings are often more pronounced in the temporal, parietal, or occipital regions, usually correlating with clinical findings. MRI abnormalities may appear as late as one week after symptom onset and seem to arise independently from the occurrence of seizures. In one case series 27% of patients developed cortical laminar necrosis in a region with previous gyral enhancement on T2 MRI images. In a similar number of patients in the same series ischemic brain lesions were seen on follow-up imaging [75].

The pathophysiology of this syndrome remains unknown. A study failed to demonstrate cerebrovascular hyper-reactivity as an explanation for the findings. Other hypotheses include endothelial damage, neuronal dysfunction, genetic susceptibility, and a postictal phenomenon [78].

Early treatment of epileptic seizures with anticonvulsants is warranted. Although unproven, antiplatelet medication, propranolol, verapamil, and statins have been used.

Conclusion

Cerebrovascular lesions occur typically as a very delayed complication of radiation therapy. The pathology is diverse. Although a causal relationship is very likely in many instances, high-quality prospective, controlled studies are lacking. Similarly, there are no controlled data on the optimal management of cerebrovascular disorders associated with RT, and often the same therapeutic stance is adopted had the vascular lesions or strokes occurred in patients who did not undergo RT. Neurovascular specialists should always take into account RT as a possible contributing factor for cerebrovascular lesions and radiation therapists or oncologists should be aware of the potentially devastating consequences of RT. A prudent approach would be to strongly advocate strict vascular risk factor management in patients who have been treated with radiotherapy.

References

1. Moller T R, Brorsson B, Ceberg J, et al. A prospective survey of radiotherapy practice 2001 in Sweden. *Acta Oncol.* 2003; **42**:387–410.

2. Slotman B, Faivre-Finn C, Kramer G, et al. Prophylactic cranial irradiation in extensive small-cell lung cancer. *N Engl J Med.* 2007; **357**:664–72.

3. Morris B, Partap S, Yeom K, et al. Cerebrovascular disease in childhood cancer survivors: A children's oncology group report. *Neurology.* 2009; **73**:1906–13.

4. Bowers D C, Liu Y, Leisenring W, et al. Late-occurring stroke among long-term survivors of childhood leukemia and brain tumors: A report from the childhood cancer survivor study. *J Clin Oncol.* 2006; **24**:5277–82.

5. Campen C J, Kranick S M, Kasner S E, et al. Cranial irradiation increases risk of stroke in pediatric brain tumor survivors. *Stroke.* 2012; **43**:3035–40.

6. Grisold W, Oberndorfer S, Struhal W. Stroke and cancer: A review. *Acta Neurol Scand.* 2009; **119**:1–16.

7. Labauge P, Laberge S, Brunereau L, Levy C, Tournier-Lasserve E. Hereditary cerebral cavernous angiomas: Clinical and genetic features in 57 French families. Societe Francaise de Neurochirurgie. *Lancet.* 1998; **352**:1892–7.

8. Gunel M, Awad I A, Finberg K, et al. A founder mutation as a cause of cerebral cavernous malformation in Hispanic Americans. *N Engl J Med.* 1996; **334**:946–51.

9. Laberge-le Couteulx S, Jung H H, Labauge P, et al. Truncating mutations in ccm1, encoding krit1, cause hereditary cavernous angiomas. *Nat Genet.* 1999; **23**:189–93.

10. Bergametti F, Denier C, Labauge P, et al. Mutations within the programmed cell death 10 gene cause cerebral cavernous malformations. *Am J Hum Genet.* 2005; **76**:42–51.

11. Nimjee S M, Powers C J, Bulsara K R. Review of the literature on de novo formation of cavernous malformations of the central nervous system after radiation therapy. *Neurosurg Focus.* 2006; **21**:e4.

12. Lew S M, Morgan J N, Psaty E, et al. Cumulative incidence of radiation-induced cavernomas in long-term survivors of medulloblastoma. *J Neurosurg.* 2006; **104**:103–7.

13. Al-Shahi Salman R, Hall J M, Horne M A, et al. Untreated clinical course of cerebral cavernous malformations: A prospective, population-based cohort study. *Lancet Neurol.* 2012; **11**:217–24.

14. Kivelev J, Niemela M, Hernesniemi J. Treatment strategies in cavernomas of the brain and spine. *J Clin Neurosci.* 2012; **19**:491–7.

15. Niranjan A, Lunsford L D. Stereotactic radiosurgery guidelines for the management of patients with intracranial cavernous malformations. *Prog Neurol Surg.* 2013; **27**:166–75.

16. Schneble H M, Soumare A, Herve D, et al. Antithrombotic therapy and bleeding risk in a prospective cohort study of patients with cerebral cavernous malformations. *Stroke.* 2012; **43**:3196–9.

17. de Weerd M, Greving J P, Hedblad B, et al. Prevalence of asymptomatic carotid artery stenosis in the general population: An individual participant data meta-analysis. *Stroke.* 2010; **41**:1294–7.

18. Compter A, van der Worp H B, Algra A, Kappelle L J. Second manifestations of AdSG. Prevalence and prognosis of asymptomatic vertebral artery origin stenosis in patients with clinically manifest arterial disease. *Stroke.* 2011; **42**:2795–800.

19. Marquardt L, Kuker W, Chandratheva A, Geraghty O, Rothwell P M. Incidence and prognosis of > or = 50% symptomatic vertebral or basilar artery stenosis: Prospective population-based study. *Brain.* 2009; **132**:982–8.

20. Feldmann E, Daneault N, Kwan E, et al. Chinese-White differences in the distribution of occlusive cerebrovascular disease. *Neurology.* 1990; **40**:1541–5.

21. Plummer C, Henderson R D, O'Sullivan J D, Read S J. Ischemic stroke and transient ischemic attack after head and neck radiotherapy: A review. *Stroke.* 2011; **42**:2410–18.

22. Scott A S, Parr L A, Johnstone P A. Risk of cerebrovascular events after neck and supraclavicular radiotherapy: A systematic review. *Radiother Oncol.* 2009; **90**:163–5.

23. Jagsi R, Griffith K A, Koelling T, Roberts R, Pierce L J. Stroke rates and risk factors in patients treated with radiation therapy for early-stage breast cancer. *J Clin Oncol.* 2006; **24**:2779–85.

24. Nilsson G, Holmberg L, Garmo H, Terent A, Blomqvist C. Increased incidence of stroke in women with breast cancer. *Eur J Cancer.* 2005; **41**:423–9.

25. Nilsson G, Holmberg L, Garmo H, Terent A, Blomqvist C. Radiation to supraclavicular and internal mammary lymph nodes in breast cancer increases the risk of stroke. *Br J Cancer.* 2009; **100**:811–16.

26. Hooning M J, Dorresteijn L D, Aleman B M, et al. Decreased risk of stroke among 10-year survivors of breast cancer. *J Clin Oncol.* 2006; **24**:5388–94.

27. Zou W X, Leung T W, Yu S C, et al. Angiographic features, collaterals, and infarct topography of symptomatic occlusive radiation vasculopathy: A case-referent study. *Stroke.* 2013; **44**:401–6.

28. Murros K E, Toole J F. The effect of radiation on carotid arteries. A review article. *Arch Neurol.* 1989; **46**:449–55.

29. O'Connor M M, Mayberg M R. Effects of radiation on cerebral vasculature: A review. *Neurosurgery*. 2000; **46**: 138–49.

30. Fokkema M, den Hartog A G, Bots M L, *et al*. Stenting versus surgery in patients with carotid stenosis after previous cervical radiation therapy: Systematic review and meta-analysis. *Stroke*. 2012; **43**:793–801.

31. Abbott A L. Carotid surgery or stenting following neck irradiation: Time to address the assumptions. *Eur J Vasc Endovasc Surg*. 2012; **43**:8–9.

32. McDonald M W, Moore M G, Johnstone P A. Risk of carotid blowout after reirradiation of the head and neck: A systematic review. *Int J Radiat Oncol Biol Phys*. 2012; **82**:1083–9.

33. Haas R A, Ahn S H. Interventional management of head and neck emergencies: Carotid blowout. *Semin Intervent Radiol*. 2013; **30**:245–8.

34. Bowers D C, Mulne A F, Reisch J S, *et al*. Nonperioperative strokes in children with central nervous system tumors. *Cancer*. 2002; **94**:1094–101.

35. Grill J, Couanet D, Cappelli C, *et al*. Radiation-induced cerebral vasculopathy in children with neurofibromatosis and optic pathway glioma. *Ann Neurol*. 1999; **45**:393–6.

36. Erridge S C, Conkey D S, Stockton D, *et al*. Radiotherapy for pituitary adenomas: Long-term efficacy and toxicity. *Radiother Oncol*. 2009; **93**:597–601.

37. Flickinger J C, Nelson P B, Taylor F H, Robinson A. Incidence of cerebral infarction after radiotherapy for pituitary adenoma. *Cancer*. 1989; **63**:2404–8.

38. Bowen J, Paulsen C A. Stroke after pituitary irradiation. *Stroke*. 1992; **23**:908–11.

39. Brada M, Burchell L, Ashley S, Traish D. The incidence of cerebrovascular accidents in patients with pituitary adenoma. *Int J Radiat Oncol Biol Phys*. 1999; **45**:693–8.

40. Bailey E L, Smith C, Sudlow C L, Wardlaw J M. Pathology of lacunar ischemic stroke in humans: A systematic review. *Brain Pathol*. 2012; **22**:583–91.

41. Millikan C, Futrell N. The fallacy of the lacune hypothesis. *Stroke*. 1990; **21**:1251–7.

42. Futrell N. Lacunar infarction: Embolism is the key. *Stroke*. 2004; **35**:1778–9.

43. Futrell N, Millikan C, Watson B D, Dietrich W D, Ginsberg M D. Embolic stroke from a carotid arterial source in the rat: Pathology and clinical implications. *Neurology*. 1989; **39**:1050–6.

44. Norrving B. Lacunar infarcts: No black holes in the brain are benign. *Pract Neurol*. 2008; **8**:222–8.

45. Patel B, Markus H S. Magnetic resonance imaging in cerebral small vessel disease and its use as a surrogate disease marker. *Int J Stroke*. 2011; **6**:47–59.

46. Kwee R M, Kwee T C. Virchow–Robin spaces at MR imaging. *Radiographics*. 2007; **27**:1071–86.

47. Gouw A A, Seewann A, van der Flier W M, *et al*. Heterogeneity of small vessel disease: A systematic review of MRI and histopathology correlations. *J Neurol Neurosurg Psychiatry*. 2011; **82**:126–35.

48. Atwood L D, Wolf P A, Heard-Costa N L, *et al*. Genetic variation in white matter hyperintensity volume in the Framingham study. *Stroke*. 2004; **35**: 1609–13.

49. Fornage M, Debette S, Bis J C, *et al*. Genome-wide association studies of cerebral white matter lesion burden: The charge consortium. *Ann Neurol*. 2011; **69**: 928–39.

50. Debette S, Markus H S. The clinical importance of white matter hyperintensities on brain magnetic resonance imaging: Systematic review and meta-analysis. *BMJ*. 2010; **341**:c3666.

51. Ebi J, Sato H, Nakajima M, Shishido F. Incidence of leukoencephalopathy after whole-brain radiation therapy for brain metastases. *Int J Radiat Oncol Biol Phys*. 2012.

52. DeAngelis L M, Delattre J Y, Posner J B. Radiation-induced dementia in patients cured of brain metastases. *Neurology*. 1989; **39**:789–96.

53. Schrag M, McAuley G, Pomakian J, *et al*. Correlation of hypointensities in susceptibility-weighted images to tissue histology in dementia patients with cerebral amyloid angiopathy: A postmortem MRI study. *Acta Neuropathol*. 2010; **119**:291–302.

54. Fazekas F, Kleinert R, Roob G, *et al*. Histopathologic analysis of foci of signal loss on gradient-echo T2*-weighted MR images in patients with spontaneous intracerebral hemorrhage: Evidence of microangiopathy-related microbleeds. *Am J Neuroradiol*. 1999; **20**:637–42.

55. Fisher M, French S, Ji P, Kim R C. Cerebral microbleeds in the elderly: A pathological analysis. *Stroke*. 2010; **41**:2782–5.

56. Schrag M, McAuley G, Pomakian J, *et al*. Correlation of hypointensities in susceptibility-weighted images to tissue histology in dementia patients with cerebral amyloid angiopathy: A postmortem MRI study. *Acta Neuropathol*. 2009.

57. Greenberg S M, Vernooij M W, Cordonnier C, *et al*. Cerebral microbleeds: A guide to detection and interpretation. *Lancet Neurol*. 2009; **8**:165–74.

58. Roob G, Schmidt R, Kapeller P, *et al*. MRI evidence of past cerebral microbleeds in a healthy elderly population. *Neurology*. 1999; **52**:991–4.

59. Vernooij M W, van der Lugt A, Ikram M A, *et al*. Prevalence and risk factors of cerebral microbleeds:

The Rotterdam scan study. *Neurology*. 2008; **70**: 1208–14.

60. Benavente O R, Hart R G, McClure L A, *et al*. Effects of clopidogrel added to aspirin in patients with recent lacunar stroke. *N Engl J Med*. 2012; **367**:817–25.

61. Brisman J L, Song J K, Newell D W. Cerebral aneurysms. *N Engl J Med*. 2006; **355**:928–39.

62. van Gijn J, Kerr R S, Rinkel G J. Subarachnoid haemorrhage. *Lancet*. 2007; **369**:306–18.

63. Vernooij M W, Ikram M A, Tanghe H L, *et al*. Incidental findings on brain MRI in the general population. *N Engl J Med*. 2007; **357**:1821–8.

64. Feigin V L, Rinkel G J, Lawes C M, *et al*. Risk factors for subarachnoid hemorrhage: An updated systematic review of epidemiological studies. *Stroke*. 2005; **36**: 2773–80.

65. Wiebers D O, Whisnant J P, Huston J, 3rd, *et al*. Unruptured intracranial aneurysms: Natural history, clinical outcome, and risks of surgical and endovascular treatment. *Lancet*. 2003; **362**:103–10.

66. Lau W Y, Chow C K. Radiation-induced petrous internal carotid artery aneurysm. *Ann Otol Rhinol Laryngol*. 2005; **114**:939–40.

67. Sciubba D M, Gallia G L, Recinos P, Garonzik I M, Clatterbuck R E. Intracranial aneurysm following radiation therapy during childhood for a brain tumor. Case report and review of the literature. *J Neurosurg*. 2006; **105**:134–9.

68. Kuroda S, Houkin K. Moyamoya disease: Current concepts and future perspectives. *Lancet Neurol*. 2008; 7:1056–66.

69. Liu W, Morito D, Takashima S, *et al*. Identification of rnf213 as a susceptibility gene for moyamoya disease and its possible role in vascular development. *PLoS One*. 2011; **6**:e22542.

70. Kamada F, Aoki Y, Narisawa A, *et al*. A genome-wide association study identifies rnf213 as the first moyamoya disease gene. *J Hum Genet*. 2011; 56:34–40.

71. Kestle J R, Hoffman H J, Mock A R. Moyamoya phenomenon after radiation for optic glioma. *J Neurosurg*. 1993; **79**:32–5.

72. Ullrich N J, Robertson R, Kinnamon D D, *et al*. Moyamoya following cranial irradiation for primary brain tumors in children. *Neurology*. 2007; **68**: 932–8.

73. Pandey P, Steinberg G K. Neurosurgical advances in the treatment of moyamoya disease. *Stroke*. 2011; **42**: 3304–10.

74. Shuper A, Packer R J, Vezina L G, Nicholson H S, Lafond D. 'Complicated migraine-like episodes' in children following cranial irradiation and chemotherapy. *Neurology*. 1995; **45**:1837–40.

75. Black D F, Morris J M, Lindell E P, *et al*. Stroke-like migraine attacks after radiation therapy (SMART) syndrome is not always completely reversible: A case series. *Am J Neuroradiol*. 2013; **34**:2298–303.

76. Tomek M, Bhavsar S V, Patry D, Hanson A. The syndrome of stroke-like migraine attacks after radiation therapy associated with prolonged unresponsiveness in an adult patient. *Neurologist*. 2015; **19**:49–52.

77. Armstrong A E, Gillan E, DiMario F J, Jr. SMART syndrome (stroke-like migraine attacks after radiation therapy) in adult and pediatric patients. *J Child Neurol*. 2014; **29**:336–41.

78. Farid K, Meissner W G, Samier-Foubert A, *et al*. Normal cerebrovascular reactivity in stroke-like migraine attacks after radiation therapy syndrome. *Clin Nucl Med*. 2010; **35**:583–5.

79. Smith G L, Smith B D, Buchholz T A, *et al*. Cerebrovascular disease risk in older head and neck cancer patients after radiotherapy. *J Clin Oncol*. 2008; **26**:5119–25.

80. Haynes J C, Machtay M, Weber R S, *et al*. Relative risk of stroke in head and neck carcinoma patients treated with external cervical irradiation. *Laryngoscope*. 2002; **112**:1883–7.

81. Dorresteijn L D, Kappelle A C, Boogerd W, *et al*. Increased risk of ischemic stroke after radiotherapy on the neck in patients younger than 60 years. *J Clin Oncol*. 2002; **20**:282–8.

82. Elerding S C, Fernandez R N, Grotta J C, *et al*. Carotid artery disease following external cervical irradiation. *Ann Surg*. 1981; **194**:609–15.

83. De Bruin M L, Dorresteijn L D, van't Veer M B, *et al*. Increased risk of stroke and transient ischemic attack in 5-year survivors of Hodgkin lymphoma. *J Natl Cancer Inst*. 2009; **101**:928–37.

84. Moser E C, Noordijk E M, van Leeuwen F E, *et al*. Long-term risk of cardiovascular disease after treatment for aggressive non-Hodgkin lymphoma. *Blood*. 2006; **107**:2912–19.

Chapter 12

Stroke after chiropractic manipulations

Lars Neeb and Uwe Reuter

Introduction

There is an ongoing controversy whether cervical manipulation – especially chiropractic manipulation – with its swift, thrusting movements is associated with an elevated stroke risk due to dissection of the carotid or vertebral artery. Cervical arterial dissection (CAD) is defined as a tear in one of the major arteries in the neck that leads to stenosis or aneurysmal dilatation. It may occur after a significant or minor trauma as well as spontaneously [1]. Spontaneous CAD accounts for only 2% of all ischemic strokes, but in patients younger than 45 years up to 10 to 25% of the cases are attributed to spontaneous CAD [2].

Anatomy and pathophysiology of cervical artery dissections

An arterial dissection can occur either in the subintimal or subadventitial tissue depending of the proximity of the dissection to the layer of the artery. As a consequence to intimal tearing blood penetrates into the vessel wall, forms an intramural hematoma, and narrows the lumen of the artery, which can result in complete vessel occlusion. Subadventitial dissection results in a dissecting aneurysm or pseudoaneurysm causing dilatation of the artery. In further course, parts of the intraluminal thrombus can break off and embolize into the cerebral vessels, leading to cerebral ischemia and stroke. Another possible mechanism of cervical dissection resulting in stroke is the distal extension of the dissection into the intracranial part with occlusion of branching vessels.

Since parts of the extracranial course of the vertebral and internal carotid artery are mobile they are potentially vulnerable to injuries due to neck movement. Most of the strokes reported in close temporal association with cervical manipulation treatment (CMT) are located in the posterior circulation and related to vertebral artery dissection (VAD).

The vertebral arteries arise on both sides of the body from the subclavian arteries and enter the transverse processes of the 6th cervical vertebra (C6). They continue upwards in the transverse foramen of the cervical vertebrae until C1. Before each of the vertebral arteries enters the base of the skull it changes its direction from a vertical path to a horizontal path (segment V3–V4) and then enters the skull. This part of the vertebral artery is the most vulnerable part for dissections.

A great fraction of spontaneous dissections are idiopathic but some patients may be suffering from predisposing connective tissue disorders such as Ehler–Danlos syndrome type IV, Marfan syndrome, autosomal-dominant polycystic kidney disease, and osteogenesis imperfecta type I. Although these conditions are found only in up to 5% of patients with spontaneous dissections, 20% of these patients are believed to suffer from clinically apparent but as yet unnamed connective tissue disorders. A positive family history with at least one family member who experienced a spontaneous dissection of the aorta or its main branches can be detected in 5% of the patients with spontaneous cervical dissections. In about 15% of patients with spontaneous dissections the non-specific abnormalities fibromuscular dysplasia and cystic medial necrosis are found. Both conditions are so far non-specific disorders associated with a variety of systemic disorders [1]. Most of the attempts to define an association between CAD and genetic factors have failed, with the exception for genetic polymorphism of intracellular adhesion molecule-1 [3] and for methylene-tetrahydrofolate reductase (MTHFR) [4]. Certain polymorphisms of these genes were significantly more prevalent in patients

Treatment-Related Stroke, ed. Alexander Tsiskaridze, Arne Lindgren and Adnan Qureshi. Published by Cambridge University Press. © Cambridge University Press 2016.

with CADs compared to healthy controls. However, in case of MTHFR no significant difference was detected between patients with MTHFR polymorphism and stroke due to cervical dissection and stroke due to other causes [4]. Two other studies with more patients did not find an association between the occurrence of CAD and MTHFR polymorphism [5,6].

Clinical manifestation of cervical artery dissection

The most common early clinical manifestation of symptomatic internal carotid and vertebral artery dissection is headache and neck pain that occurs in approximately 70 to 80% of patients [7,8].

Internal carotid artery dissection causes typically unilateral pain of the head, face, or neck, and is in approximately 50% of the cases accompanied by ipsilateral partial Horner's syndrome (oculosympathetic palsy). In some patients, the pain can also involve the entire hemicranium or the occipital area. The character of the headache is described by most of the patients as a constant steady aching, but can also be throbbing or sharp [7]. Besides oculosympathetic palsy, carotid dissection can also be associated with cranial nerve palsies, particularly of the lower cranial nerves such as the hypoglossal nerve or the oculomotor, trigeminal, and facial nerve [9]. Furthermore, a quarter of patients describe a pulsatile tinnitus [7].

The pain associated with VAD is in most cases located uni- or bilaterally in the back of the neck or head, but can also spread over the entire hemicranium or the frontal area. The headache may be throbbing or steady and sharp. The neck pain is often falsely interpreted as musculoskeletal in origin [7].

Both headaches can be mistaken for a migraine attack especially in patients with a history of migraine. Among headache patients with arterial dissection only 50% describe the pain as different from their usual headaches [7]. One study reported 8% of all patients with CAD present with pain as the only symptom [10]. No definite characteristics/criteria exist for pain associated with CAD. Therefore it is difficult to identify patients who experience a dissection without focal neurological symptoms.

Ischemic symptoms develop in 50 to 95% of patients with spontaneous dissection of the internal carotid artery and in more than 90% of patients with VAD in a certain interval (hours to weeks) from the onset of headache. Strokes in internal carotid artery

dissections are often preceded by transient ischemic attacks [11] including transient ocular blindness, whereas transient ischemic attacks are less common in vertebral artery dissections [7,8].

In VAD ischemic symptoms are typically located in the posterior circulation and involve the brain stem, thalamus, and the cerebral or cerebellar hemispheres [1,7]. Accordingly, focal neurological symptoms include dysarthria, dysphagia, ataxia, nystagmus, and visual field abnormalities. Other more unspecific symptoms associated with VAD are vertigo, unsteadiness, unilateral facial paraesthesia, and nausea and vomiting in about half of the patients [12].

Cervical artery dissections and chiropractic treatment

It remains unclear whether minor trauma or certain head and neck motions can cause cervical artery dissection. Spinal manipulation has become increasingly popular since the introduction of this technique in the eighteenth century. About 250 million office visits are made to chiropractors each year in the United States, mainly for headache and musculoskeletal disorders such as neck and back pain [13]. Cervical manipulation treatment is not only performed by chiropractors but also provided by orthopedic surgeons, physiotherapists, osteopaths, general practitioners, homeopaths, and neurologists.

Up to 70% of all visits to a chiropractor or a physician offering manual manipulation result in cervical manipulation [13,14]. During the rotation of the neck the arteries become stretched and compressed, which may cause dissection. Especially the sudden rapid movements that are used during cervical spine adjustments are believed to cause a dissection due to intense force to the tissue.

The first report of a possible association between stroke and chiropractic manipulation dates back to 1934 [15]. Most of the strokes associated with CMT are located in the posterior circulation territory and are due to vertebral artery dissection. A review of case reports and surveys found 165 vertebrobasilar accidents due to spinal manipulation until the end of 1993. Twenty-seven percent of these cases made a full recovery, while 52% suffered residual effects and 18% died. A review published in 2003 found only 13 reported cases of internal carotid dissection in temporal relation to CMT [16]. In a case series of

126 patients with CAD, chiropractic manipulation of the spine was performed in 30% of the patients with a VAD (compared to 6% with internal carotid artery dissection) [17]. However, the opinion on neck manipulations and its consequences is highly controversial between medical specialists. Neurologists have little doubt that chiropractic manipulation can cause VAD: they define dissection and stroke as a relatively frequent complication of cervical manipulative therapy [18,19]. In contrast, chiropractors find dissections after manipulation extremely rare and accuse medical literature of overreporting such cases [16,20,21].

Epidemiology and risk estimation

The annual incidence of spontaneous VAD has been estimated between 1 and 1.5/100,000 and for CAD between 2.6 and 2.9/100,000 [1,8,22,23]. However, the true incidence of CAD is unknown as some cases remain asymptomatic and mainly severe cases with clinical symptoms are seen by doctors and taken into account. The risk for severe vascular or neurological complications due to chiropractic maneuvers has been estimated in great variety between 1/585 million and 1/20,000 manipulations [14,24,25].

Association of dissection and stroke with chiropractic maneuvers was first mentioned in several case reports that reported a temporal proximity of previous cervical manipulations and discovery of dissection. The first retrospective surveys revealed the differing perception of the frequency of neurological complications of chiropractic therapy among various professions. In a survey of the 367 members of the Swiss Society for Manual Medicine the estimated rate of slight neurological complications was 1/40,000 and the rate of important complications 1/400,000 [26]. In a survey of the Danish chiropractor association, the estimated incidence of cerebrovascular events was one case per 362 chiropractor years and one case per 1.3 million cervical treatment sessions [27]. In contrast, in a survey among Californian neurologists, 177 physicians reported 101 patients with neurological complications within 24 hours of chiropractic (mainly cervical) manipulation (55 patients with a stroke, 16 with myelopathies, and 30 with radiculopathies) [18]. Haldemann *et al.* suggested a selection or referral bias as an explanation for the different opinions of neurologists and chiropractors: in a retrospective review of 23 cases

of VAD following CMT they calculated that one in 48 chiropractors was exposed to one of these patients in comparison to one in two neurologists [28].

A few other studies could show a temporal correlation of CMT and the onset of neurological symptoms. In a retrospective review of 64 medicolegal cases of stroke associated with CMT, 40 of these patients reported immediate onset of neurologic symptoms following CMT. In eight cases the onset of symptoms started 5 to 30 minutes after the procedure and in 12 cases after 30 minutes and within 48 hours. The longest delay between CMT and stroke was 11 days in this study [29]. This is in line with other studies demonstrating a highly variable interval between CMT and onset of neurological symptoms [17]. In our own retrospective study we could identify 36 patients with VAD after chirotherapy of the neck in three years in 13 university neurology centers. Clinical symptoms consistent with VAD started in 55% of patients within 12 hours after neck manipulation. A new onset of pain with different character after the procedure and the acute or subacute development of neurological deficits in this case series argued against a simple coincidence of VAD and CMT. Pain characteristics were clearly different before and after CMT [30].

Controversial results exist regarding the risk of VAD when exposure rates to CMT and the way of manipulation are considered. Two studies could not find any dose–response relationship: ischemic events did occur in patients who had never received a manipulation of the cervical spine before but also in patients who had already received over 100 manipulations, all by the same practitioner [31,32]. On the other hand, a case-control study demonstrated an association of a higher number of CMT visits with higher rate ratios for the risk of VAD [33].

It has been suggested that omitting rotation and extension of the neck during the cervical maneuver would reduce the risk of complications [24]. However, a case study showed that refraining from use of rotation and extension during the manipulation did not prevent a VAD. The authors concluded that stroke should be considered a random and unpredictable complication of any neck movement and that any manipulation carries some risk [31].

Based on these case reports and surveys it is not possible to draw conclusions on the possible risk of CAD following chiropractic manipulation. A causal relationship between VAD and CMT cannot be proven by case series. To appropriately evaluate the risk of dissection due to cervical manipulation either a randomized controlled trial or alternatively a prospective cohort study would be necessary. In addition, not only clinical symptoms should be assessed but also duplex sonography of cervical arteries should be performed to detect clinically silent dissections. However, due to the low number of dissections following cervical manipulation both trial designs need a large number of study subjects to assess the risk related to the treatment. Furthermore, designing a randomized controlled trial in a treatment paradigm involving physical activity is a challenge.

A few observational studies examined the risk of CAD in association with cervical manipulation. The first approach to this topic was a nested case-control study that identified 582 cases in Ontario, Canada with vertebrobasilar accidents. Each of these cases was age- and sex- matched to four controls with no history of stroke. The study revealed that young adults (≤45 years) with a vertebrobasilar accident were five times more likely than controls to have visited a chiropractor within one week of the accident. When they had three or more visits in the previous month the estimated rate ratio for the risk of VAD was four times higher than in controls. In the group aged >45 years no association between a vertebrobasilar accident and a visit to the chiropractor was found. The reported number of cases corresponds to an incidence of 1.3 VADs within one week after treatment per 100,000 individuals aged < 45 years undergoing chiropractic neck manipulation [33]. A North American retrospective cohort analysis among 1,157,475 Medicare B beneficiaries with neck pain aged 66 to 99 compared the hazard of vertebrobasilar stroke and any stroke at 7 and 30 days after an office visit to either a chiropractor or primary care physician for neck pain. While the overall incidence of vertebrobasilar stroke was extremely low, the adjusted risk of stroke of any type was even significantly lower at seven days in the chiropractic cohort as compared to the primary care cohort. However, at 30 days a slight risk elevation was observed for the chiropractic cohort. The small differences in risk between the two cohorts were rated by the authors as probably not clinically significant [34]. The second case-control study compared 51 patients with CAD and ischemic stroke or transient ischemia attacks (TIA) aged under 60 years and 100 control patients. The authors found a strong relationship between recent spinal manipulation

treatment (SMT) and VAD. Arterial dissection was independently associated with SMT within 30 days (odds ratio (OR), 6.62) and pain before stroke/TIA (OR, 3.76). Two of the patients in this study experienced stroke immediately after chiropractic manipulation [35].

Forty-seven patients with CAD and stroke were compared to 47 age-matched controls with ischemic stroke due to other etiologies. The authors assessed if patients had recently had CMT and if they additionally suffered from headache or neck pain, a recent infection, as well as mechanical trigger factors including mild direct or indirect neck trauma, heavy lifting, sexual intercourse, jerky head movements, and sports activity <24 hours and <7 days prior to symptom onset. No significant difference was found for any comparison between the CAD and control groups. Cervical manipulation treatment and recent infections were more frequent in the dissection group but failed to reach statistical significance, possibly due to the small sample size. However, a significant association was seen between the mechanical risk factors as a whole and CAD [36].

A study assessing the overall quality of reports of the association between CMT, CAD, and stroke demonstrated that the current literature infrequently reports useful data toward the understanding of this relation [37]. A systematic review concluded that the current evidence is not sufficient to confirm or reject an association between neck manipulation and stroke [38]. The association between CMT and VAD shown in two of these case-control studies is not sufficient to draw conclusions on a causal relationship. It is relevant to mention that an artery dissection that leads to stroke in a temporal relationship to CMT is not necessarily caused by CMT. Patients with spontaneous CAD commonly experience neck pain. This pain is often misdiagnosed as pain of musculoskeletal origin. For the treatment of neck pain these patients may seek help from a chiropractor. Cervical manipulation may then be an aggravating factor or a coincidental event precipitating ischemia in these patients [31]. Thus it cannot be ruled out that a dissection that pre-existed before cervical manipulation caused a stroke independently of treatment. However, CMT could still contribute to the risk of stroke by exacerbating the pre-existing dissection or dislodging an embolus.

One study tried to assess this question by adding a case-crossover design to the standard case-control design. Eight hundred and eighteen cases with stroke due to VAD were compared to independent control subjects from the same source population. The cases served as their own controls. In addition to the visits to chiropractors within 30 days, the authors recorded the visits to primary care physicians within 30 days prior to a VAD stroke. In accordance with the previous studies, they also found an increased association between visits to a chiropractor within 30 days and VADs in persons aged <45 years and no association in persons >45 years of age. In addition, they observed the same association between visits to primary care physicians and VADs in patient groups under and over 45 years of age. Both groups were about three times more likely to see a chiropractor or a primary care physician before their stroke than controls. Based on their results, the odds of stroke occurring within 24 hours of a visit to a primary care physician did not differ from the odds of stroke occurring within 24 hours of a visit to a chiropractor. The authors concluded that there was no excess risk of VAD stroke due to chiropractic care. As head and neck pain precede approximately 80% of VAD strokes, the authors stated that individuals with head and neck pain due to VAD seek care for these symptoms either at their primary care physician or a chiropractor [39]. However, existing case reports describe immediate onset of neurologic symptoms during or shortly after CMT. These cases also involve patients who developed VAD after a visit to a chiropractor and did not suffer from previous neck pain. These findings suggest that CMT can directly produce dissection or at least aggravate a pre-existing dissection leading to stroke.

Risk factors for cervical dissections could be helpful to exclude patients from potential disabling manipulation therapies. Proposed risk factors for cervical dissections are connective tissue diseases, age, male gender, migraine headache, hypertension, diabetes, arteriosclerotic disease, hyperhomocysteinemia, cervical spondylosis, contraception, infection, smoking, presence of abdominal or cerebral aneurysm, and a family history of arterial dissections [29,40–42]. However, CAD strokes following CMT occur mainly in younger and otherwise healthy adults [32,43]. Effectiveness of screening patients for these factors has not been convincingly demonstrated and to date no population at special risk for stroke due to chiropractic cervical treatment could be defined [13,32].

Conclusion

In summary, the controversy regarding a causal relationship between stroke due to artery dissection and CMT remains open. Existing clinical data and study results do not provide a clear answer. In our view, a randomized controlled trial or at least a prospective cohort study performed by physicians and CMT practitioners could finally provide sufficient evidence.

Patients who are evaluated for CMT should be screened for symptoms of pre-existing dissections. Due to the low incidence of CAD compared to the high number of patients seeking CMT for treatment of neck pain and headache, diagnostic imaging cannot be recommended in every patient with unilateral headache without focal neurological symptoms who is going to have CMT. However, a reliable clinical screening for dissections is a challenge, as in many cases no clear symptoms exist that can help the therapist to distinguish patients with musculoskeletal pain and neck pain associated with a pre-existing dissection. Historical factors such as known connective tissue disease or preceding symptoms of TIAs should alert the practitioner. Attention should be raised if the patient describes a sudden onset of a severe unilateral neck pain and headache, particularly if these are accompanied by neurological symptoms such as drop attacks, dysarthria, dysphagia, ataxia, numbness, or a nystagmus.

In these cases, the suspicion of previous dissection should be carefully explored prior to performing any neck manipulations. To exclude a CAD, magnetic resonance (MR) imaging or state-of-the-art vascular imaging by MR angiography with fat suppression techniques, CT angiography, or conventional digital subtraction angiography is needed. In the hands of an experienced examiner, ultrasonographic techniques with Doppler color-flow imaging can be used for screening of patients for internal carotid artery dissection as well as for VADs. However, in most of the cases confirmatory testing and visualization with MR angiography is necessary.

Cervical manipulation treatment must be avoided in patients with existing dissections, since manipulation on a dissected artery may accelerate its progression to stroke. Before performing CMT patients should be informed about the possible risk of this treatment. In detail, patients must be aware that ischemic symptoms or vascular injuries in temporal proximity to manipulation are unpredictable, inherent, and rare complications of any neck movement including cervical manipulation independent of the technique of manipulation.

References

1. Schievink W I. Spontaneous dissection of the carotid and vertebral arteries. *N Engl J Med*. 2001; **344**:898–906.

2. Ferro J M, Massaro A R, Mas J L. Aetiological diagnosis of ischaemic stroke in young adults. *Lancet Neurol*. 2010; **9**:1085–96.

3. Longoni M, Grond-Ginsbach C, Grau A J, *et al*. The ICAM-1 E469 K gene polymorphism is a risk factor for spontaneous cervical artery dissection. *Neurology*. 2006; **66**:1273–5.

4. Pezzini A, Del Zotto E, Archetti S, *et al*. Plasma homocysteine concentration, C677T MTHFR genotype, and 844ins68bp CBS genotype in young adults with spontaneous cervical artery dissection and atherothrombotic stroke. *Stroke*. 2002; **33**:664–9.

5. Gallai V, Caso V, Paciaroni M, *et al*. Mild hyperhomocyst(e)inemia: a possible risk factor for cervical artery dissection. *Stroke*. 2001; **32**:714–18.

6. Konrad C, Muller G A, Langer C, *et al*. Plasma homocysteine, MTHFR C677T, CBS 844ins68bp, and MTHFD1 G1958A polymorphisms in spontaneous cervical artery dissections. *J Neurol*. 2004; **251**:1242–8.

7. Silbert P L, Mokri B, Schievink W I. Headache and neck pain in spontaneous internal carotid and vertebral artery dissections. *Neurology*. 1995; **45**: 1517–22.

8. Lee V H, Brown R D, Jr., Mandrekar J N, Mokri B. Incidence and outcome of cervical artery dissection: a population-based study. *Neurology*. 2006; **67**:1809–12.

9. Mokri B, Silbert P L, Schievink W I, Piepgras D G. Cranial nerve palsy in spontaneous dissection of the extracranial internal carotid artery. *Neurology*. 1996;**46**:356–9.

10. Arnold M, Cumurciuc R, Stapf C, *et al*. Pain as the only symptom of cervical artery dissection. *J Neurol Neurosurg Psychiatry*. 2006; **77**:1021–4.

11. Biousse V, D'Anglejan-Chatillon J, Touboul P J, Amarenco P, Bousser M G. Time course of symptoms in extracranial carotid artery dissections. A series of 80 patients. *Stroke*. 1995; **26**:235–9.

12. Saeed A B, Shuaib A, Al-Sulaiti G, Emery D. Vertebral artery dissection: Warning symptoms, clinical features and prognosis in 26 patients. *Can J Neurol Sci*. 2000; **27**:292–6.

13. Hurwitz E L, Aker P D, Adams A H, Meeker W C, Shekelle P G. Manipulation and mobilization of the cervical spine. A systematic review of the literature. *Spine*. 1996; **21**:1746–60.

14. Haldeman S, Carey P, Townsend M, Papadopoulos C. Arterial dissections following cervical manipulation: the chiropractic experience. *CMAJ*. 2001; **165**:905–6.

15. Thornton R V. Malpractice: death resulting from chiropractic treatment of headache (medicolegal abstract). *JAMA*. 1934; **103**:1260.

16. Haneline M T, Croft A C, Frishberg B M. Association of internal carotid artery dissection and chiropractic manipulation. *Neurologist*. 2003; **9**:35–44.

17. Dziewas R, Konrad C, Drager B, *et al*. Cervical artery dissection: Clinical features, risk factors, therapy and outcome in 126 patients. *J Neurol*. 2003; **250**:1179–84.

18. Lee K P, Carlini W G, McCormick G F, Albers G W. Neurologic complications following chiropractic manipulation: a survey of California neurologists. *Neurology*. 1995; **45**:1213–15.

19. Norris J W, Beletsky V, Nadareishvili Z G. Sudden neck movement and cervical artery dissection. The Canadian Stroke Consortium. *CMAJ*. 2000; **163**:38–40.

20. Dabbs V, Lauretti W J. A risk assessment of cervical manipulation vs. NSAIDs for the treatment of neck pain. *J Manipulative Physiol Ther*. 1995; **18**:530–6.

21. Haneline M T, Lewkovich G. Identification of internal carotid artery dissection in chiropractic practice. *J Can Chiropr Assoc*. 2004; **48**:206–10.

22. Schievink W I, Mokri B, Whisnant J P. Internal carotid artery dissection in a community. Rochester, Minnesota, 1987–1992. *Stroke*. 1993; **24**:1678–80.

23. Giroud M, Fayolle H, Andre N, *et al*. Incidence of internal carotid artery dissection in the community of Dijon. *J Neurol Neurosurg Psychiatry*. 1994; **57**:1443.

24. Assendelft W J, Bouter L M, Knipschild P G. Complications of spinal manipulation: A comprehensive review of the literature. *J Fam Pract*. 1996; **42**:475–80.

25. Showalter W, Esekogwu V, Newton K I, Henderson S O. Vertebral artery dissection. *Acad Emerg Med*. 1997; **4**:991–5.

26. Dvorak J, Orelli F V. How dangerous is manipulation to the cervical spine? *Man Med*. 1985; **2**:1–4.

27. Klougart N, Leboeuf-Yde C, Rasmussen L R. Safety in chiropractic practice, Part I; The occurrence of cerebrovascular accidents after manipulation to the neck in Denmark from 1978–1988. *J Manipulative Physiol Ther*. 1996; **19**:371–7.

28. Haldeman S, Carey P, Townsend M, Papadopoulos C. Clinical perceptions of the risk of vertebral artery dissection after cervical manipulation: the effect of referral bias. *Spine J*. 2002; **2**:334–42.

29. Haldeman S, Kohlbeck F J, McGregor M. Unpredictability of cerebrovascular ischemia associated with cervical spine manipulation therapy: a review of sixty-four cases after cervical spine manipulation. *Spine*. 2002; **27**:49–55.

30. Reuter U, Hamling M, Kavuk I, Einhaupl K M, Schielke E. Vertebral artery dissections after chiropractic neck manipulation in Germany over three years. *J Neurol*. 2006; **253**:724–30.

31. Haldeman S, Kohlbeck F J, McGregor M. Stroke, cerebral artery dissection, and cervical spine manipulation therapy. *J Neurol*. 2002; **249**:1098–104.

32. Hufnagel A, Hammers A, Schonle P W, Bohm K D, Leonhardt G. Stroke following chiropractic manipulation of the cervical spine. *J Neurol*. 1999; **246**: 683–8.

33. Rothwell D M, Bondy S J, Williams J I. Chiropractic manipulation and stroke: a population-based case-control study. *Stroke*. 2001; **32**:1054–60.

34. Whedon J M, Song Y, Mackenzie T A, *et al.* Risk of stroke after chiropractic spinal manipulation in Medicare B beneficiaries aged 66 to 99 years with neck pain. *J Manipulative Physiol Ther*. 2015; **38**:93–101.

35. Smith W S, Johnston S C, Skalabrin E J, *et al.* Spinal manipulative therapy is an independent risk factor for vertebral artery dissection. *Neurology*. 2003; **60**:1424–8.

36. Dittrich R, Rohsbach D, Heidbreder A, *et al.* Mild mechanical traumas are possible risk factors for cervical artery dissection. *Cerebrovasc Dis*. 2007; **23**: 275–81.

37. Wynd S, Westaway M, Vohra S, Kawchuk G. The quality of reports on cervical arterial dissection following cervical spinal manipulation. *PLoS One*. 2013; **8**:e59170.

38. Haynes M J, Vincent K, Fischhoff C, *et al.* Assessing the risk of stroke from neck manipulation: A systematic review. *Int J Clin Pract*. 2012; **66**:940–7.

39. Cassidy J D, Boyle E, Cote P, *et al.* Risk of vertebrobasilar stroke and chiropractic care: results of a population-based case-control and case-crossover study. *J Manipulative Physiol Ther*. 2009; **32**:S201–208.

40. Guillon B, Berthet K, Benslamia L, *et al.* Infection and the risk of spontaneous cervical artery dissection: a case-control study. *Stroke*. 2003; **34**:e79–81.

41. Cagnie B, Barbaix E, Vinck E, D'Herde K, Cambier D. Atherosclerosis in the vertebral artery: an intrinsic risk factor in the use of spinal manipulation? *Surg Radiol Anat*. 2006; **28**:129–34.

42. Pezzini A, Del Zotto E, Padovani A. Hyperhomocysteinemia: a potential risk factor for cervical artery dissection following chiropractic manipulation of the cervical spine. *J Neurol*. 2002; **249**: 1401–3.

43. Frisoni G B, Anzola G P. Neck manipulation and stroke. *Neurology*. 1990; **40**:1910.

Chapter 13

Stroke due to air and fat embolism

Fernando de M. Cardoso and Gabriel R. de Freitas

Introduction

Ischemic or hemorrhagic stroke secondary to embolism of fat or air into the central nervous system is, fortunately, a rare condition. In most cases, stroke due to fat embolism is not an iatrogenic disorder, since its main cause is traumatic bone fracture. However, it may also be caused by medical interventions, including surgical and non-surgical procedures. On the other hand, air embolism to the brain is often an iatrogenic situation secondary to surgery, especially neurosurgery. In this article, we discuss these different disorders separately.

Fat embolism

Introduction

Fat embolism is a condition where drops of fat occur in the lungs or other organ systems, including the brain [1]. The first animal model of fat embolism was described over 330 years ago by Lower. The first case of fat embolism in humans was described by Zenker in 1862, in a patient with multiple bone fractures following an accident [2].

There are a large number of causes of fat embolism, both traumatic and non-traumatic (Table 13.1). However, this condition is more frequent after fracture of a long bone, especially with multiple fractures. Nevertheless, the majority of patients who have a fracture and subsequent fat emboli do not present with symptoms. Only a small number of these patients develop a fat embolism syndrome (FES).

Fat embolism syndrome (FES) is the clinical manifestation of fat embolism, resulting in a systemic inflammatory reaction, mainly of the microvascular system of the lungs, skin, and brain. Thus FES produces cutaneous manifestations, respiratory involvement,

Table 13.1 Traumatic and non-traumatic causes of fat emboli.

Long-bone fractures
Surgical procedure: intramedullary nailing of the long bones, total or partial hip arthroplasty, knee arthroplasty, cardiac surgery, liposuction
Diabetes
Severe burns
Blood transfusion
Neoplasia
Liver injury
Closed-chest cardiac massage
Bone marrow transplantation
Parenteral lipid infusion
Decompression sickness
Extracorporeal circulation
Acute hemorrhagic pancreatitis
Prolonged corticosteroid therapy
Sickle cell disease and thalassemia
Carbon tetrachloride poisoning

and neurological symptoms [3]. This latter is called cerebral fat embolism syndrome (CFES).

The signs and symptoms of FES are variable and non-specific. The diagnosis is based on clinical suspicion aided by laboratory and radiological examinations. The mainstay of treatment for FES is supportive [4]. Therefore prevention and early diagnosis are essential [5]. It is a self-limited disease, with an overall mortality rate of 5 to 15% [6].

Epidemiology

Virtually all patients with long-bone fractures develop fat emboli. Transesophageal echocardiography can

---

Treatment-Related Stroke, ed. Alexander Tsiskaridze, Arne Lindgren and Adnan Qureshi. Published by Cambridge University Press. © Cambridge University Press 2016.

detect fat emboli in more than 90% of patients who have suffered long-bone fractures [7]. Circulating fat globules can be detected in the blood in 60 to 95% of patients with bone fractures after trauma [8,9].

However, the clinical manifestation of fat embolism is relatively uncommon. Although initial reports showed a high incidence of FES after trauma [2], over the past decades its relative incidence has declined because of better control of risk factors.

Trauma with fracture of long bones is the main condition associated with fat emboli, and therefore FES. The overall incidence of FES after long-bone fractures is estimated at between 0.9 and 11% [10–12].

Several factors influence the incidence of FES. Patients with multiple bone fractures are at higher risk of FES than are patients with a single bone fracture. In a study that included 274 patients with isolated femoral fractures, the incidence of FES was 4% [13]. In contrast, in a retrospective study of 19 patients who developed FES after trauma, 79% had multiple bone fractures [14].

Another variable is the anatomy of the involved bone. Fat embolism syndrome is more common after a fracture of the femur than of the tibia. The incidence of FES after fracture of the tibia or femur and multiple fractures in a study performed in Taiwan was 0.15%, 0.78%, and 2.4%, respectively [15].

A third factor is the timing of the surgery. Early intervention is associated with a lower risk of FES. In a study that included 11 patients with isolated femoral shaft fractures who developed FES, all of them had the surgery performed more than ten hours after the injury [13]. Other studies also suggested that early intervention might prevent FES [16,17].

Etiology

A large number of situations and diseases can be complicated by FES. Most commonly, FES develops after trauma with orthopedic injuries, particularly fractures of a long bone [18] or multiple fractures [1,19]. Traumatic spine injuries may also cause FES. One report described a cerebral fat embolism after a sacral fracture that drained into an unsuspected Tarlov cyst [20].

Some surgical procedures can produce fat embolism, especially intramedullary nailing of the long bones [21], total or partial hip arthroplasty [22–25], and knee arthroplasty [26–28]. Non-orthopedic surgeries may also result in FES. For instance, one report described three patients who developed FES after cardiac surgery [29]. This condition may also occur after liposuction [30,31].

Non-traumatic causes of FES include severe burns [32], diabetes, blood transfusion, neoplasia [33], liver injury, closed-chest cardiac massage, bone marrow transplantation, parenteral lipid infusion [34], decompression sickness, extracorporeal circulation, acute hemorrhagic pancreatitis [35,36], prolonged corticosteroid therapy, sickle cell disease [37], thalassemia [38], and carbon tetrachloride poisoning [19].

Pathogenesis

The pathogenesis of cerebral fat embolism is uncertain. Since the second decade of the twentieth century, two hypotheses, one mechanical and the other biochemical, have attempted to explain it [39]. The mechanical theory proposes that free fat particles from the medullary channel of long bones, in situations that increase intramedullary pressure, enter venous sinusoids. Thus the fat particles pass into the right side of the heart where they are propelled to the lung capillary bed [40]. Fat is then able to pass into the left side of the heart through a patent foramen ovale (PFO) or an arteriovenous anastomosis in the lung, where it is embolized to the end organs [41]. This phenomenon results in vascular occlusion, primarily in the lungs and other systemic vessels, including intracranial vessels [33]. This hypothesis explains the occurrence of FE and FES after trauma with long-bone fractures and procedures such as intramedullary nailing of the long bones [42].

According to the biochemical theory, in conditions of injury, hypoxia, or hypotension, hormonal changes increase the activity of lipoprotein lipase [30]. This enzyme induces an intravascular lipolysis with the release of free fatty acids (FFAs), as chylomicrons. Free fatty acids are toxic to the pneumocytes, and produce a leukocyte-mediated inflammatory reaction, with complement activation, which leads to direct endothelial damage [43]. Coalescence of chylomicrons with platelets, blocking small capillaries, also occurs. This hypothesis accounts for the incidence of cerebral fat embolism following non-fracture pathology sepsis, burns, and pancreatitis [36]. Importantly, the mechanical and biochemical theories are not necessarily independent of each other, and these mechanisms may act simultaneously [33].

Clinical features

Fat embolism syndrome is a multisystem disorder. The lungs, skin, and brain are the organs that are most often affected. The classic triad of the FES is respiratory distress, cutaneous manifestations, and neurological symptoms [44]. However, other structures can also be damaged, such as the heart and eyes [19,45].

This syndrome develops 12 to 72 hours after injury or surgery, in the case of trauma. However, development of FES after this period of time has also been reported [46].

Neurological manifestations are common in FES, occurring in 56 to 100% of cases [40]. In one study, encephalopathy was reported in 59% of patients with FES [10]. Cerebral microembolism can be detected with transcranial Doppler (TCD) and transesophageal echocardiography (TEE) in more than 50% of patients during orthopedic surgery [47,48]. Cerebral fat embolism syndrome usually precedes respiratory involvement [49,50].

The symptoms are variable and non-specific, and include headache, seizures, confusion, somnolence, delirium, hallucinations, coma, and focal neurological signs such as paresis, apraxia, conjugate eye deviation, and pupillary involvement [51–53]. Cerebral fat embolism syndrome may be present without pulmonary and cutaneous involvement [54,55,18]. Cerebral fat embolism syndrome must be considered in all patients who are victims of trauma or surgery, and who develop coma or impairment of consciousness [56].

In a review of 12 patients with CFES [55], all developed encephalopathy with mental state disturbances such as confusion, visual hallucinations, or stupor. Four patients, besides impairment of the level of consciousness, showed focal neurological signs including motor deficits, aphasia, and pupillary abnormalities. The authors suggested that patients with focal signs and symptoms have more fulminant systemic disorder.

The respiratory symptoms are dyspnea, tachypnea, hypoxemia, and cyanosis. Approximately 10% of patients develop acute respiratory distress syndrome, with the need for ventilator support [57].

Petechial rash is present in 20 to 50% of cases. The rashes are more frequent in the superior and anterior parts of body, such as the upper limbs, and the oral mucous membranes and conjunctivae [42].

Table 13.2 Gurd criteria for diagnosis of fat embolism syndrome.

Major criteria
Axillary or subconjunctival petechia
Hypoxemia (PaO$_2$ <60 mmHg, FiO$_2$ <0.4)
Central nervous system depression disproportionate to hypoxemia, and pulmonary edema

Minor criteria
Tachycardia (>110 beats/min)
Pyrexia (>38.5°C)
Emboli in the retina on fundoscopic examination
Fat present in urine
Sudden unexplained drop in hematocrit or platelet levels
Increasing erythrocyte sedimentation rate
Fat globules in the sputum
Symptoms within 72 h of skeletal trauma
Shortness of breath
Altered mental status
Occasional long tract signs and posturing
Urinary incontinence

PaO$_2$: partial oxygen tension in blood; FiO$_2$: inspired fraction of oxygen

Diagnosis

The diagnosis of FE and FES may be difficult because the signs and symptoms are variable and non-specific, and only a few confirmatory laboratory and radiological examinations are conducted [58].

The first diagnostic criteria were proposed in 1970 by Gurd [59]. These criteria included the presence of clinical manifestations and laboratory abnormalities, which were divided into major and minor criteria (Table 13.2). The diagnosis of FES required at least two major symptoms or signs, or one major and four minor symptoms with fat macroglobulinemia.

In 1974 the diagnostic criteria for FES were refined, but the presence of at least two major criteria, or one major and four minor criteria were still required to diagnose the syndrome [8] (Table 13.3).

Other diagnostic systems can be used to help to perform the diagnosis [60,61]. An objective diagnostic

Table 13.3 Gurd and Wilson criteria for diagnosis of fat embolism syndrome.

Major criteria
Major criteria
Respiratory insufficiency
Cerebral involvement
Petechial rash
Minor criteria
Pyrexia (usually <39°C)
Tachycardia (>120 beats/min)
Retinal changes (fat or petechiae)
Jaundice
Renal changes (anuria or oliguria)
Anemia (a drop of more than 20% of the admission hemoglobin value)
Thrombocytopenia (a drop of >50% of the admission thrombocyte value)
High erythrocyte sedimentation rate (ESR >71 mm/h)
Fat macroglobulinemia

ESR: erythrocyte sedimentation rate

Table 13.5 Lindeque criteria for diagnosis of fat embolism syndrome.

A sustained PaO_2 of less than 8 kPa (FiO_2 0.21)
A sustained $PaCO_2$ of more than 7.3 kPa or pH of less than 7.3
A sustained respiratory rate of greater than 35 breaths/min even after adequate sedation
Increased work of breathing judged by dyspnea, use of accessory muscles, tachycardia, and anxiety

FiO_2: inspired fraction of oxygen; PaO_2: partial oxygen tension; $PaCO_2$: partial carbon dioxide tension

Table 13.4 Shonfeld criteria for diagnosis of fat embolism syndrome.

Clinical features	Score
Diffuse petechiae	5
Alveolar infiltrates	4
Hypoxemia (<70 mmHg)	3
Confusion	1
Fever >38°C	1
Heart rate >120/min	1
Respiratory rate >30/min	1

element is sufficient to establish the diagnosis. However, these criteria are not useful in diagnosing CFES, because these elements can be present without cerebral involvement.

Anemia, thrombocytopenia, hypofibrinogenemia, hypoxemia, hypoalbuminemia, hypocalcemia, and increased erythrocyte sedimentation are seen in FES and CFES [19]. Levels of serum lipase and phospholipase A2 rise in FE-related lung injury [64].

Fat globules may be detected in blood, urine, and sputum, but such a test is not sensitive [65], and fat globules may be seen in patients with FE but without signs and symptoms of CFES.

A chest radiography shows multiple bilateral patchy areas of consolidation, typically in the middle and upper zones [66]. Macrophages can be seen in samples obtained by bronchoscopy and bronchoalveolar lavage (BAL), especially in trauma patients [67].

Transcranial Doppler is able to detect fat particles in the vasculature in a non-invasive manner, and allows the diagnosis of right-to-left shunts (RLS) with high sensitivity in patients with gaseous emboli [68]. Transesophageal echocardiography is the gold-standard method for RLS detection; however, TCD is a non-invasive procedure and is equally as sensitive as TEE for the diagnosis of RLS [69]. The presence of an RLS detected by TCD may predict which patients will develop neurological dysfunction, indicating that paradoxical embolism is a potential participant in CFES [70].

Brain computed tomography (CT) and magnetic resonance imaging (MRI) are important tools for the diagnosis of CFES. Frequently a brain CT is normal in the acute stage [71]. In some patients it is possible to find diffuse edema, multiple low-density areas in the white matter [72,73], or hemorrhage [74]. The MRI is

criterion was created to evaluate the efficacy of corticosteroid treatment in the prophylaxis of the fat embolism syndrome in 62 patients [62]. This was a score system based on clinical picture (Table 13.4). A score higher than 5 was necessary for the diagnosis of FES.

There is a set of criteria based on respiratory parameters in patients with fracture of the tibia and/or femur [63] (Table 13.5). The presence of a single the method of choice for detecting a cerebral fat embolism, and is more sensitive than CT [75]. In the acute stages, diffusion-weighted MR imaging (DWI) has an important impact on the diagnosis because it can detect abnormalities before other methods such as T2-, fluid attenuated inversion recovery (FLAIR), and T1-weighted MRI [76,77]. Multiple areas of increased signal intensity in the cerebral white matter, causing a "starfield" pattern, are seen in DWI [78]. The presence of numerous restricted DWI lesions may be associated with poor outcomes [79]. Other MRI abnormalities include hyperintensities on T2- and FLAIR-weighted sequences, and hypointensities on T1-weighted MRI at the rostrum, splenium of the corpus callosum, subcortical white matter, basal ganglia, centrum semiovale, thalamus, brain stem, and cerebellum [33,80–82]. Enhancement of contrast-enhanced T1-weighted images is occasionally done to establish the presence of a rupture of the blood–brain barrier [83]. A follow-up MRI can show hypointensities on T2*-weighted gradient-echo MRI, reflecting the hemorrhagic features of the fat embolism, which may be associated with a poorer recovery [84].

Treatment

Currently, there is no specific treatment for CFES and FES. The mainstream therapies are prevention and supportive care [21,85], usually in an intensive care unit. Hypotension and hypoxia must be treated aggressively [5]. Some data suggest that fluid resuscitation with albumin solutions may be beneficial because albumin can bind with FFAs, thereby reducing the inflammatory reaction [19]. Dextran-40 may be used as well because it reduces platelet adhesion, reverses thrombocytopenia, and decreases cell aggregation. Respiratory distress should be managed appropriately, sometimes with mechanical ventilation to ensure protection of the airway and to maintain a normal oxygenation level (PO_2 >90 mmHg) [26,30].

The use of steroids in FES has been studied. A prospective randomized trial of prophylactic therapy using steroids or hypertonic glucose in 64 patients with femoral and/or tibial shaft fractures showed that none of the patients in the group that used methylprednisolone developed FES, vs. three in the group that used hypertonic glucose [86]. The authors concluded that methylprednisolone given prophylactically may reduce the incidence of FES

and can reduce the degree of hypoxemia. Similar results were reported in other trials [87]. However, it is important to emphasize that the sample sizes in these studies were small. A meta-analysis including seven trials indicated that the prophylactic use of steroids may prevent FES (relative risk 0.22, 95% confidence interval 43%–92%), especially in patients with multiple and long-bone fractures; but the analysis also found no differences in mortality [88]. Therefore the use of steroids remains controversial. Randomized clinical trials with larger sample sizes and better quality are necessary to establish the usefulness of steroids in FES.

Another pharmacological drug that can, at least theoretically, be beneficial in FES is heparin, because of its capacity to increase lipase activity and therefore decrease the pool of fat globules in the blood [39]. However, no controlled trials have been conducted to verify this benefit. Moreover, since patients who are at high risk for developing FES already have trauma, it may be dangerous to use heparin because of the possibility of bleeding.

There are no definitive data on the use of other drugs, including aspirin, alcohol solutions, and clofibrate, in the treatment of FES [19].

Because the treatment of FES and CFES is supportive, preventive measures are essential. In posttraumatic cases, with bone fractures, early fixation of the fractures may minimize the risk of FES [13,17]. An evaluation of the records of 132 patients found that a delay in orthopedic surgery (longer than 24 hours) was associated with a five-fold increase in the incidence of respiratory distress [89]. Insufficient data are available to determine which surgical techniques can better prevent FES and CFES [90].

Air gas embolism

Introduction

Air gas embolism (AGE) is the entry of gas into vascular structures (venous or arterial systems) [91] or the production of air bubbles in circulation due to dysbaric barotraumas [92]. Air gas embolism (AGE) is a rare condition, but is highly lethal if it is not recognized promptly and treated appropriately [93].

The true incidence of AGE is unknown, because most cases are asymptomatic [94]. This condition is almost always iatrogenic, most often resulting from surgical procedures [95]. Other procedures, such as upper endoscopy, may also cause AGE [96].

Table 13.6 Surgeries associated with air embolism.

Neurosurgical:
- sitting position craniotomies
- posterior fossa procedures
- cervical laminectomy

Neck procedures:
- radical neck dissection
- thyroidectomy

Ophthalmologic procedures

Cardiac surgery

Orthopedic procedures:
- total hip arthroplasty
- arthroscopy

Thoracic procedures:
- thoracocentesis
- excessive positive pressure, open chest wounds

Obstetrical–gynecological procedures:
- cesarean section
- laparoscopic procedures, Rubin insufflation procedures, vacuum abortion

Urology:
- prostatectomy

Gastrointestinal surgery:
- laparoscopic cholecystectomy
- liver transplantation

Table 13.7 Non-surgical conditions associated with air embolism.

Cranioencephalic trauma

Thoracic trauma

Cardiopulmonary resuscitation

Atrial–esophageal fistula

Pulmonary overpressurization syndrome or decompression illness

Upper gastrointestinal endoscopy

Central venous access accidents

Respiratory, cardiovascular, and neurological symptoms are the clinical manifestations of AGE [97]. The diagnosis can be challenging because there are no specific clinical features [94]. Initial treatment is direct, to maintain the vital signs and hemodynamic status. Hyperbaric oxygen therapy is considered the first-line therapy for systemic air embolism [98].

Epidemiology and etiology

Since most cases of AGE are subclinical, it is difficult to estimate its real incidence. It may occur after surgical or non-surgical procedures (Tables 13.6 and 13.7). It is important to recognize some factors that increase the risk of AGE, for example, surgeries performed in the sitting position, such as craniotomy [99]. Using TEE, AGE was diagnosed in 76% of all posterior fossa operations and in 25% of cervical laminectomies [100].

Air gas embolism may develop after other surgical procedures besides neurosurgery. Orthopedic procedures such as arthroscopy and hip arthroplasty are potential causes of AGE [101]. In one study, venous gas embolism was detected during total hip arthroplasty by Doppler ultrasound in 57% of patients, and 43% had hemodynamic abnormalities [102].

Obstetric–gynecological procedures are considered high-risk surgeries for the occurrence of AGE. The incidence of air embolism after a cesarean section ranged from 11 to 56%; however, one study reported an incidence of 97% [103]. Hysteroscopy may result in AGE as well [104].

Other surgical procedures that may result in AEG are: neck [105], ophthalmological [106], vascular [107], cardiac [108], thoracic [109–111], urological [112,113], and gastrointestinal surgeries [114–117].

Air gas embolism may also occur when there is a communication between the esophagus and the atrium. It may be caused by an accident after catheter ablation for atrial fibrillation secondary to esophageal ulceration [118], or in patients with pre-existing esophageal disease [119].

Cranioencephalic trauma may also result in the entry of air gases into the brain and cerebral vessels, especially when there are fractures involving the paranasal sinuses [120]. Air gas may enter venous systems through a central venous line [121,122] and can occur during cannulization, or the use of a catheter, or after its removal [123,124]. Trauma of the thoracic region, especially with blunt or penetrating injuries, is an important cause of AGE in modern society [125,126]. Cardiopulmonary resuscitation may also result in AGE [127,128].

Arterial or venous air embolism can also be part of the pulmonary overpressurization syndrome, or a decompression illness resulting in bubble formation from dissolved gas or overexpansion of air-filled cavities with secondary arterialization of gas bubbles [129]. These bubbles enter the bloodstream and form true emboli that can occlude arterial vessels [130].

Pathogenesis

For air gas to enter the vascular system (venous or arterial), it is necessary to have communication between an air source (i.e., the atmosphere) and the vasculature, as well as a pressure gradient favoring passage of air into the circulatory system [131].

When the air gas enters the venous system, it passes into the right atrium and then into the right ventricle. The amount of air is important for the consequences of AGE, because large volumes of air may obstruct the pulmonary outflow, resulting in elevated pressures in the right ventricle and atrium, and obstructing the venous return to the heart [132]. There are no data in humans regarding the exact amount of air volume that is necessary for a lethal outcome, but the volume is estimated to range from 200 to 300 ml [133].

The air gas may enter the arterial system when inoculated directly into the arterial vessel or through a communication between the pulmonary and systemic circulations, such as a PFO or pulmonary arteriovenous anastomoses. The emboli may reach the brain circulation and obstruct small arteries. In addition to this occlusive mechanism, an inflammatory response to the bubble occurs, with an increase in microvascular permeability, platelet aggregation, and the release of plasminogen activator inhibitor and endothelin-1 [131].

In the pulmonary overpressurization syndrome or a decompression illness, the sum of the dissolved-gas tensions and water vapor exceeds the local absolute pressure, resulting in the formation of intravascular and extravascular bubbles. These produce pulmonary barotrauma, resulting in impairment of pulmonary capillaries and allowing air gas to enter the arterial circulation [134].

Clinical features

The symptoms of AGE are various, and are dependent on several factors such as the nature of the vascular structure where the gas enters (artery or vein), the rate and absolute quantity of gas that enters the vessels, the area of the organ that is affected, especially the brain [91], and whether the patient is spontaneously breathing (negative thoracic pressure) or is under mechanical ventilation (positive pressure) [95].

Venous air embolisms are usually asymptomatic, but may result in respiratory and cardiac manifestations. Neurological symptoms are unusual. The air gases are directed to the pulmonary circulation. When the amount of gas is high and the rate of entry is fast, the pressure increases in the right atrium and, consequently, in the pulmonary artery, resulting in symptoms such as tachypnea, dyspnea, cyanosis, chest pain, and hypoxia [93]. Tachyarrhythmias are frequent. In severe cases, cardiac output decreases and cardiovascular collapse may occur.

Arterial air embolism produces sudden symptoms. Neurological manifestations are due to direct air embolism or a cardiovascular collapse with cerebral hypoperfusion, and include headache, seizures [93], focal neurological motor deficits [109], aphasia [135], and impairment of consciousness [136] with possible confusion, agitation, hallucinations, stupor, and coma [107]. Two types of neurological manifestations are reported in patients with cerebral air embolism: encephalopathic features, with a high mortality rate; and focal cerebral lesions, resulting in hemiparesis or hemianopia, affecting mostly the right hemisphere [137]. Cerebral air gas embolism (CAGE) must be suspected when a patient submitted to a surgical procedure associated with vascular air embolism develops altered mental status or delayed recovery of consciousness after the surgery. Respiratory and cardiovascular symptoms are usually present. Hemoptysis [138], tachypnea, dyspnea, cyanosis, chest pain, hypoxia, arrhythmia, and circulatory collapse are present at different stages [139,140]. Rarely, acute pulmonary edema may develop [141].

Diagnosis

The diagnosis of AGE is challenging because there are no specific clinical features of this syndrome. Moreover, rapid diagnosis is critical for appropriate treatment. The clinical suspicion must be established by the emergence of neurological, respiratory, and cardiovascular symptoms in a close temporal relationship to a high-risk procedure [91] or event (thoracic trauma, manipulations of central line venous catheter, diving).

Once suspected of CAGE, an image of the brain must be taken. Computed tomography scanning of the brain may reveal air bubbles (negative-density areas) at various sites in the brain such as the convexity, inside venous and arterial vessels, or in subarachnoid spaces [142,143]. Cerebral edema is

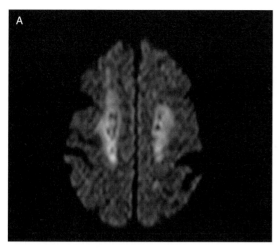 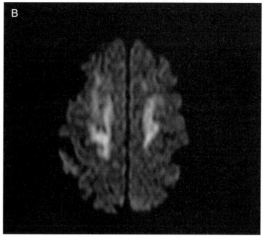

Figure 13.1 A 72-year-old woman developed coma a few hours after the performance of catheter ablation for atrial fibrillation. The diagnosis of arterial gas embolism due to an atrial–esophageal fistula was made. (A) and (B) The diffusion-weighted sequences of brain magnetic resonance imaging show bilateral, diffuse ischemic lesions on different brain slices.

common. Importantly, sometimes the pathological abnormalities are subtle and a CT scan may not show any images of AGE [91]. Cranial MRI may reveal small collections of gas within the brain and vessels [144]. Hyperintense lesions corresponding to ischemic lesions can also be detected on diffusion-weighted MRI[145] (Figure 13.1). In one report that evaluated seven cases of CAGE after diving accidents, using MRI, the lesions were large and multiple, affecting both the cortical and subcortical regions, and predominantly in the frontal and parietal lobes [146].

CAGE may be detected by using TEE or TCD to demonstrate the presence of air bubbles in the right ventricle, as well as the occurrence of PFO [147,148]. These methods are able to show micro- and macro-emboli and paradoxical arterial embolization. However, there is a concern about the possibility of AGE after a TCD or TEE "bubble test" for identification of right–left shunts. Literature sources report the occurrence of ischemic cerebrovascular complications, such as transient ischemic attacks and strokes, in patients who undergo a "bubble test" through TEE or TCD [149]. A large international multicenter study used TCD with a "bubble test" to evaluate 508 patients with acute cerebral ischemia, and identified no ischemic cerebrovascular complications, during or after TCD, showing that this method is safe [150].

Treatment

The initial therapy for AGE consists of maintenance of vital signs and respiratory protection. When there

is an evident point of entry of air, this location must be identified and treated to reduce the rate and volume, and prevent more air from entering.

It is recommended to place the patient in a partial left-lateral decubitus position ("Durant's maneuver") or in the Trendelenburg position if the patient is hemo-dynamically unstable [151], to relieve the air-lock in the right side of the heart. However, studies in animal models do not confirm the value of this strategy. In one study of induced ACE in dogs, the authors found no differences among various body positions and hemo-dynamic parameters [152]. No corresponding studies have been carried out in humans.

Oxygen should be administered in high concentrations to treat hypoxia, and to enhance washout of inert gas from the tissue and eliminate the gas in the bubbles, thus reducing the embolus volume [91].

Along with appropriate body positioning and administration of 100% oxygen, another method that may help in removing air from the right heart is aspiration of air from the right atrium, using special catheters [153,154]. Currently, no data exist to support the insertion of a catheter for air aspiration during an acute AGE.

Hyperbaric-oxygen therapy (HBO) is recommended for the treatment of AGE, for which it is considered a specific therapy [155]. In HBO a patient breathes 100% oxygen while inside a special treatment chamber [156]. The aim of HBO therapy is to increase the amount of oxygen in the plasma, and therefore to increase oxygen tension throughout the veins and arteries [157]. According to Boyle's Law, the high oxygen pressure will reduce the volume of gas and consequently of the bubbles, relieving the obstruction and restoring perfusion [158]. Hyperbaric-oxygen therapy may also raise the nitrogen partial-pressure gradient between the bubble and the surrounding tissue by eliminating the inspired nitrogen, reducing the volume of bubbles [159]. Another positive effect of HBO therapy is a decrease of edema and tissue swelling by a vaconstriction mechanism, and reduction of the permeability of blood vessels [156]. Once the diagnosis of AGE is made and the patient is stabilized, HBO therapy should be performed promptly; a delay in therapy may result in a worse outcome. In a retrospective study that evaluated 86 patients with AGE who received HBO therapy, patients treated within six hours had better outcomes [160].

Studies in animals suggest that lidocaine has a neuroprotective effect, through a reduction of the delayed deterioration of the amplitude of the somatosensory evoked potential when administered prophylactically or after an induced AGE, especially when performed in conjunction with HBO therapy [161,162]. No clinical trials have evaluated the use of lidocaine in humans in AGE. Recent data do not show a neuroprotective effect with the use of lidocaine [163].

Corticosteroids are recommended by some investigators for the treatment of decompression accidents [164]. However, in arterial or venous embolism secondary to other etiologies, their use remains controversial. Studies in animals suggest that the prophylactic use of dexamethasone may be beneficial [165].

Anticoagulant therapy with non-fractionated heparin has been studied in animals with induced AGE, due to the anti-inflammatory effect. In rabbits, a better neurological recovery was reported when this therapy was administered prophylactically [166]. However, the main concern is hemorrhagic transformation of ischemic lesions, and no data exist to support the use of heparin in AGE.

References

1. Scott A A, Welsh R P. Fat embolism: A rational approach to treatment. *Can Med Assoc J.* 1973; **109**(9): 867–71.

2. Talbot M, Schemitsch E H. Fat embolism syndrome: History, definition, epidemiology. *Injury.* 2006; **37**(Suppl 4):S3–S7.

3. Klingele K, Bhalla T, Sawardekar A, Tobias J D. Postoperative hypoxemia due to fat embolism. *Saudi J Anaesth.* 2011; **5**(3):332–4.

4. Weisz G M, Barzilai A. Fat embolism: Physiopathology, diagnosis with management. *Arch Orthop Unfall-Chir.* 1975; **82**(3):217–23.

5. Habashi N M, Andrews P L, Scalea T M. Therapeutic aspects of fat embolism syndrome. *Injury.* 2006; **37**(Suppl 4):S68–S73.

6. Fulde G W, Harrison P. Fat embolism: A review. *Arch Emerg Med.* 1991; **8**(4):233–9.

7. Christie J, Robinson C M, Pell A C, McBirnie J, Burnett R. Transcardiac echocardiography during invasive intramedullary procedures. *J Bone Joint Surg Br.* 1995; **77**(3):450–5.

8. Gurd A R, Wilson R I. The fat embolism syndrome. *J Bone Joint Surg Br.* 1974; **56B**(3):408–16.

9. Allardyce D B, Meek R N, Woodruff B, Cassim M M, Ellis D. Increasing our knowledge of the pathogenesis of fat embolism: A prospective study of 43 patients with fractured femoral shafts. *J Trauma.* 1974; **14**(11): 955–62.

10. Bulger E M, Smith D G, Maier R V, Jurkovich G J. Fat embolism syndrome. A 10-year review. *Arch Surg.* 1997; **132**(4):435–9.

11. Fabian T C, Hoots A V, Stanford D S, Patterson C R, Mangiante E C. Fat embolism syndrome: Prospective evaluation in 92 fracture patients. *Crit Care Med.* 1990; **18**(1):42–6.

12. Robert J H, Hoffmeyer P, Broquet P E, Cerutti P, Vasey H. Fat embolism syndrome. *Orthop Rev.* 1993; **22**(5):567–71.

13. Pinney S J, Keating J F, Meek R N. Fat embolism syndrome in isolated femoral fractures: Does timing of nailing influence incidence? *Injury.* 1998; **29**(2):131–3.

14. Campo-López C, Flors-Villaverde P, Calabuig-Alborch J R. Fat embolism syndrome after bone fractures. *Rev Clin Esp.* 2012; **212**(10):482–7.

15. Tsai I T, Hsu C J, Chen Y H, *et al.* Fat embolism syndrome in long bone fracture–clinical experience in a tertiary referral center in Taiwan. *J Chin Med Assoc.* 2010; **73**(8):407–10.

16. Talucci R C, Manning J, Lampard S, Bach A, Carrico C J. Early intramedullary nailing of femoral shaft fractures: A cause of fat embolism syndrome. *Am J Surg.* 1983; **146**(1):107–11.

17. Bone L B, Johnson K D, Weigelt J, Scheinberg R. Early versus delayed stabilization of femoral fractures. A prospective randomized study. *J Bone Joint Surg Am.* 1989; **71**(3):336–40.

18. Findlay J M, DeMajo W. Cerebral fat embolism. *Can Med Assoc J.* 1984; **131**(7):755–7.

19. Taviloglu K, Yanar H. Fat embolism syndrome. *Surg Today.* 2007; **37**(1):5–8.

20. Duja C M, Berna C, Kremer S, *et al.* Confusion after spine injury: Cerebral fat embolism after traumatic

rupture of a Tarlov cyst: Case report. *BMC Emerg Med.* 2010; **10**:18.

21. Powers K A, Talbot L A. Case report: Fat embolism syndrome after femur fracture with intramedullary nailing. *Am J Crit Care.* 2011; **20**:264–6.

22. Thienpont E, Kaddar S, Morrison S. Paradoxical fat embolism after uncemented total hip arthroplasty: A case report. *Acta Orthop Belg.* 2007; **73**(3):418–20.

23. Sasano N, Ishida S, Tetsu S, *et al.* Cerebral fat embolism diagnosed by magnetic resonance imaging at one, eight, and 50 days after hip arthroplasty: A case report. *Can J Anaesth.* 2004; **51**(9):875–987.

24. Rodriguez-Merchan E C, Comin-Gomez J A, Martinez-Chacon J L. Cerebral embolism during revision arthroplasty of the hip. *Acta Orthop Belg.* 1995; **61**(4):319–22.

25. Ammon J T, Khalily C, Lester D K. Fatal cerebral emboli in the absence of a cardiac arterial-venous shunt: Case report. *J Arthroplasty.* 2007; **22**(3): 477–9.

26. Chang R N, Kim J H, Lee H, *et al.* Cerebral fat embolism after bilateral total knee replacement arthroplasty: A case report. *Korean J Anesthesiol.* 2010; **59** Suppl:S207–S210.

27. Jenkins K, Chung F, Wennberg R, Etchells E E, Davey R. Fat embolism syndrome and elective knee arthroplasty. *Can J Anaesth.* 2002; **49**(1):19–24.

28. Lee S C, Yoon J Y, Nam C H, *et al.* Cerebral fat embolism syndrome after simultaneous bilateral total knee arthroplasty: A case series. *J Arthroplasty.* 2012; **27**(3):409–14.

29. Ghatak N R, Sinnenberg R J, deBlois G G. Cerebral fat embolism following cardiac surgery. *Stroke.* 1983; **14**(4):619–21.

30. Wang H D, Zheng J H, Deng C L, Liu Q Y, Yang S L. Fat embolism syndromes following liposuction. *Aesthetic Plast Surg.* 2008; **32**(5):731–6.

31. Laub D R Jr. Fat embolism syndrome after liposuction: A case report and review of the literature. *Ann Plast Surg.* 1990; **25**(1):48–52.

32. Richards R R. Fat embolism syndrome. *Can J Surg.* 1997; **40**(5):334–9.

33. Mossa-Basha M, Izbudak I, Gurda G T, Aygun N. Cerebral fat embolism syndrome in sickle cell anaemia/β-thalassemia: Importance of susceptibility-weighted MRI. *Clin Radiol.* 2012; **67**(10):1023–6.

34. Barson A J, Chistwick M L, Doig C M. Fat embolism in infancy after intravenous fat infusions. *Arch Dis Child.* 1978; **53**(3):218–23.

35. Bhalla A, Sachdev A, Lehl S S, Singh R, D'Cruz S. Cerebral fat embolism as a rare possible complication of traumatic pancreatitis. *JOP.* 2003; **4**(4):155–7.

36. Guardia S N, Bilbao J M, Murray D, Warren R E, Sweet J. Fat embolism in acute pancreatitis. *Arch Pathol Lab Med.* 1989; **113**:503–6.

37. Dang N C, Johnson C, Eslami-Farsani M, Haywood L J. Bone marrow embolism in sickle cell disease: A review. *Am J Hematol.* 2005; **79**(1):61–7.

38. Desselle B C, O'Brien T, Bugnitz M, *et al.* Fatal fat embolism in a patient with sickle-beta+ thalassemia. *Pediatr Hematol Oncol.* 1995; **12**(2):159–62.

39. ten Duis H J. The fat embolism syndrome. *Injury.* 1997; **28**(2):77–85.

40. Cox G, Tzioupis C, Calori G M, *et al.* Cerebral fat emboli: A trigger of post-operative delirium. *Injury.* 2011; **42**(S4):S6–S10.

41. Etchells E E, Wong D T, Davidson G, Houston P L. Fatal cerebral fat embolism associated with a patent foramen ovale. *Chest.* 1993; **104**(3):962–3.

42. Gossling H R, Pellegrini V D Jr. Fat embolism syndrome: A review of the pathophysiology and physiological basis of treatment. *Clin Orthop Relat Res.* 1982; **165**:68–82.

43. Butteriss D J, Mahad D, Soh C, *et al.* Reversible cytotoxic cerebral edema in cerebral fat embolism. *Am J Neuroradiol.* 2006; **27**(3):620–3.

44. Parisi D M, Koval K, Egol K. Fat embolism syndrome. *Am J Orthop.* 2002; **31**(9):507–12.

45. Adams C B. The retinal manifestations of fat embolism. *Injury.* 1971; **2**(3):221–4.

46. Murray D G, Racz G B. Fat embolism syndrome (respiratory insufficiency syndrome). A rationale for treatment. *J Bone Joint Surg.* 1974; **56**(7):1338–49.

47. Koch S, Forteza A, Lavernia C, *et al.* Cerebral fat microembolism and cognitive decline after hip and knee replacement. *Stroke.* 2007; **38**(3):1079–81.

48. Sulek C A, Davies L K, Enneking F K, Gearen P A, Lobato E B. Cerebral microembolism diagnosed by transcranial Doppler during total knee arthroplasty: Correlation with transesophageal echocardiography. *Anesthesiology.* 1999; **91**(3):672–6.

49. Van Besouw J P, Hinds C J. Fat embolism syndrome. *Br J Hosp Med.* 1989; **42**(4):304–6.

50. Finlay M E, Benson M D. Case report: Magnetic resonance imaging in cerebral fat embolism. *Clin Radiol.* 1996; **51**(6):445–6.

51. Gombar S, Dey N, Deva C. Pupillary signs in fat embolism syndrome. *Acta Anaesthesiol Scand.* 2005; **49**(5):723.

52. Manousakis G, Han D Y, Backonja M. Cognitive outcome of cerebral fat embolism. *J Stroke Cerebrovasc Dis.* 2012; **21**(8):906–8.

53. Thomas J E, Ayyar D R. Systemic fat embolism. A diagnostic profile in 24 patients. *Arch Neurol.* 1972; **26**(6):517–23.

54. Bardana D, Rudan J, Cervenko F, Smith R. Fat embolism syndrome in a patient demonstrating only neurologic symptoms. *Can J Surg.* 1998; **41**(5):398–402.

55. Jacobson D M, Terrence C F, Reinmuth O M. The neurologic manifestations of fat embolism. *Neurology.* 1986; **36**:847–51.

56. Metting Z, Rödiger L A, Regtien J G, van der Naalt J. Delayed coma in head injury: consider cerebral fat embolism. *Clin Neurol Neurosurg.* 2009; **111**(7):597–600.

57. Johnson M J, Lucas G L. Fat embolism syndrome. *Orthopedics.* 1996; **19**(1):41–8.

58. Oh W H, Mital M A. Fat embolism: Current concepts of pathogenesis, diagnosis, and treatment. *Orthop Clin North Am.* 1978; **9**(3):769–79.

59. Gurd A R. Fat embolism: An aid to diagnosis. *J Bone Joint Surg Br.* 1970; **52**(4):732–7.

60. Vedrinne J M, Guillaume C, Gagnieu M C, et al. Bronchoalveolar lavage in trauma patients for diagnosis of fat embolism syndrome. *Chest.* 1992; **102**(5):1323–7.

61. Weisz G M, Rang M, Salter R B. Posttraumatic fat embolism in children: Review of the literature and of experience in the Hospital for Sick Children, Toronto. *J Trauma.* 1973; **13**(6):529–34.

62. Schonfeld S A, Ploysongsang Y, DiLisio R, et al. Fat embolism prophylaxis with corticosteroids. A prospective study in high-risk patients. *Ann Intern Med.* 1983; **99**(4):438–43.

63. Lindeque B G, Schoeman H S, Dommisse G F, Boeyens M C, Vlok A L. Fat embolism and the fat embolism syndrome. A double-blind therapeutic study. *J Bone Joint Surg Br.* 1987; **69**(1):128–31.

64. Mellor A, Soni N. Fat embolism. *Anaesthesia.* 2001; **56**(2):145–54.

65. Shaikh N. Emergency management of fat embolism syndrome. *J Emerg Trauma Shock.* 2009; **2**(1):29–33.

66. Costa A N, Mendes D M, Toufen C, et al. Adult respiratory distress syndrome due to fat embolism in the postoperative period following liposuction and fat grafting. *J Bras Pneumol.* 2008; **34**(8):622–5.

67. Chastre J, Fagon J Y, Soler P, et al. Bronchoalveolar lavage for rapid diagnosis of the fat embolism syndrome in trauma patients. *Ann Intern Med.* 1990; **113**(8):583–8.

68. Forteza A M, Koch S, Romano J G, et al. Transcranial Doppler detection of fat emboli. *Stroke.* 1999; **30**(12):2687–91.

69. Belvis R, Leta R G, Marti-Fabregas J, et al. Almost perfect concordance between simultaneous transcranial Doppler and transesophageal echocardiography in the quantification of right-to-left shunts. *J Neuroimaging.* 2006; **16**(2):133–8.

70. Forteza A M, Koch S, Campo-Bustillo I, et al. Transcranial Doppler detection of cerebral fat emboli and relation to paradoxical embolism: A pilot study. *Circulation.* 2011; **123**(18):1947–52.

71. Gupta B, Kaur M, d'Souza N, et al. Cerebral fat embolism: A diagnostic challenge. *Saudi J Anaesth.* 2011; **5**(3):348–52.

72. Salazar J A, Romero F, Padilla F, Arboleda J A, Fernández O. Neurological manifestations of fat embolism syndrome. *Neurologia.* 1995; **10**(2):65–9.

73. Sakamoto T, Sawada Y, Yukioka T, et al. Computed tomography for diagnosis and assessment of cerebral fat embolism. *Neuroradiology.* 1983; **24**(5):283–5.

74. Beers G J, Nichols G R, Willing S J. CT demonstration of fat-embolism-associated hemorrhage in the anterior commissure. *Am J Neuroradiol.* 1988; **9**(1):212–13.

75. Stoeger A, Daniaux M, Felber S, et al. MRI findings in cerebral fat embolism. *Eur Radiol.* 1998; **8**(9):1590–93.

76. Marshall G B, Heale V R, Herx L, et al. Magnetic resonance diffusion weighted imaging in cerebral fat embolism. *Can J Neurol Sci.* 2004; **31**(3):417–21.

77. Ryu C W, Lee D H, Kim T K, et al. Cerebral fat embolism: Diffusion-weighted magnetic resonance imaging findings. *Acta Radiol.* 2005; **46**(5):528–33.

78. Aravapalli A, Fox J, Lazaridis C. Cerebral fat embolism and the 'starfield' pattern: A case report. *Cases J.* 2009; **2**:212–14.

79. Pfeffer G, Heran M K. Restricted diffusion and poor clinical outcome in cerebral fat embolism syndrome. *Can J Neurol Sci.* 2010; **37**(1):128–30.

80. Buskens C J, Gratama J W, Hogervorst M, et al. Encephalopathy and MRI abnormalities in fat embolism syndrome: A case report. *Med Sci Monit.* 2008; **14**(11):CS125–129.

81. Citerio G, Bianchini E, Beretta L. Magnetic resonance imaging of cerebral fat embolism: A case report. *Intensive Care Med.* 1995; **21**(8):679–81.

82. Yoshida A, Okada Y, Nagata Y, Hanaguri K, Morio M. Assessment of cerebral fat embolism by magnetic resonance imaging in the acute stage. *J Trauma.* 1996; **40**(3):437–40.

83. Simon A D, Ulmer J L, Strottmann J M. Contrast-enhanced MR imaging of cerebral fat embolism: Case report and review of the literature. *Am J Neuroradiol.* 2003; **24**(1):97–101.

84. Lee J. Gradient-echo MRI in defining the severity of cerebral fat embolism. *J Clin Neurol.* 2008; **4**(4):164–6.

85. Evert A Eriksson E A, Sarah E et al. Cerebral fat embolism without intracardiac shunt: A novel presentation. *Emerg Trauma Shock.* 2011; **4**(2):309–12.

86. Stoltenberg J J, Gustilo R B. The use of methylprednisolone and hypertonic glucose in the prophylaxis of fat embolism syndrome. *Clin Orthop Relat Res.* 1979; **143**:211–21.

87. Kallenbach J, Lewis M, Zaltzman M, *et al.* Low-dose corticosteroid prophylaxis against fat embolism. *J Trauma.* 1987; **27**(10):1173–6.

88. Bederman S S, Bhandari M, McKee M D, Schemitsch E H. Do corticosteroids reduce the risk of fat embolism syndrome in patients with long-bone fractures? A meta-analysis. *Can J Surg.* 2009; **52**(5): 386–93.

89. Johnson K D, Cadambi A, Seibert G B. Incidence of adult respiratory distress syndrome in patients with multiple musculoskeletal injuries: Effect of early operative stabilization of fractures. *J Trauma.* 1985; **25**(5):375–84.

90. White T, Petrisor B A, Bhandari M. Prevention of fat embolism syndrome. *Injury.* 2006; **37**(Suppl 4):S59–67.

91. Muth C M, Shank E S. Gas embolism. *N Engl J Med.* 2000; **342**(7):476–82.

92. Shaikh N, Ummunisa F. Acute management of vascular air embolism. *J Emerg Trauma Shock.* 2009; **2**(3):180–5.

93. Green B T, Tendler D A. Cerebral air embolism during upper endoscopy: Case report and review. *Gastrointest Endosc.* 2005; **61**(4):620–3.

94. Bou-Assaly W, Pernicano P, Hoeffner E. Systemic air embolism after transthoracic lung biopsy: A case report and review of literature. *World J Radiol.* 2010; **2**(5):193–6.

95. Mirski M A, Lele A V, Fitzsimmons L, Toung T J. Diagnosis and treatment of vascular air embolism. *Anesthesiology.* 2007; **106**(1):164–77.

96. Herron D M, Vernon J K, Gryska P V, Reines H D. Venous gas embolism during endoscopy. *Surg Endosc.* 1999; **13**(3):276–9.

97. Kashuk J L, Penn I. Air embolism after central venous catheterization. *Surg Gynecol Obstet.* 1984; **159**(3): 249–52.

98. Leach R M, Rees P J, Wilmshurst P. Hyperbaric oxygen therapy. *BMJ.* 1998; **317**(7166):1140–3.

99. Standefer M, Bay J W, Trusso R. The sitting position in neurosurgery: A retrospective analysis of 488 cases. *Neurosurgery.* 1984; **14**(6):649–58.

100. Papadopoulos G, Kuhly P, Brock M, *et al.* Venous and paradoxical air embolism in the sitting position. A prospective study with transoesophageal echocardiography. *Acta Neurochir.* 1994; **126**(2–4): 140–3.

101. Ngai S H, Stinchfield F E, Triner L. Air embolism during total hip arthroplasties. *Anesthesiology.* 1974; **40**(4):405–7.

102. Spiess B D, Sloan M S, McCarthy R J, *et al.* The incidence of venous air embolism during total hip arthroplasty. *J Clin Anesth.* 1988; **1**(1):25–30.

103. Lew T W, Tay D H, Thomas E. Venous air embolism during cesarean section: More common than previously thought. *Anesth Analg.* 1993; **77**(3):448–52.

104. Nishiyama T, Hanaoka K. Gas embolism during hysteroscopy. *Can J Anaesth.* 1999; **46**(4):379–81.

105. Chang J L, Skolnick K, Bedger R, Schramm V, Bleyaert A L. Postoperative venous air embolism after removal of neck drains. *Arch Otolaryngol.* 1981; **107**(8):494–6.

106. Ledowski T, Kiese F, Jeglin S, Scholz J. Possible air embolism during eye surgery. *Anesth Analg.* 2005; **100**(6):1651–2.

107. Suzuki K, Ueda M, Abe A, *et al.* Paradoxical cerebral air embolism occurred with postural change during rehabilitation, in a patient with ipsilateral internal carotid artery occlusion. *Intern Med.* 2012; **51**(9): 1107–9.

108. Timpa J G, O'Meara C, McIlwain R B, Dabal R J, Alten J A. Massive systemic air embolism during extracorporeal membrane oxygenation support of a neonate with acute respiratory distress syndrome after cardiac surgery. *J Extra Corpor Technol.* 2011; **43**(2):86–8.

109. Ueda K, Kaneda Y, Sudo M, *et al.* Cerebral air embolism during imaging of a sentinel lymphatic drainage in the respiratory tract. *Ann Thorac Surg.* 2006; **81**(2):721–3.

110. Singh A, Ramanakumar A, Hannan J. Simultaneous left ventricular and cerebral artery air embolism after computed tomographic-guided transthoracic needle biopsy of the lung. *Tex Heart Inst J.* 2011; **38**(4):424–6.

111. Le Guen M, Trebbia G, Sage E, Cerf C, Fischler M. Intraoperative cerebral air embolism during lung transplantation: Treatment with early hyperbaric oxygen therapy. *J Cardiothorac Vasc Anesth.* 2012; **26**(6):1077–9.

112. Frasco P E, Caswell R E, Novicki D. Venous air embolism during transurethral resection of the prostate. *Anesth Analg.* 2004; **99**(6):1864–6.

113. Tsou M Y, Teng Y H, Chow L H, Ho C M, Tsai S K. Fatal gas embolism during transurethral incision of the bladder neck under spinal anesthesia. *Anesth Analg.* 2003; **97**(6):1833–4.

114. Nayagam J, Ho K M, Liang J. Fatal systemic air embolism during endoscopic retrograde cholangio-pancreatography. *Anaesth Intensive Care.* 2004; **32**(2):260–4.

115. Akhtar N, Jafri W, Mozaffar T. Cerebral artery air embolism following an esophagogastroscopy: A case report. *Neurology.* 2001; **56**(1):136–7.

116. Katzgraber F, Glenewinkel F, Rittner C, Beule J. Fatal air embolism resulting from gastroscopy. *Lancet.* 1995; **346**:1714–15.

117. Lowdon J D, Tidmore T L Jr. Fatal air embolism after gastrointestinal endoscopy. *Anesthesiology.* 1988; **69**(4):622–3.

118. Zini A, Carpeggiani P, Pinelli G, Nichelli P. Brain air embolism secondary to atrial-esophageal fistula. *Arch Neurol.* 2012; **69**(6):785.

119. Williams T L, Parikh D R, Hopkin J R, *et al.* Teaching neuroimages: Cerebral air embolism secondary to atrial-esophageal fistula. *Neurology.* 2009; **72**(12): e54–55.

120. Hertz J A, Schinco M A, Frykberg E R. Extensive pneumocranium. *J Trauma.* 2002; **52**(1):188.

121. Laskey A L, Dyer C, Tobias J D. Venous air embolism during home infusion therapy. *Pediatrics.* 2002; **109**(1):1–3.

122. Grace D M. Air embolism with neurologic complications: A potential hazard of central venous catheters. *Can J Surg.* 1977; **20**(1):51–3.

123. Seeburger J, Borger M A, Merk D R, *et al.* Massive cerebral air embolism after bronchoscopy and central line manipulation. *Asian Cardiovasc Thorac Ann.* 2009; **17**(1):67–9.

124. Clark D K, Plaizier E. Devastating cerebral air embolism after central line removal. *J Neurosci Nurs.* 2011; **43**(4):193–6.

125. Yee E S, Verrier E D, Thomas A N. Management of air embolism in blunt and penetrating thoracic trauma. *J Thorac Cardiovasc Surg.* 1983; **85**(5):661–8.

126. Lai C C, Chuang C H, Chao C M, Liu W L, Hou C C. Pulmonary artery air embolism after blunt trauma. *Resuscitation.* 2011; **82**(4):369–70.

127. Hwang S L, Lieu A S, Lin C L, *et al.* Massive cerebral air embolism after cardiopulmonary resuscitation. *J Clin Neurosci.* 2005; **12**(4):468–9.

128. Arena V, Capelli A. Venous air embolism after cardiopulmonary resuscitation: The first case with histological confirmation. *Cardiovasc Pathol.* 2010; **19**(2):43–4.

129. Schwerzmann M, Seiler C. Recreational scuba diving, patent foramen ovale and their associated risks. *Swiss Med Wkly.* 2001; **131**(25–26): 365–74.

130. Spira A. Diving and marine medicine review part II: Diving diseases. *J Travel Med.* 1999; **6**(3):180–98.

131. Kapoor T, Gutierrez G. Air embolism as a cause of the systemic inflammatory response syndrome: A case report. *Crit Care.* 2003; **7**(5):98–100.

132. Alvaran S B, Toung J K, Graff T E, Benson D W. Venous air embolism: Comparative merits of external cardiac massage, intracardiac aspiration, and left lateral decubitus position. *Anesth Analg.* 1978; **57**(2): 166–70.

133. Toung T J, Rossberg M I, Hutchins G M. Volume of air in a lethal venous air embolism. *Anesthesiology.* 2001; **94**(2):360–1.

134. Vann R D, Butler F K, Mitchell S J, Moon R E. Decompression illness. *Lancet.* 2011; **377**(9760): 153–64.

135. Raju G S, Bendixen B H, Khan J, Summers R W. Cerebrovascular accident during endoscopy: Consider cerebral air embolism, a rapidly reversible event with hyperbaric oxygen therapy. *Gastrointest Endosc.* 1998; **47**(1):70–3.

136. Gursoy S, Duger C, Kaygusuz K, *et al.* Cerebral arterial air embolism associated with mechanical ventilation and deep tracheal aspiration. *Case Rep Pulmonol.* 2012; **2012**:1–2.

137. Heckmann J G, Lang C J, Kindler K, *et al.* Neurologic manifestations of cerebral air embolism as a complication of central venous catheterization. *Crit Care Med.* 2000; **28**(5):1621–5.

138. Ho A M, Ling E. Systemic air embolism after lung trauma. *Anesthesiology.* 1999; **90**(2):564–75.

139. de Blauw M H. An unusual complication of a central venous catheter placement. *Neth J Med.* 2012; **70**(1): 40–4.

140. Kuwahara T, Takahashi A, Takahashi Y, *et al.* Clinical characteristics of massive air embolism complicating left atrial ablation of atrial fibrillation: Lessons from five cases. *Europace.* 2012; **14**(2):204–8.

141. Fitchet A, Fitzpatrick A P. Central venous air embolism causing pulmonary oedema mimicking left ventricular failure. *BMJ.* 1998; **316**(7131):604–6.

142. Valentino R, Hilbert G, Vargas F, Gruson D. Computed tomographic scan of massive cerebral air embolism. *Lancet.* 2003; **361**(9372):1848.

143. Herber N, Salvolin L, Salvolini U. Changes in CT evidence of massive cerebral air embolism. *Eur J Radiol Extra.* 2004; **51**:9–10.

144. Suzuki T, Ando T, Usami A, *et al.* Cerebral air embolism as a complication of peptic ulcer in the gastric tube: case report. *BMC Gastroenterol.* 2011; **11**:139–41.

145. Griese H, Seifert D, Koerfer R. Cortical infarction following cardiosurgical procedures: Air embolism as a probable cause. *Eur Neurol.* 2009; **61**(6):343–9.

146. Gao G K, Wu D, Yang Y, *et al.* Cerebral magnetic resonance imaging of compressed air divers in diving accidents. *Undersea Hyperb Med.* 2009; **36**(1):33–41.

147. Rodriguez R A, Rubens F D, Wozny D, Nathan H J Cerebral emboli detected by transcranial Doppler during cardiopulmonary bypass are not correlated

with postoperative cognitive deficits. *Stroke*. 2010; **41**(10):2229–35.

148. Furuya H, Okumura F. Detection of paradoxical air embolism by transesophageal echocardiography. *Anesthesiology*. 1984; **60**(4):374–7.

149. Romero J R, Frey J L, Schwamm L H, *et al.* Cerebral ischemic events associated with 'bubble study' for identification of right to left shunts. *Stroke*. 2009; **40**(7):2343–8.

150. Tsivgoulis G, Stamboulis E, Sharma V K, *et al.* Safety of transcranial Doppler 'bubble study' for identification of right to left shunts: An international multicentre study. *J Neurol Neurosurg Psychiatry*. 2011; **82**(11):1206–8.

151. Orebaugh S L. Venous air embolism: Clinical and experimental considerations. *Crit Care Med*. 1992; **20**(8):1169–77.

152. Mehlhorn U, Burke E J, Butler B D, *et al.* Body position does not affect the hemodynamic response to venous air embolism in dogs. *Anesth Analg*. 1994; **79**(4):734–9.

153. Bowdle T A, Artru A A. Treatment of air embolism with a special pulmonary artery catheter introducer sheath in sitting dogs. *Anesthesiology*. 1988; **68**(1):107–10.

154. Bedford R F, Marshall W K, Butler A, Welsh J E. Cardiac catheters for diagnosis and treatment of venous air embolism: A prospective study in man. *J Neurosurg*. 1981; **55**(4):610–14.

155. Kol S, Ammar R, Weisz G, Melamed Y. Hyperbaric oxygenation for arterial air embolism during cardiopulmonary bypass. *Ann Thorac Surg*. 1993; **55**(2):401–3.

156. Sahni T, Jain M. Hyperbaric oxygen therapy: Research indications and emerging role in neurological illnesses. *Apollo Med*. 2005; **2**(1):16–20.

157. Mortensen C R. Hyperbaric oxygen therapy. *Curr Anaesth Crit Care*. 2008; **19**:333–7.

158. Murphy B P, Harford F J, Cramer F S. Cerebral air embolism resulting from invasive medical procedures. Treatment with hyperbaric oxygen. *Ann Surg*. 1985; **201**(2):242–5.

159. Newcomb A, Frawley G, Fock A, Bennett M, d'Udekem Y. Hyperbaric oxygenation in the management of cerebral arterial gas embolism during cavopulmonary connection surgery. *J Cardiothorac Vasc Anesth*. 2008; **22**(4):576–80.

160. Blanc P, Boussuges A, Henriette K, Sainty J M, Deleflie M. Iatrogenic cerebral air embolism: Importance of an early hyperbaric oxygenation. *Intensive Care Med*. 2002; **28**(5):559–63.

161. Dutka A J, Mink R, McDermott J, Clark J B, Hallenbeck J M. Effect of lidocaine on somatosensory evoked response and cerebral blood flow after canine cerebral air embolism. *Stroke*. 1992; **23**(10):1515–20.

162. McDermott J J, Dutka A J, Evans D E, Flynn E T. Treatment of experimental cerebral air embolism with lidocaine and hyperbaric oxygen. *Undersea Biomed Res*. 1990; **17**(6):525–34.

163. Mitchell S J, Merry A F, Frampton C, *et al.* Cerebral protection by lidocaine during cardiac operations: A follow-up study. *Ann Thorac Surg*. 2009; **87**(3):820–5.

164. Ballham A, Allen M J. Air embolism in a sports diver. *Br J Sports Med*. 1983; **17**(1):7–9.

165. Dutka A J, Mink R B, Pearson R R, Hallenbeck J M. Effects of treatment with dexamethasone on recovery from experimental cerebral arterial gas embolism. *Undersea Biomed Res*. 1992; **19**(2):131–41.

166. Ryu K H, Hindman B J, Reasoner D K, Dexter F. Heparin reduces neurological impairment after cerebral arterial air embolism in the rabbit. *Stroke*. 1996; **27**(2):303–9.

Stroke after discontinuation of preventive medications

Jelle Demeestere and Vincent Thijs

Introduction

The use of cardiovascular preventive medication has strongly increased in recent decades, due to the aging population and the increase in treatment options. Chronic medication is commonly interrupted or discontinued. We list several reasons for discontinuation of preventive medication in Table 14.1. Treatment complications, adverse effects, critical illness, intake difficulties, and urgent or elective surgery are the most common reasons for physician-based treatment cessation. Decisions to withdraw chronic therapy should be taken with particular care, as withdrawal may cause severe cardiovascular complications. In this chapter we describe the most commonly used cardiovascular preventive medications and the risk of cerebrovascular events (CVE) upon discontinuation.

Antiplatelet medication

Aspirin

Aspirin (acetylsalicylic acid, ASA) is one of the most successful commercial drugs and still widely used at a low dose for acute treatment or secondary prevention in patients with coronary artery disease (CAD), peripheral artery disease, or ischemic stroke. At the usual preventive dose of 80 to 160 mg per day it has few adverse effects and a low cost.

Aspirin acts by non-competitively inhibiting cyclooxygenase (COX)-1, an enzyme necessary for prostaglandin formation out of arachidonic acid [1]. COX-1 is constitutively expressed in the endoplasmic reticulum of almost all cells, including platelets. Activated platelets use prostaglandin to produce thromboxane (TX)A2, a vasoconstrictor that stimulates platelet activation and aggregation. Aspirin therefore potently inhibits

Table 14.1 Overview of the most common reasons for therapy discontinuation.

Patient driven	(Perceived) intolerance/allergy
	(Perceived) adverse effects
	Non-adherence
	Misperception about intake duration
	Financial
	Practical (out of stock, availability)
Physician driven	Adverse effects
	Treatment complications
	Intake difficulties
	Critical illness
	Surgery (urgent/elective)
	Uncertainty about chronic medication
	Medication change (e.g., oral anticoagulant)

formation of TXA2. Since circulating platelets are without nucleus and have a life span of about seven to ten days, they lose most of the ability to produce TXA2 for that period [2]. Besides inhibition of COX-1, aspirin can also acetylate fibrinogen, resulting in a molecule less likely to form fibrin and more prone to fibrinolysis [3].

A prospective trial evaluating adherence to aspirin in almost 4,000 patients with a history of transient ischemic attack (TIA) or ischemic stroke suggests a premature discontinuation rate of 18% [4]. About half of those patients quit the drug without any clear medical reason. Several retrospective observational studies suggest a connection between discontinuation of chronic aspirin therapy (sometimes used together with other antithrombotic agents) and the occurrence of ischemic stroke [5–10] (Table 14.2). Most studies describe a short interval (7 to 14 days) between aspirin

Treatment-Related Stroke, ed. Alexander Tsiskaridze, Arne Lindgren and Adnan Qureshi. Published by Cambridge University Press. © Cambridge University Press 2016.

Table 14.2 Overview of retrospective trials evaluating the relation between aspirin discontinuation and cerebral ischemic events.

Author, year	Kovich and Clark, 2003 [5]	Sibon and Orgogozo, 2004 [6]	Maulaz et al., 2005 [7]	Broderick et al., 2011 [8]	Watanabe et al., 2015 [9]	Rossini et al., 2015 [10]
Study design	Retrospective uncontrolled case survey	Retrospective cohort	Retrospective therapy-matched case-control	Retrospective cohort	Retrospective cohort	Retrospective, case-control
Setting	Perioperative, cutaneous surgery	Neurology ward admission	Stroke admission database	Stroke database cases	Perioperative, coronary artery stenting	Perioperative, coronary artery stenting
Antiplatelet medication	ASA	ASA (85%), Clop, ASA-ERDP	ASA	AT (ASA, Clop, ERDP, Ticl)	ASA, Clop, ERDP, Ticl, Cilostazole	ASA, Clop, ASA + Clop
Number of cases included	18	289	309	2,197	10,470	666
Index event	Perioperative ASA discontinuation	TIA or ischemic stroke	TIA or ischemic stroke	Verified ischemic stroke	Discontinuation of antiplatelet medication	Discontinuation of antiplatelet medication
Endpoint	All thrombotic complications[a]/TIA or ischemic stroke[b]	ASA discontinuation <1 month vs. continuation	Frequency of ASA discontinuation <4 weeks in cases[c] vs. controls[d]	Frequency of AT discontinuation ≤60 days	Definite ST, MI and stroke[e]	MCE: CD, MI or stroke[f]
Frequency of endpoint	100%[a]/72%[b]	4.5%	4%[c] vs. 1%[d]	5%	34/100 py[e]	0.5%[f]
Incidence rate ratio	–	–	–	–	1.94	–
Stroke, relative risk ratio	–	–	3.25	–	4.09	3.98 *
Mean time to event from therapy discontinuation (days)	–	7.4 ± 1.26	9 ± 7	12	–	–

AT: antithrombotic medication; ASA: aspirin, Clop: clopidogrel; ERDP: extended release dipyridamole; Ticl: ticlopidine; TIA: transient ischemic attack; ST: stent thrombosis; MI: myocardial infarction; MCE: major cardiovascular event; CD: cardiac death; py: person years.
* p = 0.51

Table 14.3 Overview of prospective trials evaluating relation between aspirin discontinuation and cerebral ischemic events.

Author, year	García Rodríguez et al., 2011 [12]	Mantz et al., 2011 [22]	Weimar et al., 2013 [13]
Study design	Prospective nested case-control	Multicenter blinded placebo-controlled RCT	Prospective case-control
Setting	Health Improvement Network UK primary care database	Perioperative, elective non-cardiac surgery	ProFESS trial database
Antiplatelet medication	ASA	ASA	ASA + ERDP
Number of cases included	6,007	291	2,843
Index event	TIA or ischemic stroke	ASA vs. placebo 10 days prior to surgery	ASA + ERDP discontinuation vs. continuation
Endpoint	ASA discontinuation recent[a] (30–180 days prior) or late[b] (180–365 days prior) vs. continuation	Stroke within 30 days post surgery	Recurrent ischemic stroke <7[e] and <30[f] days
Frequency of endpoint	10%[a] vs. 7.5%, 4.3%[b] vs. 3.7%	0% vs. 0%	–
Incidence rate ratio	–	–	5.66[e], 3.20[f]
Stroke, relative risk ratio	1.4[a]*	1	–
Mean time to event from therapy discontinuation (days)	–	–	–

* 1.97 for discontinuation 1 to 15 days prior to index event

ASA: aspirin; ERDP: extended release dipyridamole; RCT: randomized controlled trial; TIA: transient ischemic attack

withdrawal and TIA or stroke, which may be indicative of a rebound phenomenon. A similar link between aspirin withdrawal and coronary syndromes was observed, with over 10% of acute coronary syndromes following recent interruption of aspirin [11]. The mean delay of the coronary syndromes was 8.5 days, coinciding with rebound platelet activity. Two prospective studies on the subject have been published and seem to confirm the relationship between aspirin discontinuation and early stroke within the first month [12,13]. In a randomized trial the excess risk of stopping aspirin and dipyridamole led to an absolute increase of 2% in cardiovascular events within 30 days after stopping. In a prospective study of patients using low-dose aspirin for cardiovascular or cerebrovascular disease an increased relative risk of 40% within six months after stopping aspirin was observed (Table 14.3) [12].

The timing of the increased ischemic stroke risk after aspirin discontinuation suggests a rebound prothrombotic phenomenon. In vivo experiments show recovery of platelet function after aspirin withdrawal as soon as four to five days [14,15]. Animal experiments were able to demonstrate enhancement of thrombotic and thromboembolic complications eight to ten days after aspirin discontinuation [16–18]. Possible mechanisms include induction of COX-1 hyperactivity, possibly through an effect on the platelet precursor megakaryocytes, prothrombotic effects of ultra-low dose aspirin, chronic COX-2 inhibition, and increased sensitivity to various platelet agonists [17–20].

Because of this probable association of aspirin discontinuation and cardiovascular or cerebrovascular events, recent guidelines suggest perioperative maintenance of aspirin with the exception of neurosurgical and some urological procedures [21]. Although perioperative continuation is associated with an increase in bleeding complications by factor 1.5, it does not lead to a higher incidence of severe bleeding complications and does not have a negative impact on survival [9]. One must note that there are no large randomized trials that evaluate whether aspirin should be stopped prior to surgery. One randomized controlled trial of aspirin vs. placebo in a perioperative setting did not show any difference between treatment and the placebo group [22]. The trial, however, was underpowered to demonstrate a difference between the two strategies.

In conclusion, physicians should be careful about interrupting chronic aspirin use in patients. Severe intolerance, adverse effects, or major bleeding should nevertheless prompt (temporary) withdrawal until the offending etiology can be reversed.

Thienopyridines

Thienopyridines are inhibitors of the P2Y12 subtype of platelet ADP receptors. Binding of ADP to the P2Y12 receptor leads to a conformational change in another surface receptor called glycoprotein (GP) IIb/IIIa receptor. The conformational alteration promotes binding of the GP IIb/IIIa receptors with fibrinogen, thus cross-linking platelets and forming a stable platelet-rich thrombus. Platelets release ADP from dense granules upon tissue damage, hence further causing platelet activation and cross-linking [23]. The possibility of an additional anti-inflammatory effect of certain thienopyridines is the subject of debate.

Today, three types of thienopyridines are commercially available: clopidogrel, prasugrel, and ticlopidine. Clopidogrel is often used after cardiac stenting and is commonly used for secondary prevention of stroke [24]. No data exists on stroke risk after interruption of prasugrel or ticlopidine.

Limited data supports the possibility of an in vitro rebound hyperaggregability effect shortly after discontinuation of clopidogrel [25]. Several cardiological clinical trials showed an increase of stent thrombosis early after clopidogrel withdrawal [26]. Results of clinical trials investigating stroke risk early after discontinuation of clopidogrel, however, are equivocal. Most large prospective and/or placebo-controlled trials did not show a significant increase of stroke in the first weeks after clopidogrel cessation [27–29]. Three retrospective studies report a clustering of ischemic strokes the first

weeks after clopidogrel discontinuation [8,13,30]. In a randomized trial the excess risk of stopping clopidogrel led to an absolute excess of 0.40% in cardiovascular events within 30 days after stopping [13]. Because of the lack of a control group the increase might just reflect a loss of protective effect of clopidogrel treatment. However, in one trial the risk of stroke after clopidogrel discontinuation was estimated at 5% in the first three months [30]. One trial evaluated the effect of tapered clopidogrel discontinuation, thought to reduce the hypothetical rebound phenomenon on the occurrence of cardiac stent thrombosis but was unable to show superiority compared to standard withdrawal [31].

Because of uncertainty about a possible rebound prothrombotic effect discontinuation of clopidogrel should be carefully considered and avoided if possible. Although there is insufficient evidence to make recommendations about the periprocedural management of clopidogrel, most guidelines advise preoperative discontinuation of clopidogrel seven days before most surgical and therapeutic endoscopic procedures [21]. Since the risk of cardiac stent thrombosis within one year after placement is probably higher, non-acute surgery or invasive procedures should be deferred in those patients. In a recent study that tested continuation vs. stopping thienopyridines (clopidogrel or prasugrel) in patients who had received a DES stent and were treated for 30 months with dual antiplatelet therapy, an excess risk of MI and stent thrombosis was observed in the first three months compared to the three months prior to discontinuation [32].

Other

No data exists on the risk of ischemic stroke after discontinuation of glycoprotein IIb/IIIa inhibitors (abciximab, eptifibatide, and tirofiban) or the nucleoside analog ticagrelor.

Anticoagulation therapy

Vitamin K antagonists

Vitamin K antagonists (VKA) are a group of substances originally developed as rat poison. By competitively inhibiting the enzyme vitamin K epoxide reductase, they interfere with recycling of vitamin K. Depletion of vitamin K leads to reduction of the vitamin K-dependent gamma-carboxylation of coagulation factors II, VII, IX, and X, which are crucial factors of the intrinsic and extrinsic coagulation pathways. Furthermore VKA also inhibits vitamin K-dependent gamma-carboxylation of protein C and protein S, potent anticoagulant proteins that inhibit activated factor V and VIII. VKA, especially warfarin, have a long half-life. Since normal coagulation factors first have to be cleared from the circulation, the peak anticoagulant effect of VKA is usually reached only after 36 to 72 hours after intake. Steady-state concentrations of the vitamin K-dependent coagulation factors, and therefore the anticoagulant effect of VKA, are reached about one week after intake.

The most commonly used VKA are warfarin, acenocoumarol, and fenprocoumon.

VKA are typically prescribed for prevention of cardiac embolization in patients with atrial fibrillation or prosthetic (mechanical) heart valves. They are also used the first months after deep venous thrombosis and/or pulmonary embolism.

Many mechanical heart valves are strongly thrombogenic. Therefore anticoagulation with VKA is mandatory, since the risk of brain embolization is estimated at 4% per patient year [33]. The risk of stroke and systemic emboli in atrial fibrillation is variable. A scoring system with the acronym CHA_2DS_2-VASc is used to determine the chance of brain embolization (Table 14.4). A patient with atrial fibrillation receives a score of 0 to a maximum of 9, matching a yearly stroke risk of 0 to 15.2% respectively [34]. Most guidelines recommend treatment with oral anticoagulation from a score of 2 or greater.

Table 14.4 CHA_2DS_2-VASc scoring system.

Risk factor	CHA_2DS_2-VASc score (points, maximum = 9)
Congestive heart failure or LVEF <40%	1
Hypertension	1
Diabetes	1
Vascular disease	1
Age 65–74	1
Age ≥75	2
Female sex	1
Previous stroke/TIA	2

LVEF: left ventricle ejection fraction; TIA: transient ischemic attack.

Since invasive procedures and surgery during VKA therapy carry a high risk of serious bleeding complications, most guidelines recommend discontinuation five days before the procedure [35]. In high-risk patients bridging therapy with low molecular weight heparins (LMWH) is recommended from two days after VKA withdrawal until the morning of the procedure [35]. When feasible (e.g., for catheter ablation of atrial fibrillation) patients might benefit from continuation of oral anticoagulation, since limited data suggest an increased thromboembolic risk even with LMWH bridging compared to VKA continuation [36].

Several retrospective cohort studies reveal that adherence to VKA is rather low, with at least one in four patients discontinuing the medication in the first year after prescription in spite of few serious adverse events [37]. Furthermore there seems to be substantial underprescription of VKA especially in the elderly probably out of fear for bleeding complications [38].

Most studies seem to confirm an increased risk of thromboembolic stroke after VKA discontinuation [39–41]. The risk of arterial thromboembolism and death is estimated to increase by three-fold in the first three months after discontinuation [40]. Only one trial did not show a heightened incidence of thromboembolic events after discontinuing VKA [42]. However, the number of thrombotic events was small and in most patients the medication was discontinued for a period shorter than five days. A few studies mention a clustering of events in the first three months after withdrawal, suggesting a rebound hypercoagulation phenomenon [40]. The biological evidence for a hypercoagulable state is, however, limited, with only one clinical trial showing an increase in deep venous thrombosis recurrence shortly after discontinuation of VKA [43], and one in vitro study of a hypercoagulable state after VKA cessation [44].

Current guidelines do not recommend stopping VKA after successful ablation or surgery for atrial fibrillation, as good-quality data are lacking and subclinical recurrence of AF is difficult to detect without reliance on insertable cardiac monitoring devices.

Because most thrombi in atrial fibrillation originate from the left atrial appendage (LAA), percutaneous closure of the LAA is a new technique to prevent thromboembolism. The device is increasingly used in patients with high risk of hemorrhage on oral anticoagulation. In a randomized study that compared percutaneous LAA closure with the Watchman device with warfarin, superiority was shown after almost four years of follow-up [45]. Echocardiographic follow-up, however, suggests increasing gaps within the device over time [46]. Furthermore, to date no randomized controlled trials compared with new oral anticoagulants exist. Therefore cessation of oral anticoagulation should still be carefully considered in those patients.

Direct oral anticoagulants (DOAC)

Direct oral anticoagulants (DOAC) are a group of products that directly inhibit factor Xa or IIa (thrombin). Three products are commercially available and widely used for prevention of cardio-embolic stroke in patients with atrial fibrillation. Dabigatran is a direct thrombin inhibitor while rivaroxaban and apixaban are factor Xa inhibitors. All products have at least proven non-inferiority to warfarin in randomized controlled trials.

Although there is no need for regular monitoring and the anticoagulant effect is more easily controlled, adherence to DOAC is comparable to that of VKA, at least in the context of clinical trials in which the efficacy data were not yet widely known [47]. One study with dabigatran showed a higher persistence after two years of treatment [48].

Only expert opinion-based guidelines exist on the appropriate preoperative or preprocedural management of DOACs. Most experts discontinue DOACS two to four days before surgery, depending on the type of surgery, the bleeding risk, and kidney function [49,50]. Bridging with LMWH is not generally recommended unless the bridging period exceeds two days.

Very few data exist on stroke risk after interruption of DOAC. Post-hoc analysis of the Rivaroxaban vs. Warfarin for Prevention of Ischemic Stroke in Atrial Fibrillation (ROCKET-AF trial) suggested an increased risk of stroke in the first 30 days after permanent discontinuation of rivaroxaban (and transition to warfarin) compared to the warfarin group, but not after temporary interruptions or early permanent discontinuation [51]. These results probably reflect a poor management of warfarin dosing rather than a hypercoagulant effect of rivaroxaban discontinuation [52]. In this trial the incidence rate after early permanent discontinuation of rivaroxaban was 25.6 per 100 patient-years, comparable with that of warfarin discontinuation [51]. A similar phenomenon was seen after transition from apixaban to warfarin in the ARISTOTLE (Apixaban for Reduction in Stroke and Other Thromboembolic Events in Atrial Fibrillation) trial [53] and probably has a similar explanation [54].

In trials that were open label, such as the Randomized Evaluation of Long-term Anticoagulant Therapy (RE-LY) [55] or trials that paid close attention to this issue (Effective Anticoagulation with Factor Xa Next Generation in Atrial Fibrillation, ENGAGE [56]) there was no evidence for an early excess risk after discontinuation of study drug.

Statin therapy

Statins are competitive inhibitors of hydroxymethylglutaryl coenzyme A (HMG-CoA) reductase. HMG-CoA serves as a rate-limiting enzyme of the mevalonate pathway of cholesterol synthesis. By inhibiting the function of this enzyme liver cholesterol content drops, which in turn triggers a negative-feedback loop, upregulating low-density lipoprotein (LDL) receptors. This causes a reduction in total blood cholesterol levels. Several studies show that statins exert pleiotropic effects. Inhibition of HMG-CoA also reduces the synthesis of intermediate metabolites with certain biological functions. This results in up-regulation of endogenous nitric oxide (eNOS) synthesis, anti-inflammatory effects, antioxidant effects, stabilization of atheromatous plaques, and improved endothelial function [57].

The Stroke Prevention by Aggressive Reduction in Cholesterol Levels (SPARCL) trial in 2006 resulted in a significant reduction of 16% of fatal or non-fatal stroke relapse over five years follow-up in stroke patients without ischemic heart disease or known atrial fibrillation [58]. Since then, high-dose statin therapy is routinely used for secondary prevention of stroke. As with most medical treatments, however, discontinuation rates are high [59]. Therapy is often discontinued because of adverse effects – in the case of statins most often myalgia – or because of poor judgment after normalization of blood cholesterol levels. In the hospital setting the most compelling reason to discontinue statins is dysphagia, often the result of acute stroke.

There is mounting evidence that discontinuation of statins, especially in the setting of acute ischemic stroke, can be hazardous. Discontinuation of statin therapy after stroke is an independent risk factor for all-cause mortality at 12 months [59]. During acute ischemic stroke the effect of abrupt discontinuation of chronic statin therapy on stroke outcome is even more pronounced [60,61]. In a prospective randomized controlled trial, withdrawal of chronic statin treatment in the acute phase of stroke was associated with a near five-fold increase in the risk of death or dependency and a near nine-fold increase in the risk of early neurological deterioration [60]. Mean infarct sizes were significantly larger in the discontinuation group [60]. When compared to statin-naive patients, the risk of early neurological deterioration in the withdrawal group was 19-fold [60]. The findings were independent of blood cholesterol levels. The mechanism of the harmful effect of statin discontinuation on acute stroke outcome is still unclear. Animal and human experiments suggest a proinflammatory and prothrombotic state after statin withdrawal, with suppression of endothelial nitric oxide synthase (eNOS) production (limiting blood flow), production of reactive oxygen species, and impaired endothelium function [62–64]. These results advocate continuation of statin therapy, especially during the acute phase of stroke. If necessary, a nasogastric tube should be placed in dysphagic patients on chronic statin therapy with acute stroke.

In hemorrhagic stroke, patients who discontinued statin therapy in the acute phase had a worse outcome [65]. However, no prospective randomized data are available, so the observed deleterious association may only just be a marker for poor prognosis.

Antihypertensive and antidiabetic treatment

There are no high-quality studies examining the relationship between discontinuation of antihypertensive treatment and (hemorrhagic) stroke. Two trials have assessed whether antihypertensive treatment should be continued in acute stroke patients or should be stopped. In the Continue Or Stop post-Stroke Antihypertensives Collaborative Study (COSSACS) neutral results were observed [66]. In the Efficacy of Nitric Oxide in Stroke (ENOS) trial, apart from randomization into treatment with or without transdermal glyceryl trinitrate, patients on antihypertensive treatment were also randomized to either continuation or stopping of the treatment. They noted higher in-hospital mortality, together with increased rates of pneumonia, disability, and cognitive dysfunction in patients who continued antihypertensive therapy

[67]. All in all, there does not seem to be a major reason to continue antihypertensive therapy during the acute phase of ischemic stroke.

Antidiabetic treatment

There are no trials examining the relationship between discontinuation of antidiabetic treatment and occurrence of stroke. Excessive hyperglycemia, but also hypoglycemia in the acute phase of ischemic stroke, however, have a harmful effect on stroke size and outcome [68,69]. Continuation of antidiabetic treatment in combination with careful monitoring or starting a continuous intravenous insulin drip with careful titration in patients with excessive hyperglycemia and acute stroke is therefore recommended.

Conclusion

Discontinuation of preventive cardiovascular therapy may be the result of a patient's decision or ordered by a physician. Stopping a preventive drug may expose the patient to a higher risk of cerebrovascular events, even if there are good reasons for stopping. Decisions to discontinue preventive treatment agents therefore should be taken with particular care.

References

1. Vane J R. Inhibition of prostaglandin synthesis as a mechanism of action for aspirin-like drugs. *Nat New Biol.* 1971; **231**:232–5.

2. Evangelista V, Manarini S, Di Santo A, *et al.* De novo synthesis of cyclooxygenase-1 counteracts the suppression of platelet thromboxane biosynthesis by aspirin. *Circ Res.* 1998; 593–5.

3. Bjornsson T D, Schneider D E, Berger H. Aspirin aetylates fibrinogen and enhances fibrinolysis. Fibrinolytic effect is independent of changes in plasminogen activator levels. *J Pharmacol Exp Ther.* 1989; **250**:154–61.

4. De Schryver E L L M, van Gijn J, Kappelle L J, Koudstaal P J, Algra A. Non-adherence to aspirin or oral anticoagulants in secondary prevention after ischaemic stroke. *J Neurol.* 2005;**252**:1316–21.

5. Kovich O, Clark C O. Thrombotic complications related to discontinuation of warfarin and aspirin therapy perioperatively for cutaneous operation. *J Am Acad Dermatol.* 2003; **48**:233–7.

6. Sibon I, Orgogozo J-M. Antiplatelet drug discontinuation is a risk factor for ischemic stroke. *Neurology.* 2004; **62**:1187–9.

7. Maulaz A B, Bezerra D C, Michel P, Bogousslavsky J. Effect of discontinuing aspirin therapy on the risk of brain ischemic stroke. *Arch Neurol.* 2005; **62**:1217–20.

8. Broderick J P, Bonomo J B, Kissela B M, *et al.* Withdrawal of antithrombotic agents and its impact on ischemic stroke occurrence. *Stroke.* 2011; **42**:2509–14.

9. Watanabe H, Morimoto T, Natsuaki M, *et al.* Antiplatelet therapy discontinuation and the risk of serious cardiovascular events after coronary stenting: Observations from the CREDO-Kyoto Registry Cohort-2. *PLoS One.* 2015; **10**(4):e0124314.

10. Rossini R, Musumeci G, Capodanno D, *et al.* Perioperative management of oral antiplatelet therapy and clinical outcomes in coronary stent patients undergoing surgery. Results of a multicentre registry. *Thromb Haemost.* 2015; **113**(2):272–82.

11. Burger W, Chemnitius J M, Kneissl G D, Rücker G. Low-dose aspirin for secondary cardiovascular prevention – cardiovascular risks ater its perioperative withdrawal versus bleed risks with its continuation – review and meta-analysis. *J Int Med.* 2005; **257**:399–414.

12. García Rodríguez L A, Soriano L C, Hill C, Johansson S. Increased risk of stroke after discontinuation of acetylsalicylic acid: a UK primary care study. *Neurology.* 2011; **76**:740–6.

13. Weimar C, Cotton D, Sha N, *et al.* Discontinuation of antiplatelet study medication and risk of recurrent stroke and cardiovascular events: results from the PRoFESS study. *Cerebrovasc Dis.* 2013; **35**:538–43.

14. Lee J, Kim J K, Kim J H, *et al.* Recovery time of platelet function after aspirin withdrawal. *Curr Ther Res Clin Exp.* 2014; **76**:26–31.

15. Le Manach Y, Kahn D, Bachelot-Loza C, *et al.* Impact of aspirin and clopidogrel interruption on platelet function in patients undergoing major vascular surgery. *PLoS One.* 2014; **9**(8):e104491.

16. Aguejouf O, Belougne-Malfatti E, Doutremepuich F, Belon P, Doutremepuich C. Thromboembolic complications several days after a single-dose administration of aspirin. *Thromb Res.* 1998; **89**(3):123–7.

17. Doutremepuich C, Aguejouf O, Eizayaga F X, Desplat V. Reverse effect of aspirin: is the prothrombotic effect after aspirin discontinuation mediated by cyclooxygenase 2 inhibition? *Pathophysiol Haemost Thromb.* 2007; **36**:40–4.

18. Aguejouf O, Eizayaga F, Desplat V, Belon P, Doutremepuich C. Prothrombotic and hemorrhagic effects of aspirin. *Clin Appl Thromb Hemost.* 2009; **15**(5):523–8.

19. Vial J H, McLeod L J, Roberts M S. Rebound elevation in urinary thromboxane B2 and 6-keto-PGF1 alpha excretion after aspirin withdrawal. *Adv Prostatglandin Thromboxane Leukot Res.* 1991; **21**:157–60.

20. Moussa S A, Forsythe M S, Bozarth J M, Reilly T M. Effect of single oral dose of aspirin on human platelet functions and plasma plasminogen activator inhibitor-1. *Cardiology.* 1993; **83**:367–73.

21. Armstrong M J, Gronseth G, Anderson D C, *et al.* Summary of evidence-based guideline: Periprocedural management of antithrombotic medications in patients with ischemic cerebrovascular disease: Report of the guideline development subcommittee of the American Academy of Neurology. *Neurology.* 2013; **80**:2065–9.

22. Mantz J, Samama C M, Tubach F, *et al.* Impact of preoperative maintenance or interruption of aspirin on thrombotic and bleeding events after elective non-cardiac surgery: The multicentre, randomized, blinded, placebo-controlled, STRATAGEM trial. *Br J Anaesth.* 2011; **107**(6):899–910.

23. Dorsam R T, Kunapuli S P. Central role of the P2Y12 receptor in platelet activation. *J Clin Invest.* 2004; **113**(3):340–5.

24. CAPRIE Steering Committee. A randomised, blinded, trial of clopidogrel versus aspirin in patients at risk of ischaemic events (CAPRIE). *Lancet.* 1996; **348**(9038):1329–39.

25. Diehl P, Halscheid C, Olivier C, *et al.* Discontinuation of long term clopidogrel therapy induces platelet rebound hyperaggregability between 2 and 6 weeks post cessation. *Clin Res Cardiol.* 2011; **100**:765–71.

26. Sambu N, Warner T, Curzen N. Clopidogrel withdrawal: is there a "rebound" phenomenon? *Thromb Haemost.* 2011; **105**:211–20.

27. Collet J-P, Montalescot G, Steg P G, *et al.* Clinical outcomes according to permanent discontinuation of clopidogrel or placebo in the CHARISMA trial. *Arch Cardiovasc Dis.* 2009; **102**:485–96.

28. Geraghty O C, Paul N L M, Chandratheva A, Rothwell P M. Low risk of rebound events after a short course of clopidogrel in acute TIA or minor stroke. *Neurology.* 2010; **74**:1891–6.

29. Ford I, Scott N W, Herd V, *et al.* A randomized controlled trial of platelet activity before and after cessation of clopidogrel therapy in patients with stable cardiovascular disease. *J Am Coll Cardiol.* 2014; **63**:233–9.

30. Rossen J D, Chalouhi N, Wassef S N, *et al.* Incidence of cerebral ischemic events after discontinuation of clopidogrel in patients with intracranial aneurysms treated with stent-assisted techniques. *J Neurosurg.* 2012; **117**:929–33.

31. Fiedler A K, Mehilli J, Kufner S, *et al.* Randomised, double-blind trial on the value of tapered discontinuation of clopidogrel maintenance therapy

after drug-eluting stent implantation. *Thromb Haemost.* 2014; **111**:1041–9.

32. Mauri L, Kereiakes D J, Yeh R W, *et al.* Twelve or 30 months of dual antiplatelet therapy after drug-eluting stents. *N Engl J Med.* 2014;Nov 16 (Epub ahead of print).

33. Vongpatanasin W, Hillis L D, Lange R A. Prosthetic heart valves. *N Engl J Med.* 1996; **335**:407–16.

34. The Task Force for the Management of Atrial Fibrillation of the European Society of Cardiology (ESC). Guidelines for the management of atrial fibrillation. *Eur Heart J.* 2010; **31**:2369–429.

35. Douketis J D, Berger P B, Dunn A S, *et al.* The perioperative management of antithrombotic therapy. American College of Chest Physicians evidence-based clinical practice guidelines (8th edition). *Chest.* 2008; **133**:299–339S.

36. Di Biase L, Burkhardt J D, Santangeli P, *et al.* Periprocedural stroke and bleeding complications in patients undergoing catheter ablation of atrial fibrillation with different anticoagulation management. Results from the role of coumadin in preventing thromboembolism in atrial fibrillation patients undergoing catheter ablation (COMPARE) randomized trial. *Circulation.* 2014; **129**:2638–44.

37. Fang M C, Go A S, Chang Y, Borowsky L H, *et al.* Warfarin discontinuation after starting warfarin for atrial fibrillation. *Circ Cardiovasc Qual Outcomes.* 2010; **3**:624–31.

38. Tulner L R, Van Campen J P C M, Kuper I M J A, *et al.* Reasons for undertreatment with oral anticoagulants in frail geriatric outpatients with atrial fibrillation. A prospective, descriptive study. *Drugs Aging.* 2010; **27**(1):39–50.

39. Blacker D J, Wijdicks E F M, McClelland R L. Stroke risk in anticoagulated patients with atrial fibrillation. *Neurology.* 2003; **61**:964–8.

40. Raunsø J, Selmer C, Olesen J B, *et al.* Increased short-term riks of thrombo-embolism or death after interruption of warfarin treatment in patients with atrial fibrillation. *Eur Heart J.* 2012; **33**(15):1886–92.

41. Di Biase L, Gaita F, Toso E, *et al.* Does periprocedural anticoagulation management of atrial fibrillation affect the prevalence of silent thromboembolic lesion detected by diffusion cerebral magnetic resonance imaging in patients undergoing radiofrequency atrial fibrillation ablation with open irrigated catheters? Results from a prospective multicenter study. *Heart Rhythm.* 2014; **11**(5):791–8.

42. Garcia D A, Regan S, Henault L E, *et al.* Risk of thromboembolism with short-term interruption of warfarin therapy. *Arch Intern Med.* 2008; **168**(1):63–9.

43. Cundiff D K. Clinical evidence for rebound hypercoagulability after discontinuing oral anticoagulants for venous thromboembolism. *Medscape J Med.* 2008; **10**(11):258.

44. Genewein U, Haeberli A, Straub P W, Beer J H. Rebound after cessation of oral anticoagulant therapy: The biochemical evidence. *Br J Haematol.* 1996;**92**:479–85.

45. Reddy V Y, Sievert H, Halperin J, *et al.* Percutaneous left atrial appendage closure vs warfarin for atrial fibrillation: A randomized clinical trial. *JAMA.* 2014; **312**(19):1988–98.

46. Bai R, Horton R P, Di Biase L, *et al.* Intraprocedural and long-term incomplete occlusion of the left atrial appendage following placement of the Watchman device: A single center experience. *J Cardiovasc Electrophysiol.* 2012; **23**(5):455–61.

47. Chatterjee S, Sardar P, Giri J S, Ghosh J, Mukherjee D. Treatment discontinuations with new oral agents for long-term anticoagulation: Insights from a meta-analysis of 18 randomized trials including 101,801 patients. *Mayo Clin Proc.* 2014; **89**(7):896–907.

48. Zalesak M, Siu K, Francis K, *et al.* Higher persistence in newly diagnosed nonvalvular atrial fibrillation patients treated with dabigatran versus warfarin. *Circ Cardiovasc Qual Outcomes.* 2013; **6**(5):567–74.

49. Nascimento T, Birnie D H, Healey J S, *et al.* Managing novel oral anticoagulants in patients with atrial fibrillation undergoing device surgery: Canadian survey. *Can J Cardiol.* 2014; **30**(2):231–6.

50. Watanabe M, Siddiqui F M, Qureshi A I. Incidence and management of ischemic stroke and intracerebral hemorrhage in patients on dabigatran etexilate treatment. *Neurocrit Care.* 2012; **16**:203–9.

51. Patel M R, Hellkamp A S, Lokhnygina Y, *et al.* Outcomes of discontinuing rivaroxaban compared with warfarin in patients with nonvalvular atrial fibrillation: Analysis from the ROCKET AF trial (Rivaroxaban Once-Daily, Oral, Direct Factor Xa Inhibition Compared With Vitamin K Antagonism for Prevention of Stroke and Embolism Trial in Atrial Fibrillation). *J Am Coll Cardiol.* 2013; **61**(6):651–8.

52. Reynolds M R. Discontinuation of rivaroxaban: Filling in the gaps. *J Am Coll Cardiol.* 2013;**61**(6):659–60.

53. Granger C B, Alexander J H, McMurray J J, *et al.* Apixaban versus warfarin in patients with atrial fibrillation. *N Engl J Med.* 2011; **365**(11):981–92.

54. Granger C B, Lopes R D, Hanna M, *et al.* Clinical events after transitioning from apixaban versus warfarin to warfarin at the end of the apixaban for reduction in stroke and other thromboembolic events in atrial fibrillation (ARISTOTLE) trial. *Am Heart J.* 2015; **169**(1):25–30.

55. Connolly S J, Ezekowitz M D, Yusuf S, *et al.* Dabigatran versus warfarin in patients with atrial fibrillation. *N Engl J Med.* 2009; **361**(12):1139–51.

56. Giugliano R P, Ruff C T, Braunwald E, *et al*. Edoxaban versus warfarin in patients with atrial fibrillation. *N Engl J Med*. 2013; **369**(22):2093–104.

57. Davignon J, Leiter L A. Ongoing clinical trials of the pleiotropic effects of statins. *Vasc Health Risk Manag*. 2005; **1**(1):29–40.

58. Amarenco P, Bogousslavsky J, Callahan A, *et al*. High-dose atorvastatin after stroke or transient ischemic attack: The Stroke Prevention by Aggressive Reduction in Cholesterol Levels (SPARCL) investigators. *N Eng J Med*. 2006; **355**:549–59.

59. Colvicchi F, Bassi A Santini M, Caltagirone C. Discontinuation of statin therapy and clinical outcome after ischemic stroke. *Stroke*. 2007; **38**:2652–7.

60. Blanco M, Nombela F, Castellanos M, *et al*. Statin treatment withdrawal in ischemic stroke: a controlled randomized study. *Neurology*. 2007; **69**:904–10.

61. Fuentes B, Martínez-Sánchez P, Díez-Tejedor E. Lipid-lowering drugs in ischemic stroke prevention and their influence on acute stroke outcome. *Cerebrovasc Dis*. 2009; **27**(1):126–33.

62. Endres M. Statins and stroke. *J Cereb Blood Flow Metab*. 2005; **25**(9):1093–110.

63. Li J-J, Li Y-S, Chu J-M, *et al*. Changes of plasma inflammatory markers after withdrawal of statin therapy in patients with hyperlipidemia. *Clinica Chimica Acta*. 2006; **366**:269–73.

64. Rosengarten B, Auch D, Kaps M. Effects of initiation and acute withdrawal of statins on the neurovascular coupling mechanism in healthy, normocholesterolemic humans. *Stroke*. 2007; **38**:3193–7.

65. Dowlatshahi D, Demchuk A M, Fang J, *et al*. Association of statins and statin discontinuation with poor outcome and survival after intracerebral hemorrhage. *Stroke*. 2012; **43**:1518–23.

66. Robinson T G, Potter J F, Ford G A, *et al*. Effects of antihypertensive treatment after acute stroke in the Continue or Stop Post-Stroke Antihypertensives Collaborative Study (COSSACS): A prospective, randomised, open, blinded-endpoint trial. *Lancet Neurol*. 2010; **9**(8):767–75.

67. Bath *et al*. Efficacy of nitric oxide, with or without continuing antihypertensive treatment, for management of high blood pressure in acute stroke (ENOS): A partial-factorial randomised controlled trial. *Lancet*. 2014; 22 October: Epub ahead of print.

68. Baird T A, Parsons M W, Phan T, *et al*. Persistent poststroke hyperglycemia is independently associated with infarct expansion and worse clinical outcome. *Stroke*. 2003; **34**:2208–14.

69. Rosso C, Corvol J C, Pires C, *et al*. Intensive versus subcutaneous insulin in patients with hyperacute stroke: Results from the randomized INSULINFARCT trial. *Stroke*. 2012; **43**(9):2343–9.

Chapter 15

Intracranial hemorrhage: complication of endovascular therapy for acute stroke

Muhib Alam Khan and Rushna Ali

Introduction

Ischemic stroke is the leading cause of death and disability in developed nations. About 800,000 people in the United States experience a stroke each year resulting in a significant burden on health care systems. Intravenous (IV) thrombolysis is the mainstay of treatment for acute stroke since the publication of major US and European trials [1,2].

The time window from symptoms onset to treatment is narrow despite extension to 4.5 hours recently [3].

Therefore only a small portion of patients presenting with acute ischemic stroke are eligible for IV thrombolysis. Moreover, functional improvement, especially in patients with large-vessel occlusions is dismal. This has led to exploration of endovascular approaches to extend the therapeutic window and improve functional outcomes.

The most dreaded complication of acute stroke treatment is intracerebral hemorrhage (ICH). Intravenous thrombolysis can result in ICH, with significant morbidity and mortality [4].

Similarly, endovascular interventions carry a high risk of ICH. The idea of opening up a blocked vessel in the event of acute stroke comes from the coronary revascularization technique for acute myocardial infarction. The high risk of ICH associated with cerebral revascularization has plagued this field for nearly a decade and is a cause of concern. In this chapter, we review predictors and management of ICH secondary to endovascular revascularization approaches in acute ischemic stroke patients.

Definition

The hemorrhagic transformation (HT) of acute ischemic stroke is usually defined based on clinical and radiological evaluation. The goal for any stroke treatment is to prevent death and disability, so some HT types are less relevant if they do not lead to significant clinical sequelae.

The National Institute of Neurological Disorders and Stroke (NINDS) rt-PA trial divided HT radiologically into two categories: hemorrhagic cerebral infarctions and intracerebral hematomas [4]. Hemorrhagic cerebral infarction was defined as CT findings of acute infarction with punctate or variable hypodensity/hyperdensity with an indistinct border within the vascular territory. Intracerebral hematoma was defined as CT findings of a typical homogeneous, hyperdense lesion with a sharp border, with or without edema or mass effect within the brain. This hyperdense lesion could arise at a site remote from the vascular territory of the ischemic stroke or within but not necessarily limited to the territory of the presenting cerebral infarction. Hemorrhage with an intraventricular extension was considered an intracerebral hematoma. Clinically these HTs could be symptomatic (sICH) if associated with any neurological deterioration or asymptomatic if there was no neurological deterioration.

The European Cooperative Acute Stroke Study (ECASS I, II, and III) defined the HT radiologically as: hemorrhagic infarction type 1 (HI-1) (small petechiae along the margins of the infarct); hemorrhagic infarction type 2 (HI-2) (confluent petechiae within the infarcted area, but without space-occupying effect); parenchymal hematoma type 1 PH-1 (a hematoma in 30% of the infarcted area with some slight space-occupying effect); parenchymal hematoma type 2 PH-2 (a dense hematoma in 30% of the infarcted area with substantial space-occupying effect, or as any hemorrhagic lesion outside the infarcted area) [2–3,5]. Clinically these HTs could be symptomatic (sICH) if associated with worsening in NIHSS score

Treatment-Related Stroke, ed. Alexander Tsiskaridze, Arne Lindgren and Adnan Qureshi. Published by Cambridge University Press. © Cambridge University Press 2016.

by ≥4 points or asymptomatic if there was no neurological deterioration.

The Prolyse in Acute Cerebral Thromboembolism (PROACT I and PROACT II) trials, which were intra-arterial thrombolysis trials, defined sICH as HT associated with any neurological deterioration within 24 hours of treatment [6–7].

The Interventional Management of Stroke (IMS I and IMS II) trials, which used combination IV thrombolysis with intra-arterial (IA) thrombolysis, defined sICH as HT associated with any neurological deterioration within 36 hours of treatment [8–9].

The Mechanical Embolus Removal in Cerebral Ischemia MERCI, Multi MERCI, and Penumbra Pivotal trials, which were mechanical thrombectomy trials, defined sICH as HT associated with worsening in NIHSS score by ≥4 points within 24 hours of treatment [10–12].

Recently published Solitaire Flow Restoration Device vs. the Merci Retriever in Patients with Acute Ischemic Stroke (SWIFT) and Trevo vs. Merci Retrievers for Thrombectomy Revascularisation of Large Vessel Occlusions in Acute Ischemic Stroke (TREVO 2) trials defined sICH as HT associated with worsening in NIHSS score by ≥4 points within 24 hours of treatment [13–14].

The Interventional Management of Stroke (IMS III) trial comparing the benefit of endovascular therapy in addition to IV thrombolysis defined sICH as an intracranial hemorrhage temporally related to a decline in neurological status as well as new or worsening neurologic symptoms in the judgment of the clinical investigator and which may warrant medical intervention. A ≥4 point increase in the NIHSS score from baseline to subsequent CT scan at the time of potential worsening can be used as a guide by the clinical investigator for what represents a significant change in neurologic status. The imaging definitions of ICH used were similar to the ECASS III [15]. A randomized trial of intra-arterial treatment for acute ischemic stroke (MR CLEAN) defined sICH as a neurologic deterioration (a ≥4 point increase in the score on the NIHSS) and evidence of intracranial hemorrhage on imaging studies. Radiological characterization of ICH was similar to ECASS III [16]. The randomized assessment of rapid endovascular treatment of ischemic stroke (ESCAPE) and endovascular therapy for ischemic stroke with perfusion-imaging selection (EXTEND-IA) trials had similar definitions of sICH and radiological ICH [17,18].

It is evident that the definition of sICH varies from trial to trial. In spite of this variability, it has been noted that sICH leads to high mortality ranging from 45% in NINDS rt-PA trial, 83% in PROACT-II, and 28% in IMS I [4,7–8].

Frequency

The sICH rate in endovascular therapy trials is higher than in the IV thrombolysis trials. A fair comparison is not possible since usually a combination of IV thrombolysis therapy with endovascular recannalization approaches is used, leading to an additive risk of sICH. Moreover, most of the patients treated in endovascular therapy trials have high risk profiles due to failure of response to IV thrombolysis or ineligibility for it. These patients are usually out of the conventional IV t-PA window, have high National Institute of Health Stroke Scale (NIHSS) scores and have large vessel occlusions, which all translate into high periprocedural risk of developing sICH.

Intravenous thrombolysis trials NINDS rt-PA and ECASS reported sICH rates of 6.4 to 8.8% and became the benchmark for the future trials [1,2]. PROACT I and II revealed much higher sICH rates of 10.2 to 15.4% and faced a lot of criticism [6,7]. It is to be noted that PROACT trials focused on middle cerebral artery occlusion, which already has a high baseline hemorrhage risk regardless of the treatment utilized. IMS I and IMS II trials, which were IV/IA t-PA combination trials, reported lower sICH (6.3 to 9.9%) as compared to PROACT [8–9]. Mechanical thrombectomy trials MERCI, Multi MERCI and Penumbra Pivotal reported sICH rates of 7.8 to 11.2%, which are higher than the IV thrombolysis trials, but again we need to keep in mind the high risk profile of the patients enrolled in these trials [10–12].

The newer stent retriever trials SWIFT and TREVO 2 report sICH rates of 2% and 7% respectively, which are promising, highlighting the fact that the mechanical thrombectomy devices are improving with time in their safety profile [13,14]. It is also to be noted that these trials enrolled patients within eight hours of onset of symptoms, which has extended the window of treatment significantly as compared to the IV t-PA trials.

Recently published endovascular therapy trials with a bridging approach with IV t-PA have shown better outcomes as compared to IV t-PA alone. sICH rates have been between 3 to 7% [16–18]. These rates were not higher than the IV t-PA group, emphasizing that endovascular therapy can be safely performed for the selected group of large-vessel occlusion ischemic stroke patients. This safety profile improvement is mainly due to an expedited reperfusion timeline with process improvements and the use of stent retrievers [15–18]. Stent retrievers were used in 80 to 100% of patients in the endovascular groups in these trials. The median onset to revascularization time was between 51 and 260 minutes [16–18].

Pathophysiology

Complex mechanisms are involved in ICH associated with endovascular treatment. Blood–brain barrier alteration triggered by ischemia is frequently implicated, which leads to spontaneous hemorrhagic transformation seen frequently in strokes due to major artery occlusion [19]. This hemorrhagic transformation leads to parenchymal injury through mechanical compression, ischemia, and toxicity of blood products [20]. Free radicals produced both due to initial ischemia and subsequent endovascular reperfusion activate inflammatory cytokines. These cytokines start an inflammatory cascade with concurrent activation of proteolytic enzymes such as matrix metalloproteinases (MMP). MMP eventually degrade basal lamina of the blood–brain barrier resulting in hematoma formation and vasogenic edema [21].

Moreover, endovascular therapy introduced factors such as wire and catheter manipulation that cause direct damage to the endothelial wall. It has been shown that microcatheter contrast injections during IA thrombolysis also increase hemorrhagic risk, potentially due to degradation of the basal lamina of the blood–brain barrier [22].

Clinical predictors

Predictors of HT are extensively analysed in IV thrombolysis trials and similar factors have been shown to predict HT in endovascular therapy. Age, admission NIHSS, baseline blood pressure, serum glucose, and lytic dose are all predictors of HT in these patients. We will focus on the predictors of HT pertinent to endovascular recanalization therapy.

Clinical stroke severity as defined by NIHSS score has been shown to predict HT in the NINDS rt-PA trial [4]. It is to be noted that patients enrolled in

endovascular trials mostly have high NIHSS scores, providing a potential explanation for the higher rates of ICH in these trials as compared to IV thrombolysis trials.

Elevated systemic blood pressure frequently has been shown to lead to HT and should be well controlled in patients undergoing endovascular therapy similar to the IV thrombolysis treatment protocols [4].

Hyperglycemia leads to blood–brain barrier damage and leads to higher HT after endovascular therapy. The optimal glucose range is not well established but a range between 80 and 110 is suitable [23–24].

Concurrent anticoagulation with thrombolysis increases HT rates as shown in the PROACT II trial [7]. Lower intensity heparin regimens are being used now to avoid HT.

The timing of actual recanalization may predict sICH rates. Serial transcranial Dopplers (TCD) showed that sICH were more common in late recanalizers as compared to early recanalizers [25].

Radiographic predictors

Non-contrast cranial CT scan is the most widely used diagnostic modality to triage patients for IV thrombolysis. It has been demonstrated that early ischemic changes, especially hypodensity on a non-contrast CT scan, predict HT [26].

Several scoring scales have been proposed for evaluation of non-contrast images when estimating risk of hemorrhagic transformation. Alberta Stroke Program Early CT Score (ASPECTS), a ten-point grading system dividing the MCA territory into ten regions of interest, has been shown to predict the HT related to thrombolysis [27]. Subcortical structures are allotted 3 points; MCA cortex is allotted 7 points; and 1 point is subtracted for each area displaying early ischemic change. Patients with ASPECTS score below 8 are at substantially higher risk of thrombolysis-related ICH [28]. PROACT II found a correlation between low ASPECTS scores and higher symptomatic hemorrhage rates [29]. Similar results have been shown when attempting combined IV and IA t-PA treatment [30]. Therefore early ischemic changes on non-contrast CT should always be taken into account before attempting endovascular recanalization. However, IMS III did not find a correlation between ASPECTS score and sICH in the endovascular therapy group [31].

Non-contrast CT scan also provides information on the baseline substrate of the brain parenchyma in patients, especially chronic ischemic changes in the white matter. Presence of leukoaraiosis on CT has also been shown to predict HT and poor outcomes [32,33].

Computed tomography perfusion is being extensively used at multiple centers to provide rapid assessment of hemodynamic parameters of the brain and extend the intervention window. Advancement in technology enables perfusion maps of the whole brain to be obtained in minutes [34].

Cerebral blood volume (CBV), cerebral blood flow (CBF), and mean transit time (MTT) are calculated with the help of IV contrast. When only CBF or MTT is compromised but CBV is preserved, indicating salvageable tissue known as "penumbra," recanalization techniques can reverse ischemic damage to the brain tissue. Identification of brain regions with decreased CBV in combination with the ASPECTS grading system can help identify patients who are at high risk for HT from recanalization [35].

Larger infarct core size, which is characterized by significant loss of CBV, is a strong predictor of hemorrhage and poor outcomes. CBV <1.8 mL/100 g has been shown to predict HT in patients undergoing IA thrombolysis [36].

Computed tomography angiography (CTA) collateral score has been used recently to select patients for endovascular therapy. However, the ability of CTA collateral score to predict sICH is unclear at this point and further analyses are needed [37].

MRI has been shown to detect HT before any therapy is attempted in an acute stroke setting with greater sensitivity than CT [38]. Moreover, MRI is more sensitive in detecting microbleeds on gradient-echo imaging. These microbleeds are of questionable clinical significance for consideration of IV thrombolysis and IA therapy [39–41]. Similar to CT, leukoariaosis on MRI is predictive of sICH in patients undergoing endovascular therapy [42].

Gadolinium-enhanced MRI has the potential of identifying areas of blood–brain barrier disruption, which is a surrogate marker of increased vulnerability to HT [43]. It is defined as hyperintense acute reperfusion marker (HARM). HARM is associated with a higher risk of HT [44]. This MRI finding, however, has been correlated with an increased risk of asymptomatic hemorrhagic transformation. Moreover, HARM is observed with serial MRI imaging after treatment. Therefore this technique may identify patients who need targeted blood-pressure and glycemic control after reperfusion therapy.

MRI diffusion-weighted imaging (DWI) can be used for volumetric measurement of infarcted tissue. The Diffusion and Perfusion Imaging Evaluation for Understanding Stroke Evolution (DEFUSE) study identified a significant increase in risk of sICH associated with infarct lesion size [45]. Applying ASPECTS to DWI provides a good prediction of sICH after thrombolysis [46]. This technique can be used to select patients for endovascular therapy who have large-vessel occlusion [47].

Large perfusion-weighted imaging (PWI) volumes on MRI have been shown to predict HT in the DEFUSE study. This modality when combined with DWI has a potential to select patients for endovascular therapy beyond the conventional time windows and is a rapidly evolving field of acute stroke imaging [46].

Intracerebral hematomas in the setting of endovascular interventions can sometimes be mistaken for contrast medium. Early differentiation is clinically important when deciding whether to continue systemic anticoagulation therapy or treatment with antiplatelet agents. Contrast enhancement usually clears up rapidly on follow-up CT scans and does not produce any mass effect. Disruption of the blood–brain barrier is believed to be the underlying mechanism of extensive contrast extravasation [48].

Medical management

Platelet transfusion and cryoprecipitate are recommended to reverse coagulopathy secondary to systemic administration of t-PA [49].

Endovascular therapy often utilizes heparin periprocedurely in which case protamine sulfate can be used to reverse the systemic effect of heparin. Aggressive blood-pressure management should be employed in cases of thrombolysis complicated by large parenchymal hematomas. Smaller petechial hemorrhages might benefit from a less aggressive approach allowing higher blood pressure to preserve blood perfusion to tissue at risk of ischemia. Blood pressures above the recommended 180/105 can lead to hematoma expansion [50]. Moreover, large variations in blood pressure not only increase the size but also contribute to incidence of HT [51].

No clear treatment protocols are available and literature is limited on use of any particular agent to reduce hematoma expansion. These hematomas expand at a high rate and effective modalities are needed to reduce mortality associated with HT [52].

Surgical management

Surgical management of endovascular therapy-related ICH is not defined in the literature. The Surgical Trial in Intracerebral Hemorrhage (STICH) only enrolled patients with spontaneous ICH, so application of its results on revascularization-related ICH is not feasible [53].

Cases have been reported in the literature showing variable results of surgical evacuation of the hematoma in these patients and no clear inference can be derived [54–56]. There is a growing need for further studies to evaluate different management strategies for these patients, as the number of patients undergoing acute ischemic stroke intervention is increasing, with long-term financial and social impact on society.

References

1. The National Institute of Neurological Disorders and Stroke rt-PA Stroke Study Group. Tissue plasminogen activator for acute ischemic stroke. *N Engl J Med.* 1995; **333**:1581–7.

2. Hacke W, Kaste M, Fieschi C, *et al.* Randomised double-blind placebo-controlled trial of thrombolytic therapy with intravenous alteplase in acute ischaemic stroke (ECASS II). *Lancet.* 1998; **352**:1245–51.

3. Hacke W, Kaste M, Bluhmki E, *et al.* ECASS Investigators. Thrombolysis with alteplase 3 to 4.5 hours after acute ischemic stroke. *N Engl J Med.* 2008; **359**(13): 1317–29.

4. The National Institute of Neurological Disorders and Stroke rt-PA Stroke Study Group. Intracerebral hemorrhage after intravenous t-PA therapy for ischemic stroke. *Stroke.* 1997; **28**:2109–18.

5. Fiorelli M, Bastianello S, von Kummer R, *et al.* Hemorrhagic transformation within 36 hours of a cerebral infarct: relationships with early clinical deterioration and 3-month outcome in the European Cooperative Acute Stroke Study I (ECASS I) cohort. *Stroke.* 1999; **30**:2280–4.

6. del Zoppo G J, Higashida R T, Furlan A J, *et al.* PROACT: a phase II randomized trial of recombinant pro-urokinase by direct arterial delivery in acute middle cerebral artery stroke. PROACT Investigators. Prolyse in Acute Cerebral Thromboembolism. *Stroke.* 1998; **29**:4–11.

7. Furlan A, Higashida R, Wechsler L, *et al.* Intra-arterial prourokinase for acute ischemic stroke. The PROACT II study: a randomized controlled trial. Prolyse in Acute Cerebral Thromboembolism. *JAMA.* 1999; **282**:2003–11.

8. IMS Study Investigators. Combined intravenous and intraarterial recanalization for acute ischemic stroke: The Interventional Management of Stroke Study. *Stroke.* 2004; **35**:904–11.

9. IMS II Trial Investigators. The Interventional Management of Stroke (IMS) II Study. *Stroke.* 2007; **38**:2127–35.

10. Smith W S, Sung G, Starkman S, *et al.* Safety and efficacy of mechanical embolectomy in acute ischemic stroke: results of the MERCI trial. *Stroke.* 2005; **36**:1432–8.

11. Smith W S, Sung G, Saver J, *et al.* Mechanical thrombectomy for acute ischemic stroke: Final results of the Multi MERCI trial. *Stroke.* 2008; **39**:1205–12.

12. Penumbra Pivotal Stroke Trial Investigators. The penumbra pivotal stroke trial: Safety and effectiveness of a new generation of mechanical devices for clot removal in intracranial large vessel occlusive disease. *Stroke.* 2009; **40**:2761–8.

13. Saver J L, Jahan R, Levy E I, *et al.* SWIFT Trialists. Solitaire Flow Restoration Device versus the Merci Retriever in Patients with Acute Ischaemic Stroke (SWIFT): A randomised, parallel-group, non-inferiority trial. *Lancet.* 2012; **380**(9849):1241–9.

14. Nogueira R G, Lutsep H L, Gupta R, *et al.* TREVO 2 Trialists. Trevo versus Merci retrievers for thrombectomy revascularisation of large vessel occlusions in acute ischaemic stroke (TREVO 2): A randomised trial. *Lancet.* 2012; **380**(9849):1231–40.

15. Broderick J P, Palesch Y Y, Demchuk A M, *et al.* Interventional Management of Stroke (IMS) III Investigators. Endovascular therapy after intravenous t-PA versus t-PA alone for stroke. *N Engl J Med.* 2013; **368**(10):893–903.

16. Berkhemer O A, Fransen P S, Beumer D, *et al.* MR CLEAN Investigators. A randomized trial of intraarterial treatment for acute ischemic stroke. *N Engl J Med.* 2015; **372**(1):11–20.

17. Goyal M, Demchuk A M, Menon B K, *et al.* ESCAPE Trial Investigators. Randomized assessment of rapid endovascular treatment of ischemic stroke. *N Engl J Med.* 2015; **372**(11):1019–30.

18. Campbell B C, Mitchell P J, Kleinig T J, *et al.* EXTEND-IA Investigators. Endovascular therapy for ischemic stroke with perfusion-imaging selection. *N Engl J Med.* 2015; **372**(11):1009–18.

19. Alexandrov A V, Black S E, Ehrlich L E, Caldwell C B, Norris J W. Predictors of hemorrhagic transformation occurring spontaneously and on anticoagulants in patients with acute ischemic stroke. *Stroke.* 1997; **28**:1198–202.

20. Wang X, Lo E H. Triggers and mediators of hemorrhagic transformation in cerebral ischemia. *Mol Neurobiol.* 2003; **28**:229–44.

21. Gasche Y, Copin J C, Sugawara T, Fujimura M, Chan P H. Matrix metalloproteinase inhibition prevents

oxidative stress-associated blood–brain barrier disruption after transient focal cerebral ischemia. *J Cereb Blood Flow Metab.* 2001; 21:1393–400.

22. Khatri R, Khatri P, Khoury J, *et al.* Microcatheter contrast injections during intra-arterial thrombolysis increase intracranial hemorrhage risk. *J Neurointerv Surg.* 2010; **2**:115–19.

23. Demchuk A M, Morgenstern L B, Krieger D W, *et al.* Serum glucose level and diabetes predict tissue plasminogen activator-related intracerebral hemorrhage in acute ischemic stroke. *Stroke.* 1999; **30**:34–9.

24. Natarajan S K, Dandona P, Karmon Y, *et al.* Prediction of adverse outcomes by blood glucose level after endovascular therapy for acute ischemic stroke. *Clinical Article J Neurosurg.* 2011; **114**:1785–99.

25. Molina C A, Alvarez-Sabin J, Montaner J, *et al.* Thrombolysis-related hemorrhagic infarction: A marker of early reperfusion, reduced infarct size, and improved outcome in patients with proximal middle cerebral artery occlusion. *Stroke.* 2002; **33**:1551–6.

26. Dubey N, Bakshi R, Wasay M, Dmochowski J. Early computed tomography hypodensity predicts hemorrhage after intravenous tissue plasminogen activator in acute ischemic stroke. *J Neuroimaging.* 2001; **11**:184–8.

27. Barber P A, Demchuk A M, Zhang J, Buchan A M. Validity and reliability of a quantitative computed tomography score in predicting outcome of hyperacute stroke before thrombolytic therapy. ASPECTS Study Group. Alberta Stroke Programme Early CT Score. *Lancet.* 2000; **355**:1670–4.

28. Dzialowski I, Hill M D, Coutts S B, *et al.* Extent of early ischemic changes on computed tomography (CT) before thrombolysis: prognostic value of the Alberta Stroke Program Early CT Score in ECASS II. *Stroke.* 2006; **37**:973–8.

29. Hill M D, Rowley H A, Adler F, *et al.* PROACT-II Investigators. Selection of acute ischemic stroke patients for intra-arterial thrombolysis with pro-urokinase by using ASPECTS. *Stroke.* 2003; **34**: 1925–31.

30. Hill M D, Demchuk A M, Tomsick T A, Palesch Y Y, Broderick J P. Using the baseline CT scan to select acute stroke patients for IV-IA therapy. *Am J Neuroradiol.* 2006; **27**:1612–16.

31. Hill M D, Demchuk A M, Goyal M, *et al.* IMS3 Investigators. Alberta Stroke Program early computed tomography score to select patients for endovascular treatment: Interventional Management of Stroke (IMS)-III Trial. *Stroke.* 2014; **45**(2):444–9.

32. Whiteley W N, Slot K B, Fernandes P, Sandercock P, Wardlaw J. Risk factors for intracranial hemorrhage in acute ischemic stroke patients treated with recombinant tissue plasminogen activator: a systematic review and meta-analysis of 55 studies. *Stroke.* 2012; **43**(11):2904–9.

33. Henninger N, Lin E, Baker S P, *et al.* Leukoaraiosis predicts poor 90-day outcome after acute large cerebral artery occlusion. *Cerebrovasc Dis.* 2012; **33**(6):525–31.

34. Orrison W W Jr, Snyder K V, Hopkins L N, *et al.* Whole-brain dynamic CT angiography and perfusion imaging. *Clin Radiol.* 2011; **66**:566–74.

35. Gasparotti R, Grassi M, Mardighian D, *et al.* Perfusion CT in patients with acute ischemic stroke treated with intra-arterial thrombolysis: Predictive value of infarct core size on clinical outcome. *Am J Neuroradiol.* 2009; **30**:722–7.

36. Bhatt A, Vora N A, Thomas A J, *et al.* Lower pre-treatment cerebral blood volume increases hemorrhagic risks after intra-arterial revascularization in acute stroke. *Neurosurgery.* 2008; **63**:874–9.

37. Liebeskind D S, Tomsick T A, Foster L D, *et al.* IMS III Investigators. Collaterals at angiography and outcomes in the Interventional Management of Stroke (IMS) III trial. *Stroke.* 2014;**45**(3):759–64.

38. Kidwell C S, Chalela J A, Saver J L, *et al.* Comparison of MRI and CT for detection of acute intracerebral hemorrhage. *JAMA.* 2004; **292**:1823–30.

39. Kakuda W, Thijs V N, Lansberg M G, *et al.* DEFUSE Investigators. Clinical importance of microbleeds in patients receiving IV thrombolysis. *Neurology.* 2005; **65**:1175–8.

40. Fiehler J, Albers G W, Boulanger J M, *et al.* MR Stroke Group. Bleeding risk analysis in stroke imaging before thrombolysis. *Stroke.* 2007; **38**:2738–44.

41. Soo Y O, Siu D Y, Abrigo J, *et al.* Risk of intracerebral hemorrhage in patients with cerebral microbleeds undergoing endovascular intervention. *Stroke.* 2012; **43**(6):1532–6.

42. Shi Z S, Loh Y, Liebeskind D S, Saver J L, *et al.* Leukoaraiosis predicts parenchymal hematoma after mechanical thrombectomy in acute ischemic stroke. *Stroke.* 2012; **43**(7):1806–11.

43. del Zoppo G J, von Kummer R, Hamann G F. Ischaemic damage of brain microvessels: inherent risks for thrombolytic treatment in stroke. *JNNP.* 1998; **65**:1–9.

44. Warach S, Latour L L. Evidence of reperfusion injury, exacerbated by thrombolytic therapy, in human focal brain ischemia using a novel imaging marker of early blood–brain barrier disruption. *Stroke.* 2004; **35**(suppl I):2659–61.

45. Lansberg M G, Thijs V N, Bammer R, *et al.* DEFUSE Investigators. Risk factors of symptomatic intracerebral hemorrhage after tPA therapy for acute stroke. *Stroke.* 2007; **38**:2275–8.

46. Singer O C, Kurre W, Humpich M C, *et al.* MR Stroke Study Group Investigators. Risk assessment of symptomatic intracerebral hemorrhage after thrombolysis using DWI-ASPECTS. *Stroke.* 2009; **40**(8):2743–8.

47. Deguchi I, Dembo T, Fukuoka T, *et al.* Usefulness of MRA-DWI mismatch in neuroendovascular therapy for acute cerebral infarction. *Eur J Neurol.* 2012; **19**(1):114–20.

48. Yoon W, Seo J J, Kim J K, *et al.* Contrast enhancement and contrast extravasation on computed tomography after intra-arterial thrombolysis in patients with acute ischemic stroke. *Stroke.* 2004; **35**:876–81.

49. Broderick J, Connolly S, Feldmann E, *et al.* Guidelines for the management of spontaneous intracerebral hemorrhage in adults: 2007 update: a guideline from the American Heart Association/American Stroke Association Stroke Council, High Blood Pressure Research Council, and the Quality of Care and Outcomes in Research Interdisciplinary Working Group. *Stroke.* 2007; **38**:2001–23.

50. Mokin M, Kass-Hout T, Kass-Hout O, Zivadinov R, Mehta B. Blood pressure management and evolution of thrombolysis-associated intracerebral hemorrhage in acute ischemic stroke. *J Stroke Cerebrovasc Dis.* 2012; **21**(8):852–9.

51. Ko Y, Park J H, Yang M H, *et al.* The significance of blood pressure variability for the development of hemorrhagic transformation in acute ischemic stroke. *Stroke.* 2010; **41**:2512–18.

52. Goldstein J N, Marrero M, Masrur S, *et al.* Management of thrombolysis-associated symptomatic intracerebral hemorrhage. *Arch Neurol.* 2010; **67**:965–9.

53. Mendelow A D, Gregson B A, Fernandes H M, *et al.* STICH investigators. Early versus initial conservative treatment in patients with spontaneous supratentorial intracerebral haematomas in the International Surgical Trial in Intracerebral Haemorrhage (STICH): A randomised trial. *Lancet.* 2005; **365**:387–97.

54. Williams A, Sittampalam M, Barua N, Mohd Nor A. Case series of post-thrombolysis patients undergoing hemicraniectomy for malignant anterior circulation ischaemic stroke. *Cardiovasc Psychiatry Neurol.* 2011; 254569.

55. Alshekhlee A, Horn C, Jung R, Alawi A A, Cruz-Flores S. In-hospital mortality in acute ischemic stroke treated with hemicraniectomy in US hospitals. *J Stroke Cerebrovasc Dis.* 2011; **20**:196–201.

56. Fargen K M, Hoh B L, Fautheree G L, *et al.* Aggressive intervention to treat a young woman with intracranial hemorrhage following unsuccessful intravenous thrombolysis for left middle cerebral artery occlusion. Case report. *J Neurosurg.* 2011; **115**:359–63.

Chapter 16

Intracranial hemorrhage: complication of intravenous thrombolysis

Norbert Nighoghossian

Introduction

Treatment of ischemic stroke dramatically changed after the introduction of thrombolytic therapy in 1995 [1]. Although therapy improves functional outcome through reperfusion salvage of threatened tissue, symptomatic intracerebral hemorrhage (SICH) still represents the most feared complication of thrombolysis. With intravenous thrombolysis (IVT), about 6% of patients have SICH [2–8]. The ECASS II study showed that only the PH-2 type parenchymal hematomas were independently associated with clinical deterioration [3].

The objective of this chapter is to review the clinical, biological, and imaging predictors of SICH.

Clinical predictors

Age

In a collaboration study by the Safe Implementation of Treatments in Stroke International Stroke Thrombolysis Registry (SITS-ISTR) and the Virtual International Stroke Trials Archive (VISTA) [9], the SICH rate was slightly increased in patients over 80 years compared with those below 80 years. But the association between thrombolysis and improved outcome was maintained in very old people. There was no increase in severe intracerebral hemorrhage after IV t-PA in very old patients but, in general, outcome was worse as compared with younger patients. There is no evidence to exclude ischemic stroke patients from thrombolysis based on a predefined age threshold.

Clinical severity

In the NINDS study [10], patients with an NIHSS score >20 at admission were 11 times more likely to

endure a SICH than patients with an NIHSS score <5. The iScore [11] is a recently developed and validated risk score that can be used to estimate the risk of short- and long-term mortality after an acute ischemic stroke. A cohort of patients with stroke treated at 154 centers in Ontario was used for external validation. Outcome between patients receiving and not receiving t-PA was assessed. Patients were stratified into three a priori defined groups according to stroke severity using the iScore. Among 12,686 patients with an acute ischemic stroke, 1,696 (13.4%) received IV thrombolysis. Higher iScores were associated with poor outcomes in both the t-PA and non-t-PA groups (P <0.001). The incident risk of neurological deterioration and hemorrhagic transformation (any or symptomatic) with t-PA increased with the iScore risk [12].

A relevant predictive score of hemorrhagic transformation has also been established from the SITS-ISTR. The outcome measure was SICH as per the SITS-MOST definition: a type 2 parenchymal hemorrhage with deterioration in NIHSS score of ≥4 points or death. Nine independent risk factors for SICH were identified: (1) baseline NIHSS score, (2) serum glucose, (3) systolic blood pressure, (4) age, (5) body weight, (6) stroke onset to treatment time, (7) aspirin treatment, (8) combined aspirin and clopidogrel treatment, and (9) history of hypertension. The overall rate of SICH was 1.8%. The risk score ranged from 0 to 12 points and showed a >70-fold graded increase in the rate of SICH for patients with a score ≥10 points (14.3%) compared with a score of 0 points (0.2%) [13].

Comparison of risk-scoring systems in predicting symptomatic intracerebral hemorrhage after intravenous thrombolysis is still a challenging issue. Mazya *et al.* have recently performed an external validation of the SEDAN score for prediction of intracerebral hemorrhage in stroke thrombolysis. The performance

Treatment-Related Stroke, ed. Alexander Tsiskaridze, Arne Lindgren and Adnan Qureshi. Published by Cambridge University Press. © Cambridge University Press 2016.

of the score in predicting SICH as per the ECASS II and SITS-MOST definitions in the SITS-ISTR was assessed. In this very large data set, the predictive and discriminatory performances of the SEDAN score were only moderate for SICH as per the ECASS II and low for SICH as per the SITS-Monitoring Study [14].

Door-to-needle time

Door-to-needle time is a critical determinant of SICH. A recent study [8] showed that SICH is less frequent (4.7% vs. 5.6%; P< 0.0017) for patients with door-to-needle times ≤60 minutes compared with patients with door-to-needle times >60 minutes.

Blood pressure (BP)

In the EPITHET study [15], the temporal profile of BP in the post-treatment period was different for patients who developed SICH. Patients with SICH had significantly higher weighted average systolic and diastolic BP, compared with those without bleeding.

Previous treatments

According to Diedler *et al.* a previous use of antiplatelet drugs may have no influence on SICH occurrence or stroke outcome after t-PA [16]. The influence of statins on the results of IV thrombolysis for ischemic stroke is controversial. A recent meta-analysis [17] suggests that previous use of statin was neither related to long-term functional outcome nor mortality, but it was a risk factor for SICH. However, prospective studies are needed to confirm this safety concern.

Dose of t-PA and weight

The maximum dose of 90 mg alteplase is sufficient for patients with ischemic stroke weighing >100 kg. Symptomatic ICH in SITS-MOST occurred significantly more often in patients >100 kg [18].

Level of blood glucose

Hyperglycemia (≥8.0 mmol/L) during 48 hours after IV thrombolysis of ischemic stroke is strongly associated with SICH as demonstrated by Putaala and colleagues from the Helsinki Stroke Registry [19].

Stroke etiology

The Helsinki Registry showed that patients with small-vessel disease were spared from bleeding complications. These results may be related to the small size of ischemic lesion with lower risk of bleeding [20]. In addition, the intracranial hemorrhage rates did not differ between patients with ischemic stroke, with or without underlying dissection, who received thrombolytic treatment (6.9% vs. 6.4%) [21].

Remote or extra-ischemic intracerebral hemorrhage

Intracerebral hemorrhage after treatment with intravenous recombinant t-PA for ischemic stroke can occur in local relation to the infarct, parenchymal hemorrhage (PH), as well as in brain areas remote from infarcted tissue, remote parenchymal hemorrhage (PHr). In the SITS Registry remote bleeding occurred in 970 patients (2.2%), whereas 2,325 (5.3%) patients had PH and 438 (1.0%) both PH and PHr, and 39,761 (91.4%) no PH or PHr. Previous stroke (P = 0.023) and higher age (P <0.001) were independently associated with PHr, but not with PH. Atrial fibrillation, computed tomographic hyperdense cerebral artery sign, and elevated blood glucose were associated with PH, but not with PHr. Female sex had a stronger association with PHr than with PH. Functional independence at three months was more common in PHr than in PH (34% vs. 24%; P <0.001), whereas three-month mortality was lower (34% vs. 39%; P <0.001).

Differences between risk factor profiles indicate an influence of previous vascular pathology in PHr and acute large-vessel occlusion in PH. Additional research is needed on the effect of pre-existing cerebrovascular disease on complications of recanalization therapy in acute ischemic stroke [22].

Biomarkers of SICH

Many encouraging molecular candidates have been found after stroke. However, whether these putative biomarkers may indeed have direct clinical utility remains to be quantitatively validated for routine use in clinical prediction of SICH. To date, a high serum level of cellular fibronectin and matrix metalloproteinase-9 may predict symptomatic parenchymatous hemorrhage [23].

Magnetic resonance imaging predictors of SICH

It has been suggested that MRI could improve patient selection for thrombolysis and lead to a safer use of t-PA. Three main factors may be considered to predict the hemorrhagic risk: lesion size, hemodynamic parameters such as cerebral blood volume (CBV) decrease, and microbleeds.

Lesion size

In the DEFUSE study [24], patients with large baseline diffusion-weighted imaging (DWI) lesion volumes who achieved early reperfusion appeared to be at greatest risk of t-PA-related SICH. The EPITHET study has confirmed the predictive value of the lesion size [25].

MRI hemodynamic markers

The predictive value of CBV was recently assessed by Campbell *et al.* [25] who reported that a low CBV indicates a collapse of the vascular bed and a failure of collaterality. The risk of hemorrhage was greater in areas with low CBV.

Markers of small arterial disease: microbleeds and leukoencephalopathy

The presence of microbleeds on MRI represents a marker of microangiopathy and may increase the risk of hemorrhagic transformation. However, in a recent pooled analysis of 570 patients [26], the presence of microbleeds (detected in 86 patients) was not predictive of symptomatic ICH after thrombolysis. As suggested by recent data [27–30], signs of cerebral small vessel disease (SVD) on conventional MRI, either microbleeds or leukoencephalopathy, remain controversial in their ability to predict hemorrhagic transformation and stroke outcome in the elderly.

Mechanical thrombectomy in addition to IV thrombolysis and bleeding risk

Three trials evaluating endovascular therapy, published in 2013 – IMS III (Interventional Management of Stroke III), MR RESCUE (Mechanical Retrieval and Recanalization of Stroke Clots Using Embolectomy) and SYNTHESIS (Local versus Systemic Thrombolysis for Acute Ischemic Stroke) – reported neutral results on clinical outcome and bleeding risk. Possible explanations for failure to demonstrate superiority of endovascular therapy over IVT were long delay between symptom onset and treatment, inadequate patient selection, less than desired recanalization rates, and

use of older generation devices. IMS III showed no difference in safety and clinical outcomes compared to IVT [31–33].

Conversely, the MR CLEAN trial (Multicenter Randomized Clinical trial of Endovascular Treatment in the Netherlands), using stent retrievers in 97% of the cases, showed benefit of endovascular therapy up to six hours after stroke onset in the proximal anterior circulation in addition to best medical therapy (IVT up to 4.5 hours in most patients). Onset to IVT was 85 to 87 minutes in both intervention and control groups and onset time to arterial puncture was 260 minutes. The endovascular procedure was associated with a shift to improved function at 90 days, as reflected in more patients in the lower modified Rankin Score (mRS) categories, with an adjusted common odds ratio (acOR) of 1.67 (95% confidence interval [CI], 1.21–2.30). Secondary outcome parameters (NIHSS at 24 hours and one week, recanalization at 24 hours and final infarct at one week) were all statistically significant favoring the intervention group. Treatment effect was consistent in all predefined subgroups [34].

The ESCAPE trial [35] (Endovascular Treatment for Small Core and Anterior Circulation Proximal Occlusion with Emphasis on Minimizing CT to Recanalization Times) was prematurely halted after randomization of 316 patients due to a positive interim analysis. To be randomized, patients needed to have an NIHSS >5, a CT angiography (CTA) confirmed occlusion of the carotid T or the middle cerebral artery (MCA, M1, or large M2 segment), good collaterals on multiphase CTA, a CT-ASPECTS >5, and had to be enrolled <12 hours. rt-PA before randomization was given if patients were eligible. Results: the adjusted risk ratio for an mRS shift with thrombectomy at 90 days was 3.1 (CI, 2.0–4.7). A favorable 95% mRS of 0 to 2 at 90 days was seen in 53.0% in thrombectomy vs. 29.3% in controls (Numbers Needed to Treat, NNT = 4), and reduction of mortality was significant. All subgroups of patients had similar benefit, including the elderly and patients treatable after six hours from onset time. About 75% of patients received IVT and stent retrievers were used in 86.1%.

The SWIFT PRIME trial [36] (Solitaire™ with the Intention for Thrombectomy as Primary Treatment for Acute Ischemic Stroke) was prematurely stopped after a positive interim analysis of the first 196 patients. To be randomized, all patients needed to have received IVT <4.5 hours, an NIHSS between 8 and 29, a CTA or MR angiography showing an occlusion of the intracranial carotid or M1 segment of the MCA without extracranial carotid occlusion, a CT-ASPECTS >6, and CT hypodensity (or MRI hyperintensity) <1/3 of the MCA territory, and treatable <6 hours. Results (two co-primary endpoints): the OR for an mRS shift at 90 days with thrombectomy using the Solitaire™ FR stent retriever was highly significant (p <0.001), and mRS 0 to 2 at 90 days was 60.2% in thrombectomy patients vs. 35.5% in controls (p <0.001, NNT = 4). There was a trend for reduced mortality. The onset-to-arterial-puncture delay was 252 minutes. All subgroups of patients had similar benefit.

The EXTEND-IA trial [37] (Extending the Time for Thrombolysis in Emergency Neurological Deficits with Intra-Arterial Therapy), a phase II trial looking at early reperfusion and neurological improvement on day 3, was prematurely stopped because of a positive interim analysis of the first 70 randomized patients. To be randomized, all patients needed to have received IVT <4.5 hours, a CT or MR angiography showing an occlusion of the intracranial carotid, M1 or M2 segment of the MCA, significant mismatch and limited core on MR- or CT perfusion (using the RAPID® software), and had to be treatable <6 hours. Results (two co-primary endpoints): early reperfusion of the ischemic tissue at 24 hours with thrombectomy with the Solitaire™ FR stent retriever was 100% vs. 37% in the control group (p <0.001), an NIHSS reduction ≥ 8 points or NIHSS 0 to 1 at three days with thrombectomy was 80% vs. 37% in the control group (p <0.001). mRS 0 to 2 at 90 days was 71% in thrombectomy patients and 40% in controls (p <0.01, NNT = 3). There was a trend towards reduction of mortality. The onset-to-arterial-puncture delay was 210 minutes.

In summary, in all these new trials the risk of bleeding in proximal occlusion was not increased by a mechanical approach when compared to t-PA alone arms. However, it is possible that in these studies the absence of increased risk of bleeding may be related to the exclusion of patients with too large lesions, and a faster therapeutic approach associated with safer devices.

Poor collateral vessels and bleeding risk

Collateral vessels sustain the ischemic penumbra, which limits the growth of the infarct core before recanalization. The angiographic grade of collateral flow strongly influences the rate of HT after therapeutic recanalization for acute ischemic stroke. Poor baseline collaterals may limit effective reperfusion, and recanalization upstream from the regions of severe hypoperfusion may enhance hemorrhagic conversion. Consequently, poor baseline collaterals may result in a high frequency of HT with worsened clinical neurological status [38].

Blood–brain barrier changes and bleeding

Post-ischemic increase in the blood–brain barrier (BBB) permeability may increase the risk of hemorrhagic transformation after t-PA therapy [39,40]. The resulting disruption of the BBB and the impairment of the autoregulatory capacity of the cerebral vasculature predispose to blood extravasation when the ischemic tissue is eventually reperfused. Importantly, the degree of anatomical and physiological disruption appears highly dependent on the duration of ischemia and usually BBB changes occurred after three hours of treatment onset as demonstrated in a recent acute sequential MRI monitoring study [41].

Conclusions

Adherence to the inclusion criteria of the NINDS study remains the key to a favorable benefit–risk ratio in the routine use of t-PA for stroke.

However, these inclusion criteria do not take into account the diagnostic and prognostic input of pre-therapeutic MRI.

The input of multimodal MRI sequences and of the new biomarkers of ICH risk in the appreciation of the benefit–risk ratio is very important to consider as demonstrated in recent successful endovascular trials.

References

1. The National Institute of Neurological Disorders and Stroke tPA Stroke Study Group. Tissue plasminogen activator for acute ischemic stroke. *N Engl J Med*. 1995; **333**:1581–7.

2. Hacke W, Kaste M, Fieschi C, *et al*. Intravenous thrombolysis with recombinant tissue plasminogen activator for acute hemispheric stroke. The European Cooperative Acute Stroke Study (ECASS). *JAMA*. 1995; **13**:1017–25.

3. Hacke W, Kaste M, Fieschi C, *et al*. Second European-Australasian Acute Stroke Study Investigators. Randomised double-blind placebo-controlled trial of

thrombolytic therapy with intravenous alteplase in acute ischaemic stroke (ECASS II). *Lancet*. 1998; **352**:1245–51.

4. Hacke W, Donnan G, Fieschi C, *et al.* Association of outcome with early stroke treatment: Pooled analysis of ATLANTIS, ECASS, and NINDS rt-PA stroke trials. *Lancet*. 2004; **363**:768–74.

5. Hacke W, Kaste M, Bluhmki E, *et al.* Thrombolysis with alteplase 3 to 4.5 hours after acute ischemic stroke. *N Engl J Med*. 2008; **359**:1317–29.

6. Albers G W, Clark W M, Madden K P, Hamilton S A. ATLANTIS trial: results for patients treated within 3 hours of stroke onset. Alteplase Thrombolysis for Acute Noninterventional Therapy in Ischemic Stroke. *Stroke*. 2002; **33**:493–5.

7. Wahlgren N, Ahmed N, Eriksson N, *et al.* Safe Implementation of Thrombolysis in Stroke-Monitoring Study Investigators. Multivariable analysis of outcome predictors and adjustment of main outcome results to baseline data profile in randomized controlled trials: Safe Implementation of Thrombolysis in Stroke-Monitoring STudy (SITS-MOST). *Stroke*. 2008; 3316–22.

8. Fonarow G C, Smith E E, Saver J L, *et al.* Timeliness of tissue-type plasminogen activator therapy in acute ischemic stroke: Patient characteristics, hospital factors, and outcomes associated with door-to-needle times within 60 minutes. *Circulation*. 2011; **7**:750–8.

9. Mishra N K, Ahmed N, Andersen G, *et al.* VISTA collaborators; SITS collaborators. Thrombolysis in very elderly people: Controlled comparison of SITS International Stroke Thrombolysis Registry and Virtual International Stroke Trials Archive. *BMJ*. 2010; **341**:c6046. doi:10.1136.

10. Intracerebral haemorrhage after intravenous t-PA therapy for ischemic stroke. The NINDS t-PA Stroke Study Group. *Stroke*. 1997; **11**: 2109–18.

11. Saposni G, Raptis S, Kapral M K, *et al.* Investigators of the Registry of the Canadian Stroke Network and the Stroke Outcome Research Canada Working Group. The iScore predicts poor functional outcomes early after hospitalization for an acute ischemic stroke. *Stroke*. 2011; **12**:3421–8.

12. Saposnik G, Fang J, Kapral M K, *et al.* Investigators of the Registry of the Canadian Stroke Network (RCSN); Stroke Outcomes Research Canada (SORCan) Working Group. The iScore predicts effectiveness of thrombolytic therapy for acute ischemic stroke. *Stroke*. 2012; **5**:1315–22.

13. Mazya M, Egido J A, Ford G A, *et al.* SITS Investigators. Predicting the risk of symptomatic intracerebral hemorrhage in ischemic stroke treated with intravenous alteplase: Safe Implementation of Treatments in Stroke (SITS) symptomatic

intracerebral hemorrhage risk score. *Stroke*. 2012; **43**:1524–31.

14. Mazya M V, Bovi P, Castillo J, *et al.* External validation of the SEDAN score for prediction of intracerebral hemorrhage in stroke thrombolysis. *Stroke*. 2013; **44**: 1595–600.

15. Butcher K, Christensen S, Parsons M, *et al.* EPITHET Investigators. Postthrombolysis blood pressure elevation is associated with hemorrhagic transformation. *Stroke*. 2010; **1**:72–7.

16. Diedler J, Ahmed N, Sykora M, *et al.* Safety of intravenous thrombolysis for acute ischemic stroke in patients receiving antiplatelet therapy at stroke onset. *Stroke*. 2010; **2**:288–94.

17. Martinez-Ramirez S, Delgado-Mederos R, Marín R, *et al.* Statin pretreatment may increase the risk of symptomatic intracranial haemorrhage in thrombolysis for ischemic stroke: Results from a case-control study and a meta-analysis. *J Neurol*. 2012; **1**:111–18.

18. Diedler J, Ahmed N, Glahn J, *et al.* Is the maximum dose of 90 mg alteplase sufficient for patients with ischemic stroke weighing >100 kg? *Stroke*. 2011; **6**:1615–20.

19. Putaala J, Sairanen T, Meretoja A, *et al.* Post-thrombolytic hyperglycemia and 3-month outcome in acute ischemic stroke. *Cerebrovasc Dis*. 2011; **1**:83–92.

20. Mustanoja S, Meretoja A, Putaala J, *et al.* Helsinki Stroke Thrombolysis Registry Group. Outcome by stroke etiology in patients receiving thrombolytic treatment: descriptive subtype analysis. *Stroke*. 2011; **1**:102–6.

21. Qureshi A I, Chaudhry S A, Hassan A E, *et al.* Thrombolytic treatment of patients with acute ischemic stroke related to underlying arterial dissection in the United States. *Arch Neurol*. 2011; **12**:1536–42.

22. Mazya M V, Ahmed N, Ford G A, *et al.* Remote or extraischemic intracerebral hemorrhage – an uncommon complication of stroke: Results from the Safe Implementation of Treatments in Stroke – International Stroke Thrombolysis Register. *Stroke*. 2014; **45**:1657–63.

23. Castellanos M, Sobrino T, Millán M, *et al.* Serum cellular fibronectin and matrix metalloproteinase-9 as screening biomarkers for the prediction of parenchymal hematoma after thrombolytic therapy in acute ischemic stroke: A multicenter confirmatory study. *Stroke*. 2007; **6**:1855–914.

24. Albers G W, Thijs V N, Wechsler L, *et al.* DEFUSE Investigators. Magnetic resonance imaging profiles predict clinical response to early reperfusion: The Diffusion and Perfusion Imaging Evaluation for

Understanding Stroke Evolution (DEFUSE) study. *Ann Neurol.* 2006; **5**:508–17.

25. Campbell B C, Christensen S, Butcher K S, *et al.* EPITHET Investigators. Regional very low cerebral blood volume predicts hemorrhagic transformation better than diffusion-weighted imaging volume and thresholded apparent diffusion coefficient in acute ischemic stroke. *Stroke.* 2010; **1**:82–8.

26. Fiehler J, Albers G W, Boulanger J M, *et al.* MR STROKE Group. Bleeding Risk Analysis in Stroke Imaging before thromboLysis (BRASIL): Pooled analysis of T2*-weighted magnetic resonance imaging data from 570 patients. *Stroke.* 2007; 2738–44.

27. Dannenberg S, Scheitz J F, Rozanski M, *et al.* Number of cerebral microbleeds and risk of intracerebral hemorrhage after intravenous thrombolysis. *Stroke.* 2014; **10**:2900–5.

28. Gratz P P, El-Koussy M, Hsieh K, *et al.* Preexisting cerebral microbleeds on susceptibility-weighted magnetic resonance imaging and post-thrombolysis bleeding risk in 392 patients. *Stroke.* 2014; **6**:1684–8.

29. Jung S, Mono M L, Findling O, *et al.* White matter lesions and intra-arterial thrombolysis. *J Neurol.* 2012; **7**:1331–6.

30. Neumann-Haefelin T, Hoelig S, Berkefeld J, *et al.* Leukoaraiosis is a risk factor for symptomatic intracerebral hemorrhage after thrombolysis for acute stroke. *Stroke.* 2006; 37: 2463–6.

31. Broderick J P, Palesch Y Y, Demchuk A M, *et al.* Endovascular therapy after intravenous t-PA versus t-PA alone for stroke. *N Engl J Med.* 2013; **368**:893–903.

32. Kidwell C S, Jahan R, Saver J L. Endovascular treatment for acute ischemic stroke. *N Engl J Med.* 2013; **368**:2434–5.

33. Ciccone A, Valvassori L, Nichelatti M, *et al.* Endovascular treatment for acute ischemic stroke. *N Engl J Med.* 2013; **368**:904–13.

34. Berkhemer O A, Fransen P S, Beumer D, *et al.* MR CLEAN Investigators. A randomized trial of intraarterial treatment for acute ischemic stroke. *N Engl J Med.* 2015; **1**:11–20.

35. Goyal M, Demchuk A M, Menon B K, *et al.* ESCAPE Trial Investigators. Randomized assessment of rapid endovascular treatment of ischemic stroke. *N Engl J Med.* 2015; **11**:1019–30.

36. Saver J L, Goyal M, Bonafe A, *et al.* SWIFT PRIME Investigators. Solitaire™ with the Intention for Thrombectomy as Primary Endovascular Treatment for Acute Ischemic Stroke (SWIFT PRIME) trial: Protocol for a randomized, controlled, multicenter study comparing the Solitaire revascularization device with IV tPA with IV tPA alone in acute ischemic stroke. *Int J Stroke.* 2015; **3**:439–48.

37. Campbell B C, Mitchell P J, Kleinig T J, *et al.* EXTEND-IA Investigators. Endovascular therapy for ischemic stroke with perfusion-imaging selection. *N Engl J Med.* 2015; **11**:1009–18.

38. Bang O Y, Saver J L, Kim S J, *et al.* Collateral flow averts hemorrhagic transformation after endovascular therapy for acute ischemic stroke. *Stroke.* 2011; **42**: 2235–9.

39. Warach S, Latour L L. Evidence of reperfusion injury, exacerbated by thrombolytic therapy, in human focal brain ischemia using a novel imaging marker of early blood–brain barrier disruption. *Stroke.* 2004; **35**: 2659–61.

40. Khatri R, McKinney A M, Swenson B, *et al.* Blood–brain barrier, reperfusion injury, and hemorrhagic transformation in acute ischemic stroke. *Neurology.* 2012; **79**:S52–7.

41. Giraud M, Cho T H, Nighoghossian N, *et al.* Early blood brain barrier changes in acute ischemic stroke: A sequential MRI study. *J Neuroimaging.* 2015; **25**:959–63.

Chapter

17

Intracranial hemorrhages secondary to antiplatelet treatment

Shraddha Mainali

Introduction

Intracranial hemorrhage (ICH) can be defined as the pathological accumulation of blood within the cranial vault. It may occur within brain parenchyma or the surrounding meningeal spaces. Intracranial hemorrhage can be divided into traumatic or non-traumatic based on the etiology. Non-traumatic ICH most commonly results from hypertensive damage to blood vessel walls (e.g., hypertension, eclampsia, substance abuse), but it may also be due to autoregulatory dysfunction with enhanced cerebral blood flow (e.g., reperfusion injury, hemorrhagic transformation, cold exposure), rupture of an aneurysm or arteriovenous malformation (AVM), arteriopathy (e.g., cerebral amyloid angiopathy, moyamoya), altered hemostasis (e.g., bleeding diathesis, secondary to antiplatelet or anticoagulant medication), hemorrhagic necrosis (e.g., tumor, infection), venous outflow obstruction (e.g., cerebral venous thrombosis), or iatrogenic from antithrombotic therapies [1]. Intracranial hemorrhage and accompanying edema may disrupt or compress adjacent brain tissue, leading to neurological dysfunction. Substantial mass effect on the brain parenchyma may increase intracranial pressure (ICP) and potentially lead to fatal herniation syndromes.

In this chapter, we will discuss some of the commonly used antiplatelet agents in the management of cerebrovascular diseases and their associated risk of ICH. We will also briefly discuss the management of ICH.

Antiplatelet treatment

Antiplatelet treatment remains the mainstay in preventing aberrant platelet activation in pathophysiological conditions such as myocardial infarction (MI), peripheral arterial ischemia, and ischemic stroke. Currently available antiplatelet agents predominantly act on four major pathways of platelet activation: (1) the cyclooxygenase-1 (COX-1) inhibitor aspirin; (2) the adenosine diphosphate receptor (P2Y12) inhibitors clopidogrel, ticlopidine, and prasugrel; (3) the phosphodiesterase (PDE) inhibitors cilostazol and dipyridamole; and (4) the glycoprotein IIb/IIIa inhibitors abciximab, eptifibatide, and tirofiban.

On average, these agents reduce the relative risk of stroke, MI, or death by about 22% but are associated with an increased risk of hemorrhagic complications [2]. The incidence ranges between 0.2 and 0.4 cases per 1,000 individuals per year [3,4]. Hematoma volume is the critical determinant of death and functional outcome after ICH [5], and it appears to be the result of a dynamic process, with continuous bleeding and/or rebleeding over several hours [6,7]. About 30% of total ICH occurs in patients on antithrombotic treatment. The relative risk of ICH in patients on antithrombotic therapy is estimated to be about 11- to 16-fold greater than in untreated subjects [8–10].

Although antiplatelet treatment has been shown to be a risk factor for spontaneous ICH as well as increased ICH volume and increased mortality, the exact increase has not been consistently demonstrated for any specific drug among many reports [11–17].

Aspirin

Aspirin is an inhibitor of the platelet cyclooxygenase and results in an irreversible inhibition of platelet-dependent thromboxane formation. Aspirin has been evaluated in the doses of 50 to 1,500 mg/day in various trials. It is rapidly metabolized within minutes, and its metabolite is ineffective. Thus newly produced platelets have normal function. Ten percent of platelets are

Treatment-Related Stroke, ed. Alexander Tsiskaridze, Arne Lindgren and Adnan Qureshi. Published by Cambridge University Press. © Cambridge University Press 2016.

produced every day; therefore in a patient with a platelet count of 200×10^9/L, 20,000 would be produced daily. If the patient had last ingested aspirin three days earlier, then he would have an estimated 60,000 normally functioning platelets. As such, aspirin induces only mild to moderate platelet dysfunction because all platelet glycoprotein receptors and other biochemical pathways are still intact.

The risk for ICH appears to be dose dependent with aspirin, but exists with other agents as well [12,13,18–23]. Studies have suggested that aspirin treatment increases the relative risk of ICH by approximately 40%, with estimates ranging from 24 to 84% [24]. It is estimated that approximately 4,000 of the 60,000 ICHs occurring annually in the United States are associated with the use of aspirin [24].

The increased risk of ICH associated with aspirin treatment has been observed in a few primary intervention studies and several large secondary prevention trials among patients with a history of stroke or transient ischemic attack [25–29]. Low-dose aspirin has been used in primary [25] and secondary [26] prevention trials, which together suggested a 4.0- to 4.8-fold increase in risk of ICH, which would substantially reduce the net benefit of aspirin treatment for primary prevention in low-risk populations. A meta-analysis of 16 randomized, placebo-controlled clinical trials showed that treatment with aspirin was associated with a relative risk (RR) of hemorrhagic stroke of 1.84 (p = 0.001) [27]. Across studies, the risk of hemorrhagic stroke associated with aspirin therapy ranged between 0.1 to 0.4 cases/1,000 annually [27,28]. There is some evidence that higher doses of aspirin may increase the risk of ICH [29]. In the elderly population, long-term aspirin use has been shown to increase the incidence of ICH, but the magnitude of increase is small (about 1/2,000 aspirin users per year for elderly persons). Furthermore, aspirin use at the time of ICH may increase the risk of death and disability [30].

In a meta-analysis of nine trials [31] the incidence rates of subdural hemorrhage (SDH) ranged from 0.02 per 1,000 patient-years to 1 to 2 per 1,000 patient-years in patients on aspirin therapy. Overall the 1.6-fold increased risk of SDH associated with aspirin therapy was not statistically significant compared with non-users. The absolute rate of SDH among healthy middle-aged health professionals taking aspirin was extremely low (0.02/1,000 patient-years). However, the risk was substantially higher in older patients

(average age of 70 years) with atrial fibrillation (1 to 2 per 1,000 patient-years).

Dipyridamole and aspirin combination

Dipyridamole inhibits the activity of adenosine deaminase and phosphodiesterase, which causes an accumulation of adenosine, adenine nucleotides, and cyclic AMP; these mediators then inhibit platelet aggregation and may cause vasodilation; they may also stimulate release of prostacyclin or prostaglandin D2. There are six clinical trials comparing the effects of aspirin and dipyridamole with aspirin alone in patients with ischemic stroke and/or TIAs for secondary stroke prevention [20]. No significant difference in major hemorrhagic events was noted between the two groups [20–22]. There is no evidence to suggest that use of dipyridamole alone increases the risk of ICH.

Ticlopidine

Ticlopidine is a platelet adenosine diphosphate (ADP) receptor antagonist that has been evaluated in randomized trials of patients with cerebrovascular disease comparing it with aspirin (TASS, the Ticlopidine Aspirin Stroke Study) [32] and placebo (CATS, the Canadian American Ticlopidine Study in thromboembolic stroke) [33].

Ticlopidine was superior to placebo and has comparable benefit to aspirin in prevention of cerebrovascular disease. No significant differences in risk for stroke, MI, or vascular death were found at long-term follow-up. Risk of neutropenia and TTP limit the widespread use of this medication. Limited data exist regarding the risk of ICH associated with ticlopidine.

P2Y12 adenosine diphosphate receptor inhibitors

The drugs clopidogrel, prasugrel, and ticagrelor are the available antiplatelet agents in this category. Clopidogrel is the most widely used and studied drug in this group and is discussed in detail below.

Data regarding ICH with prasugrel is limited; however, one study of dual antiplatelet treatment using prasugrel and aspirin in patients with clopidogrel resistance suggested higher incidence of hemorrhagic complications including ICH in this group compared to antiplatelet treatment with aspirin and clopidogrel [18]. Similarly direct comparison of prasugrel with clopidogrel suggested higher bleeding complications [34].

In the PLATO (Platelet Inhibition and Patient Outcomes) trial [35], ticagrelor was compared to clopidogrel in the treatment of acute coronary syndrome and was found to have a higher rate of ICH, although total major bleeds and fatal bleeding complications were noted to be similar between the two groups. Limited data exist regarding the use of ticagrelor in the management of cerebrovascular disease.

Clopidogrel

Clopidogrel is a thienopyridine inhibitor of the platelet P2Y12 ADP receptor. Clopidogrel is an agent that irreversibly inhibits ADP-induced platelet aggregation. The interaction of ADP with the platelet P2Y12 receptor induces platelet shape change, reversible aggregation, initial glycoprotein (GP) IIb/IIIa activation, phospholipase C activation, and calcium flux, all of which is inhibited with clopidogrel. Inhibition of platelet aggregation is concentration-dependent and irreversible, and maximal inhibition is achieved in 4–7 days, after which higher doses cannot produce additional inhibition. Regular use of clopidogrel (75 mg daily) can produce 40 to 50% inhibition of ADP-induced platelet aggregation. This function makes it one of the drugs of choice for secondary stroke prevention, and also part of dual antiplatelet therapy in patients undergoing angioplasty and/or stent placement and acute coronary syndromes [36]. In most patients, platelet function returns to normal five to seven days after discontinuing the medication [37].

As a single agent, clopidogrel has been evaluated for secondary stroke prevention in two major trials, one comparing it with aspirin (CAPRIE, Trial of Clopidogrel vs. Aspirin in Patients at Risk of Ischemic Events) [38], and another comparing it with combination aspirin/dipyridamole (ASA-DP) (PRoFESS, Prevention Regimen for Effectively Avoiding Second Strokes) [39]. In each trial, rates of primary outcomes were similar between the treatment groups. The ProFESS trial demonstrated no significant difference in efficacy or safety between clopidogrel and aspirin combined with extended release dipyridamole, although ASA-DP was associated with a higher risk of major hemorrhages, including ICH (HR 1.15; 95% CI 1.00–1.32) [40].

The CAPRIE trial [38] assessed the relative efficacy of a once-daily regimen of either 75 mg of clopidogrel or 325 mg of aspirin in reducing the incidence of ischemic stroke, MI, or vascular death in nearly 20,000 patients who had recent ischemic stroke, MI, or symptomatic peripheral arterial disease. Patients treated with clopidogrel had an annual 5.32% risk of ischemic stroke, myocardial infarction, or vascular death compared with 5.83% in patients treated with aspirin (RR reduction 8.7%; p = 0.043, CI 0.3–16.5). Although there were no significant differences in terms of safety, hemorrhagic complications were slightly more frequent in the aspirin group than in the clopidogrel group (ICH 0.47% vs. 0.33% and GI hemorrhage 0.72% vs. 0.52% respectively). However, in a retrospective comparison of patients presenting with ICH on aspirin or clopidogrel, Campbell et al. [41] noted larger ICH size, decreased chance of discharge to home, and increased trend to mortality in the clopidogrel group compared to the aspirin group.

Proton pump inhibitors (PPI), such as esomeprazole, reduce the effectiveness of clopidogrel and its co-administration may lead to increased risk for major cardiovascular events, including stroke and MI. When antacid therapy is required in a patient on clopidogrel, an H2 blocker may be preferable to a PPI. In addition, functional genetic variants in CYP genes can affect the effectiveness of platelet inhibition in patients taking clopidogrel. Carriers of at least one CYP2C19 reduced-function allele had a relative reduction of 32% in plasma exposure to the active metabolite of clopidogrel compared with non-carriers.

Combination of clopidogrel and aspirin

Combination of clopidogrel and aspirin is commonly used in secondary prevention of cardiovascular and cerebrovascular diseases to provide synergistic inhibition of platelet aggregation. Naidech et al. [42–44] demonstrated that increased platelet inhibition (as measured with VerifyNow ASA and P2Y12 tests for aspirin and clopidogrel, respectively), correlated with increased ICH volume growth at 12 hours, increased volume of intraventricular hemorrhage (IVH), increased chance of death at 14 days, and poor outcome at three months.

Combination of clopidogrel and aspirin in secondary stroke prevention has been studied in several trials.

Trials such as CHARISMA (Clopidogrel for High Atherothrombotic Risk and Ischemic Stabilization, Management, and Avoidance) [45]; MATCH (Aspirin and Clopidogrel Compared with Clopidogrel Alone after Recent Ischemic Stroke or Transient Ischemic Attack in High-Risk Patients) [46]; and FASTER (Fast Assessment of Stroke and Transient Ischemic Attack to Prevent Early Recurrence) [54], examined the role of monotherapy vs. combination antiplatelet treatment for secondary prevention of non-cardioembolic strokes. Other trials like CHANCE (Clopidogrel in High-Risk Patients with Acute Non-Disabling Cerebrovascular Events) [48] and ongoing trials like POINT (Platelet-Oriented Inhibition in New TIA and Minor Ischemic Stroke) [49] have studied the benefits of short-term dual antiplatelet therapy in patients with minor stoke or TIA. Trials including SPS3 (Secondary Prevention of Small Subcortical Strokes) [50], SAMMPRIS (Stenting vs. Aggressive Medical Management for Preventing Recurrent Stroke in Intracranial Stenosis) [51]; and CLAIR (Clopidogrel plus aspirin vs. aspirin alone for reducing embolization in patients with acute symptomatic cerebral or carotid artery stenosis) [52] have investigated the role of anti-platelet treatment for secondary stroke prevention in patients with specific stroke mechanisms.

In the MATCH trial (Aspirin and Clopidogrel Compared with Clopidogrel Alone after Recent Ischemic Stroke or Transient Ischemic Attack in High-risk Patients) [46], which randomized 7,599 patients within three months of ischemic stroke or TIA to aspirin 81 to 162 mg daily and clopidogrel 75 mg daily vs. only clopidogrel 75 mg daily, there was no excess of bleeding in the antiplatelet treatment group during the first month of treatment, though an increased bleeding risk in the aspirin/clopidogrel group became apparent after three months of therapy. Overall the combination therapy showed an increased trend of ICH by 61% (p = 0.06) compared with clopidogrel alone. The CHANCE (Clopidogrel in High-risk Patients with Acute Non-disabling Cerebrovascular Events) trial randomized 5,100 patients within 24 hours of stroke or TIA to aspirin/clopidogrel for 21 days, followed by clopidogrel alone, vs. aspirin alone. Results suggest a large benefit in stroke reduction at 90 days with use of combination therapy within 24 hours of minor stroke or TIA. In this study, hemorrhagic stroke occurred in eight patients in each of the two study groups (0.3% of each group). All vascular deaths (including death from hemorrhagic stroke) occurred in six patients (0.2%) in the clopidogrel/aspirin group and in five (0.2%) in the aspirin group [53].

The pooled effects of treatment with single (aspirin, clopidogrel or dipyridamole) vs. dual (aspirin/clopidogrel or aspirin/dipyridamole) antiplatelet therapy in the acute peri-ischemic period were examined in a meta-analysis [54]. A total of twelve randomized trials including 3,766 subjects were analyzed. Only trials with randomization within 72 hours of acute stroke or TIA were included. Only five studies (24% of patients) used a combination of aspirin/clopidogrel as dual antiplatelet therapy. Despite the different combinations, there was no heterogeneity in any of the analyses. Stroke recurrence was significantly reduced (3.3% vs. 5.0%, RR 0.67, 95% CI 0.56–0.91) in the dual antiplatelet group, as were total major vascular events. There was no difference with regards to overall mortality. However, dual therapy was associated with a non-significant increase in major bleeding (0.9% vs. 0.4%, RR 2.09, 95% CI 0.86–5.06).

Dual antiplatelet therapy for secondary stroke prevention in patients with small-vessel and large-vessel diseases

The SPS3 trial enrolled 3,020 subjects with MRI-confirmed small subcortical (lacunar) infarcts within six months of stroke. Patients were followed for a mean of 3.4 years. Patients were randomized to either daily aspirin 325 mg/placebo or aspirin 325 mg/clopidogrel 75 mg and were further randomized to systolic blood pressure targets of either <130 mmHg or 130–149 mmHg [50]. Primary outcomes were all recurrent strokes, secondary outcomes included acute myocardial infarction and death (vascular, non-vascular, or unknown) and the primary safety outcome was major extracranial hemorrhage. The risk of recurrent stroke was not significantly reduced in the dual antiplatelet group. The risk of all major hemorrhage was almost doubled with dual antiplatelet therapy (2.1% per year) compared with aspirin alone (1.1% per year) (p<0.001). However, the increase in ICH with dual antiplatelet therapy was not significant (hazard ratio 1.52; 95% CI 0.79–2.93). There was no significant interaction between the antiplatelet therapies and the systolic blood pressure targets (p = 0.46).

In the SAMMPRIS trial [51], patients with recent TIA or stroke secondary to stenosis of 70–99% of the diameter of a major intracranial artery were randomly assigned to aggressive medical management (90 days of dual antiplatelet therapy using aspirin and clopidogrel as well as risk factor modification) or aggressive medical management plus percutaneous transluminal angioplasty and stenting (PTAS) with use of the Wingspan stent system. It was concluded that, in patients with intracranial arterial stenosis, aggressive medical management was superior to PTAS, both because the risk of early stroke after PTAS was high and because the risk of stroke with aggressive medical therapy alone was lower than expected.

Two trials, CLAIR [52] and CARESS [55], assessed aspirin vs. aspirin/clopidogrel in patients with large-vessel disease and both studies measured microembolic signals on transcranial Doppler as primary outcomes. Although both of these studies suggested lower incidence of microemboli in the dual antiplatelet group, no significant difference in rates of bleeding was noted between the two groups.

Dual antiplatelet therapy for secondary stroke prevention in patients with atrial fibrillation

In the ACTIVE-A trial (Atrial Fibrillation Clopidogrel Trial with Irbesartan for Prevention of Vascular Events – Aspirin), 7,554 subjects were randomized to aspirin 75 to 100 mg daily/clopidogrel 75 mg daily vs. aspirin alone [56]. There was an overall reduction of combined vascular events with dual antiplatelet therapy but the benefit was marginal when rates of major bleeding were taken into account (2.0% vs. 1.3% per year, RR 1.57, 95% CI 1.29–1.92). ACTIVE-W (Atrial Fibrillation Clopidogrel Trial with Irbesartan for Prevention of Vascular events – Warfarin) assigned 6,706 participants to aspirin 75 to 100 mg daily/clopidogrel 75 mg daily vs. dose-adjusted warfarin (target INR 2.0–3.0) [57]. The trial was stopped after 1.3 years due to clear superiority in the warfarin group for reduction of combined vascular endpoints. There was no significant difference in major bleeding rates (2.4% vs. 2.2%), although there were significantly more bleeding events overall in the warfarin group (15.4% vs. 13.2%).

Based on current evidence, it can be inferred that in high-risk populations with a sufficiently high frequency of coronary artery disease, the benefit of long-term dual antiplatelet therapy lies in a reduction of MI. However, it is counteracted by morbidity and mortality secondary to increased incidences of moderate to fatal hemorrhages, especially with long-term dual

antiplatelet use. Patients with overall low mortality rates and low frequencies of coronary artery disease may have increased mortality with >90 days of antiplatelet treatment because the absolute reduction in coronary events does not offset death related directly or indirectly to bleeding complications. However, more recent studies have suggested benefits of "short-term" dual antiplatelet therapy in patients with minor stroke or TIAs. In patients with intracranial atherosclerotic disease, aggressive medical management including short-term dual antiplatelet therapy along with lifestyle modification is superior to intracranial stenting. Other ongoing trials with antiplatelet treatment for secondary stroke prevention in small-vessel disease can further elucidate the risk/benefit of aspirin/clopidogrel therapy in this group of patients.

Glycoprotein IIb/IIIa inhibitors

Glycoprotein IIb/IIIa (GPIIb IIIa) complexes mediate platelet aggregation by binding fibrinogen or von Willebrand factor (vWF), protein cofactors that form bridges between adjacent platelets. The cross-linked adhesive proteins assemble platelets into the aggregate [58]. Agents that block the function of the GPIIb-IIIa complex of platelets constitute a powerful generation of antithrombotic drugs. Abciximab, eptifibatide and tirofiban fall under this category. These agents are available in intravenous formulation and are primarily used in the setting of acute coronary syndrome and during percutaneous coronary interventions [59,60]. The use of abciximab was first evaluated in the EPIC trial [61], which was a prospective, randomized, double-blind trial consisting of 2,099 patients undergoing high-risk coronary intervention. This study showed a beneficial effect of abciximab in reducing rates of death and myocardiac infarction primarily in patients with unstable angina. However, increased bleeding complications and transfusions were noted in the treatment group. Among all study patients, six patients had ICH. Of these, one patient had received an abciximab bolus, and two patients had received the abciximab bolus and infusion.

In the neurointerventional setting, they are used as an adjunct for carotid artery stents or as a rescue agent to manage thrombotic complications of endovascular procedures. The evidence regarding safety of abciximab and eptifibatide is limited to case reports and case series, and has mixed results regarding use for neurointervention [62–65]. In 2002, Qureshi *et al.* published a compiled report based on the clinical experience of neurointerventionists at three academic medical centers between 1999 and 2000 [66]. This study suggested a higher rate of intracerebral hemorrhage associated with neurointerventional procedures compared to coronary interventional procedures. It suggests that the use of intravenous abciximab in conjunction with aspirin, clopidogrel, and heparin as an adjunct to neurointerventional procedures can result in rapidly progressive intracerebral hemorrhages. Due to such safety concerns, it is not used as the first-line antithrombotic agent.

Information regarding risk of tirofiban is also limited; however, it has been shown to increase the risk of fatal intracerebral hemorrhage and poor outcome in patients with endovascular stroke therapy [67].

Cilostazol

Cilostazol inhibits phosphodiesterase III, leading to increase in cyclic adenosine monophosphate (cAMP), which in turn inhibits platelet aggregation. It also reduces the number of circulating, partially activated, or preconditioned platelets, by reducing the surface expression of adhesive molecules in endothelial cells interacting with circulating platelets. Additionally, it causes vasodilation, especially in femoral vascular beds.

The effect of cilostazol in secondary prevention of stroke was studied in the cilostazol and stroke prevention study [68]. Cilostazol is found to have minimal bleeding risk as compared to other antiplatelet agents and is not considered to be a significant risk for ICH [75].

Factors associated with increased risk for intracranial hemorrhage with antithrombotic use

Clinical factors associated with an increased ICH risk during antithrombotic therapy include age, previous stroke, and severe hypertension [24]. Brain-imaging studies using CT suggest that leukoaraiosis is a risk factor for ICH in patients taking warfarin but there have been few studies of imaging risk factors for aspirin-related ICH [70,71]. Other factors associated with increased risk of ICH are discussed below.

Evidence of microhemorrhages on MRI

Microbleeds detected on MRI may be considered a biomarker of bleeding prone small-vessel diseases, in particular hypertensive small-vessel arteriopathy and cerebral amyloid angiopathy (CAA). MRI-demonstrated microbleeds are not uncommon in patients with stroke or TIA [72] and in asymptomatic elderly individuals (up to 40%) [73]. Several studies in patients with stroke have suggested an association between microbleeds and an increased risk of ICH [74,75]. Studies have also suggested an association between microbleeds and antiplatelet use [76], and between microbleeds and the risk of antithrombotic-related ICH with a dose-dependent effect [77]. Pathogenetically, antithrombotic therapies may exaggerate the underlying risk of spontaneous ICH [78].

Previous autopsy and MRI studies have established that lobar microbleeds are indicative of CAA [79,80]. In CAA, amyloid β-protein is deposited in the walls of superficial cortical and leptomeningeal vessels, causing them to become brittle and prone to bleeding. CAA may account for a large proportion of spontaneous ICH in older people and has been suggested as a risk factor for ICH associated with warfarin and aspirin [81], as well as with ICH after thrombolysis for ischemic stroke. In a study by Gregoire *et al.* [82], the prevalence and distribution of microbleeds in antiplatelet users with symptomatic ICH was compared with matched antiplatelet users without ICH. Because microbleeds are known to be associated with ICH regardless of antiplatelet use, a case to case comparison study between antiplatelet users with ICH and patients with spontaneous ICH was also conducted. Microbleeds were more prevalent and numerous in antiplatelet users who developed symptomatic ICH compared with matched antiplatelet users who did not develop ICH. The microbleed number was strongly associated with ICH risk, even after controlling for the presence of leukoaraiosis and other potential confounding factors. In separate regression analyses adjusted for the presence of leukoaraiosis, lobar (but not deep) microbleeds were a statistically significant predictor of antiplatelet therapy-related ICH. Available data suggests that CAA is an important risk factor for ICH related to antithrombotic therapy, and careful consideration of the risks and benefits should be undertaken prior to prescribing any antithrombotic agents to this group of patients.

Concurrent anticoagulant use

Concurrent anticoagulant use increases the risk of anti-platelet therapy-associated ICH [83]. In younger patients with prosthetic cardiac valves or coronary artery disease who have inherently low ICH risks, absolute rates of ICH during combined warfarin/aspirin therapy are likely low [24]. In older patients or with target INRs >3, addition of aspirin to anticoagulation should be performed only after careful consideration of the benefit/risk ratio because of increased risk of ICH.

Co-administration of warfarin and aspirin for thromboembolism prevention appears to be of benefit in patients with some mechanical heart valves and is sometimes necessary in patients with strong coincident indications for warfarin and arterial stent placement [84]. Evidence supporting co-administration in settings such as concurrent atrial fibrillation and coronary disease is, however, lacking, as the risk of bleeding is significantly increased [85].

Platelet function tests

Platelet activity and levels of inhibition can be measured in a variety of ways including conventional platelet count, in vivo bleeding time, or many different types of platelet function assays. The in vivo bleeding time is poorly reproducible, invasive, insensitive, and time consuming [86] and a normal bleeding time does not predict safety of surgical procedures. Hence its use is limited only to initial screening test to identify patients with severe hemostatic defects [87,88]. There are multiple additional laboratory and point-of-care testing systems available and results are reported in units of time, change in light transmission, platelet count, surface area covered, and flow cytometry [89]. On many of these systems, high platelet inhibition has been associated with bleeding events and low platelet inhibition with in-stent thrombosis after coronary artery stenting [90,91]. Nonetheless, multiple comparison studies have been unable to establish a correlation between the results of the various testing systems [92–97]. Furthermore, point-of-care testing tends to have greater inaccuracy than hematology lab testing [89]. There is currently no established standard to define inappropriate platelet activity [89].

Reversal of antiplatelet therapy

Although there is no specific antidote, the aspirin effect can be reversed by platelet transfusion.

In experimental studies, rFVIIa has been shown to reverse the in vitro inhibition of thrombin generation caused by aspirin [98]. In case reports researchers have successfully used deamino-d-arginine-vasopressin (DDAVP) to reverse the aspirin effect [99,100]. It may be a valuable option for rapid intraoperative control of bleeding.

Like aspirin, clopidogrel lacks a specific antidote. Platelet transfusion, rFVIIa, and DDAVP have also been tried for clopidogrel reversal with reported success. Platelet dysfunction due to clopidogrel is more severe than that with aspirin; thus, for neurosurgical bleeding, generally two doses of platelets (two single donor or ten pooled concentrates) transfusion is recommended [101]. Ticlopidine has a bleeding profile similar to clopidogrel, and similar strategies are used to reverse its effect [101].

Reversal of glycoprotein IIb/IIIa inhibitors can be achieved by discontinuation and allowing time for clearance. Abciximab has an approximate 12-hour pharmacologic effective half-life. The half-life of eptifibatide and tirofiban is much shorter (i.e., two to four hours). Platelet transfusion can also be used to overcome the antiplatelet effect of a glycoprotein IIb/IIIa receptor antagonist [102,103].

When considering antiplatelet-related ICH, the exact role that antiplatelet agents play in ICH formation, growth, and outcome as well as the role for antiplatelet reversal in patients with ICH is unclear. Currently, there is no well-supported algorithm for reversing these agents. The decision to stop all antiplatelet medication needs to be carefully considered, weighing the size and morbidity of the ICH against the reason the agents were initiated. The value of platelet function assays in patients presenting with ICH is uncertain at this time. Reversing antiplatelet medication with transfusion, desmopressin, or other factors is not currently supported by clinical evidence and should be considered investigational [101]. According to ASA/AHA guidelines, the usefulness of platelet transfusions in ICH patients with a history of antiplatelet use is unclear and is considered investigational (Class IIb; Level of Evidence: B) [104–106]. A randomized trial is currently underway to evaluate antiplatelet agent reversal in ICH (PATCH, Platelet Transfusion in Cerebral Hemorrhage trial) [107].

Management of intracranial hemorrhage

Management of ICH is principally focused on supportive measures to minimize injury and stabilize the patient. Certain evidence-based quality indicators have been identified in the management of ICH [108]. A summary of ICH management is outlined below.

Acute management in the emergency department

Initial diagnosis

In patients with concern for acute stroke, evaluation by emergency department (ED) physician and hemodynamic monitoring within 10 minutes of patient arrival is an important first step. Acquisition of neuroimaging within 25 minutes and interpreting a CT scan within 45 minutes is key to timely diagnosis and is consistent with the recommendations of the National Symposium on Rapid Identification and Treatment of acute stroke as well as the Brain Attack Coalition.

Airway protection

In patients requiring intubation, a timely controlled intubation within 30 minutes, as opposed to a rushed intubation within 5 to 10 minutes, is preferred to minimize complications such as oropharyngeal injury, aspiration, glottic edema, and esophageal intubation.

Reversal of anticoagulation

In patients with concomitant anticoagulation use, rapid reversal of INR within two hours of first elevated INR >1.4 reduces the extent of hematoma growth. Multiple guidelines suggest that patients diagnosed with anticoagulant-related life-threatening hemorrhage, including ICH, should receive emergent therapy to lower their INR [109]. Increasing intensity of anticoagulation is strongly associated with increasing mortality. A combination of IV vitamin K, PCC, or FFP and fVIIa is usually recommended without clear evidence for superiority of one regimen over another. Rapid reversal of INR also permits urgent surgical evacuations in neurologically deteriorating patients with anticoagulant-related ICH. In patients with novel anticoagulant use, dabigatran reversal can be achieved by use of recently FDA approved reversal agent idarucizumab [110]. Rivaroxaban and apixaban do not have specific reversal agents, are likely to benefit from PCC administration and are unlikely to benefit from hemodialysis [101].

Blood pressure management

Prompt management of acute hypertensive response by lowering blood pressure is necessary, especially in the first 24 hours. Systolic blood pressure (SBP) >200 mmHg has been associated with hematoma expansion and increased mortality [111,112]. Persistently higher SBP is also associated with perihematoma brain edema formation [113]. The Intensive Blood Pressure Reduction in Acute Cerebral Hemorrhage Trial (INTERACT-2) showed a trend toward lower relative and absolute growth in hematoma volumes from baseline to 24 hours in the intensive treatment group (<140 mmHg) compared with the control group (<180 mmHg) [114]. In addition, there was no excess of neurological deterioration or other adverse events related to intensive BP lowering. Another study, the Antihypertensive Treatment in Acute Cerebral Hemorrhage (ATACH-I) trial also suggested the feasibility and safety of early rapid BP lowering in ICH [115], although the Phase III trial (ATACH-II) was stopped early and final results are awaited. The Intracerebral Hemorrhage Acutely Decreasing Arterial Pressure Trial (ICH ADAPT) [116] evaluated the theory of ischemic vulnerability in the perihematoma region with rapid BP reduction in patients with ICH. The investigators used two systolic BP targets of <150 mmHg vs. <180 mmHg (baseline SBP 182±20 mmHg vs. 184±25 mmHg respectively) in patients with moderate ICH volume. The investigators found no difference in perihematoma cerebral blood flow (CBF) between the two groups using CT perfusion studies within two hours of randomization, despite significant difference in mean BP reduction between the two groups. As per current ASA/AHA recommendations, in patients presenting with a systolic BP of 150 to 220 mmHg, acute lowering of systolic BP to 140 mmHg is probably safe (Class IIa; Level of Evidence: B). Judicious lowering is recommended in patients with high ICP to maintain cerebral perfusion pressure (CPP) >60.

Treatment of mass effect

In patients with intracranial mass effect or transtentorial herniation (TTH), prompt medical and surgical intervention should be undertaken as it represents a usually fatal consequence [117]. Medical management includes use of hyperosmolar agents including mannitol and hypertonic saline in addition to ICP lowering maneuvers like head elevation and hyperventilation. Surgical intervention such as placement of an external ventricular drain (EVD) and decompressive hemicraniectomy may be performed. Persistent clinically significant intracranial mass effect or intracranial hypertension is common after the first episode of intracranial hypertension or TTH and requires additional treatment including intraventricular drainage, hypertonic saline infusion, repeated mannitol boluses, and neurosurgical evaluation.

Intensive care unit care

Once ICH has been recognized and prompt management initiated, admission to a dedicated ICU is recommended due to the high risk of neurologic deterioration, cardiovascular instability, and the possible need for intubation. Hourly assessment of neurological status with use of a standard evaluation such as the Glasgow Coma Scale (GCS) score is necessary for detection of deterioration. In addition to continuing the care initiated in the ED, the following management plans have to be implemented.

Seizure monitoring

Convulsive or non-convulsive status epilepticus in the ICU patient is associated with high mortality. Patients with ICH have a high likelihood of seizures. In one study, up to 28% of patients on continuous EEG monitoring were found to have electrographic seizures within 72 hours of admission [118]. Timely management of seizures is important as status epilepticus becomes progressively less responsive to treatment. Cessation of seizure activity within 20 minutes of therapy and no return within the next 40 minutes defines initial treatment success. No recurrence of overt or subtle seizure 12 hours after the first seizure indicates sustained treatment success.

Blood pressure management

In patients with persistently elevated BP, oral antihypertensive medications can be initiated at 24 to 48 hours after symptom onset [119].

Glucose monitoring

Elevated serum glucose has been associated with hematoma expansion [19] and poor clinical outcomes [120] in clinical studies. The first 72 hours after onset represents a period of increased vulnerability to both primary and secondary (recurrent) hyperglycemia and prompt glucose management is indicated. Hypoglycemia should be avoided.

Fever and infection control

Hyperpyrexia in the first 12 to 24 hours after stroke onset is associated with poor functional outcome [121]. Identification of fever source as well as initiation of appropriate therapy is indicated.

Patients with ICH are prone to hospital-acquired infections and prompt management is indicated. Administration of IV antibiotics within 24 hours of first persistent fever when meeting other criteria for hospital-acquired or ventilator-associated pneumonia (VAP) is important as delay in treatment can be associated with increased mortality [122].

Deep venous thrombosis prophylaxis

Prevalence of deep venous thrombosis (DVT) is high among patients with ICH [123]. The first 48 hours after symptom onset was considered the appropriate time to initiate DVT prophylaxis based on consistent safety and effectiveness data provided by clinical trials in ICH patients [124,125]. There is no specific recommendation regarding the method of DVT prophylaxis; however, heparin and low molecular weight heparin should be avoided in patients with bleeding diathesis, severe cerebral edema, deep coma, and marked hypertensive response.

Gastric ulcer prophylaxis

Gastric prophylaxis is indicated in patients with ICH due to the relatively high prevalence of gastric ulcers in this group of patients. The first 48 hours after symptom onset is considered the appropriate time to initiate prophylaxis based on safety and effectiveness data provided by clinical trials in ICH patients [126,127].

Initiation of diet

Dysphagia screening should be performed within 72 hours of symptom onset and appropriate enteral feeding should be initiated within this period. Poor nutrition has been documented to adversely affect functional outcomes after strokes [128].

Plan for tracheostomy and percutaneous endoscopic gastrostomy placement

The decision regarding tracheostomy should be ideally performed by day 8 of mechanical ventilation because of the low probability of subsequent extubation or in-hospital death [129]. In a systematic review of 12 prospective studies [130], the timing of tracheostomy did not alter mortality significantly but led to a reduced duration of ventilation and shorter stays in the ICU.

In patients who fail their dysphagia screen, feeding should be initiated via a nasogastric (NG) or orogastric tube. Placement of a percutaneous endoscopic gastrostomy (PEG) tube should be considered in those patients who continue to be on tube feeds beyond two to three weeks of presentation. In one multicenter randomized controlled trial comparing NG vs PEG tube in the early phase (within three days of enrollment) PEG feeding was associated with an absolute increase in risk of death by 1% and an almost eight-fold increased risk of death or poor outcome [131].

Declaration of do not resuscitate status

It is found that early care limitations with do not resuscitate (DNR) status are independently associated with both short- and long-term all-cause mortality after ICH despite adjustment for expected predictors of ICH mortality [132]. Withdrawal of care within 24 hours of admission is considered premature and an adverse parameter. Withdrawal of care between 24 hours and 7 days of admission without documentation of appropriate justification is also considered an adverse parameter. Reliance on objective data only available at the time of presentation is frequently insufficient to preclude withdrawal of care. However, a DNR decision may be appropriate when any two of the following three clinical criteria are present: severe stroke; life-threatening brain damage; and significant comorbidities.

Conclusions

Antiplatelet therapy is widely used for the prevention of cerebrovascular conditions. It is important to recognize that antiplatelet use can be associated with increased risk of intracranial hemorrhage in certain patients. Careful consideration of the patient profile is important in initiating antiplatelet therapy. Furthermore, combination of antiplatelet therapy is associated with higher risk of hemorrhagic complications. However, risk of ICH should not preclude the use of antiplatelet agents if overall benefit outweighs the risk in these patients.

References

1. Qureshi A I, Mendelow A D, Hanley D F. Intracerebral haemorrhage. *Lancet.* 2009; 373:1632–44.

2. Trialists' Collaboration. A collaborative meta-analysis of randomised trials of antiplatelet therapy for prevention of death, myocardial infarction, and stroke in high risk patients. *British Medical Journal.* 2002; 324:71–86.

3. Sudlow C L M, Warlow C P; International Stroke Incidence C. Comparable studies of the incidence of stroke and its pathological types: Results from an international collaboration. *Stroke.* 1997; 28:491–9.

4. Carolei A, Marini C, Di Napoli M, et al. High stroke incidence in the prospective community-based l'Aquila registry (1994–1998): First year's results. *Stroke.* 1997; 28:2500–6.

5. Dennis M S. Outcome after brain haemorrhage. *Cerebrovascular Diseases.* 2003; 16(suppl 1):9–13.

6. Kothari R U, Brott T, Broderick J P, et al. The ABCs of measuring intracerebral hemorrhage volumes. *Stroke.* 1996; 27:1304–5.

7. Broderick J P, Brott T G, Duldner J E, Tomsick T, Huster G. Volume of intracerebral hemorrhage. A powerful and easy-to-use predictor of 30-day mortality. *Stroke.* 1993; 24:987–93.

8. Palareti G, Leali N, Coccheri S, et al. Bleeding complications of oral anticoagulant treatment: An inception-cohort, prospective collaborative study (ISCOAT). *Lancet.* 1996; 348:423–8.

9. Nicolini A, Ghirarduzzi A, Iorio A, et al. Intracranial bleeding: Epidemiology and relationships with antithrombotic treatment in 241 cerebral hemorrhages in Reggio Emilia. *Haematologica.* 2002; 87:948–56.

10. Rosand J, Eckman M H, Knudsen K A, Singer D E, Greenberg S M. The effect of warfarin and intensity of anticoagulation on outcome of intracerebral hemorrhage. *Archives of Internal Medicine.* 2004; 164:880–4.

11. Campbell P G, Sen A, Yadla S, Jabbour P, Jallo J. Emergency reversal of antiplatelet agents in patients presenting with an intracranial hemorrhage: A clinical review. *World Neurosurgery.* 2010; 74:279–85.

12. Cantalapiedra A, Gutierrez O, Tortosa J I, *et al*. Oral anticoagulant treatment: Risk factors involved in 500 intracranial hemorrhages. *Journal of Thrombosis and Thrombolysis*. 2006; **22**:113–20.

13. Caso V, Paciaroni M, Venti M, *et al*. Effect of on-admission antiplatelet treatment on patients with cerebral hemorrhage. *Cerebrovascular Diseases*. 2007; **24**:215–18.

14. Foerch C, Sitzer M, Steinmetz H, Neumann-Haefelin T. Pretreatment with antiplatelet agents is not independently associated with unfavorable outcome in intracerebral hemorrhage. *Stroke*. 2006; **37**:2165–7.

15. Roquer J, Campello A R, Gomis M, *et al*. Previous antiplatelet therapy is an independent predictor of 30-day mortality after spontaneous supratentorial intracerebral hemorrhage. *Journal of Neurology*. 2005; **252**:412–16.

16. Sansing L H, Messe S R, Cucchiara B L, *et al*. Prior antiplatelet use does not affect hemorrhage growth or outcome after ICH. *Neurology*. 2009; **72**:1397–402.

17. Toyada K, Okada Y, Minematsu K, *et al*. Antiplatelet therapy contributes to acute deterioration of intracerebral hemorrhage. *Neurology*. 2005; **65**:1000–4.

18. Akbari S H, Reynolds M R, Kadkhodayan Y, Cross D T, Moran C J. Hemorrhagic complications after prasugrel (Effient) therapy for vascular neurointerventional procedures. *Journal of Neurointerventional Surgery*. 2012.

19. Broderick J P, Diringer M N, Hill M D, *et al*. Determinants of intracerebral hemorrhage growth: an exploratory analysis. *Stroke*. 2007; **38**:1072–5.

20. Lacut K, Le Gal G, Seizeur R, *et al*. Antiplatelet drug use preceding the onset of intracerebral hemorrhage is associated with increased mortality. *Fundamental & Clinical Pharmacology*. 2007; **21**:327–33.

21. Roquer J. Previous antiplatelet treatment and mortality in patients with intracerebral hemorrhage. *Stroke*. 2007; **38**:863.

22. Sorimachi T, Fujii Y, Morita K, Tanaka R. Predictors of hematoma enlargement in patients with intracerebral hemorrhage treated with rapid administration of antifibrinolytic agents and strict blood pressure control. *Journal of Neurosurgery*. 2007; **106**:250–4.

23. Thrift A G, McNeil J J, Forbes A, Donnan G A. Risk of primary intracerebral haemorrhage associated with aspirin and non-steroidal anti-inflammatory drugs: Case-control study. *British Medical Journal*. 1999; **318**:759–64.

24. Hart R G, Tonarelli S B, Pearce L A. Avoiding central nervous system bleeding during antithrombotic therapy: recent data and ideas. *Stroke*. 2005; **36**:1588–93.

25. Hennekens C. Final report on the aspirin component of the ongoing physicians health study. *New England Journal of Medicine*. 1989; **321**:129–35.

26. The SALT Collaborative Group. Swedish Aspirin Low-dose Trial (SALT) of 75 mg aspirin as secondary prophylaxis after cerebrovascular ischaemic events. *Lancet*. 1991; **338**:1345–19.

27. He J, Whelton P, Vu B, Klag M. Aspirin and risk of hemorrhagic stroke. *Journal of the American Medical Association*. 1998; **280**:1930–5.

28. Sudlow C. *Antithrombotic Treatment: Clinical Evidence*. London: BMJ Publishing Group; 2001.

29. Thrift A G, McNeil J J, Forbes A, Donnan G A. Risk of primary intracerebral haemorrhage associated with aspirin and non-steroidal anti-inflammatory drugs: Case-control study. *British Medical Journal*. 1999; **318**:759.

30. Baldi G, Altomonte F, Altomonte M, *et al*. Intracranial haemorrhage in patients on antithrombotics: Clinical presentation and determinants of outcome in a prospective multicentric study in Italian emergency departments. *Cerebrovascular Diseases*. 2006; **22**:286–93.

31. Connolly B J, Pearce L A, Kurth T, Kase C S, Hart R G. Aspirin therapy and risk of subdural hematoma: Meta-analysis of randomized clinical trials. *Journal of Stroke and Cerebrovascular Diseases*. 2013.

32. Hass W K, Easton J D, Adams Jr H P, *et al*. Ticlopidine Aspirin Stroke Study Group. A randomized trial comparing ticlopidine hydrochloride with aspirin for the prevention of stroke in high-risk patients. *New England Journal of Medicine*. 1989; **321**:501–7.

33. Gent M, Donald Easton J, Hachinski V, *et al*. The Canadian American Ticlopidine Study (CATS) in thromboembolic stroke. *Lancet*. 1989; **333**:1215–20.

34. Montalescot G, Wiviott S D, Braunwald E, *et al*. Prasugrel compared with clopidogrel in patients undergoing percutaneous coronary intervention for ST-elevation myocardial infarction (triton-timi 38): Double-blind, randomised controlled trial. *Lancet*. 2009; **373**:723–31.

35. Becker R C, Bassand J P, Budaj A, *et al*. Bleeding complications with the p2y12 receptor antagonists clopidogrel and ticagrelor in the Platelet Inhibition and Patient Outcomes (PLATO) trial. *European Heart Journal*. 2011; ehr422.

36. Cordina S M, Hassan A E, Ezzeddine M A. Prevalence and clinical characteristics of intracerebral hemorrhages associated with clopidogrel. *Journal of Vascular and Interventional Neurology*. 2009; **2**:136.

37. Weber A A, Braun M, Hohlfeld T, *et al*. Recovery of platelet function after discontinuation of clopidogrel treatment in healthy volunteers. *British Journal of Clinical Pharmacology*. 2001; **52**:333–6.

179

38. Gent M, Beaumont D, Blanchard J, *et al.* CAPRIE Steering Committee. A randomised, blinded, trial of clopidogrel versus aspirin in patients at risk of ischaemic events (CAPRIE). *Lancet.* 1996; **348**:1329–39.

39. Diener H-C, Sacco R L, Yusuf S, *et al.* Effects of aspirin plus extended-release dipyridamole versus clopidogrel and telmisartan on disability and cognitive function after recurrent stroke in patients with ischaemic stroke in the prevention regimen for effectively avoiding second strokes (PROFESS) trial: A double-blind, active and placebo-controlled study. *Lancet Neurology.* 2008; 7:875–84.

40. Sacco R L, Diener H-C, Yusuf S, *et al.* Aspirin and extended-release dipyridamole versus clopidogrel for recurrent stroke. *New England Journal of Medicine.* 2008; **359**:1238–51.

41. Campbell P G, Yadla S, Sen A N, Jallo J, Jabbour P. Emergency reversal of clopidogrel in the setting of spontaneous intracerebral hemorrhage. *World Neurosurgery.* 2011; **76**:100–4.

42. Naidech A M, Bendok B R, Garg R K, *et al.* Reduced platelet activity is associated with more intraventricular hemorrhage. *Neurosurgery.* 2009; **65**: 684–8.

43. Naidech A M, Bernstein R A, Levasseur K, *et al.* Platelet activity and outcome after intracerebral hemorrhage. *Annals of Neurology.* 2009; **65**:352–6.

44. Naidech A M, Jovanovic B, Liebling S, *et al.* Reduced platelet activity is associated with early clot growth and worse 3-month outcome after intracerebral hemorrhage. *Stroke.* 2009; **40**:2398–401.

45. Berger P B, Bhatt D L, Fuster V, *et al.* Bleeding complications with dual antiplatelet therapy among patients with stable vascular disease or risk factors for vascular disease: results from the clopidogrel for high atherothrombotic risk and ischemic stabilization, management, and avoidance (CHARISMA) trial. *Circulation.* 2010; **121**:2575–83.

46. Diener H-C, Bogousslavsky J, Brass L M, *et al.* Aspirin and Clopidogrel Compared with Clopidogrel Alone after Recent Ischaemic Stroke or Transient Ischaemic Attack in High-risk Patients (MATCH): Randomised, double-blind, placebo-controlled trial. *Lancet.* 2004; **364**:331–7.

47. Kennedy J, Hill M D, Ryckborst K J, *et al.* Fast Assessment of Stroke and Transient Ischaemic Attack to Prevent Early Recurrence (FASTER): A randomised controlled pilot trial. *Lancet Neurology.* 2007; **6**:961–9.

48. Wang Y, Wang Y, Zhao X, *et al.* Clopidogrel with aspirin in acute minor stroke or transient ischemic attack. *New England Journal of Medicine.* 2013; **369**:11–19.

49. Johnston S C, Easton J D, Farrant M, *et al.* Platelet-oriented inhibition in new TIA and minor ischemic stroke (POINT) trial: rationale and design. *International Journal of Stroke.* 2013; **8**:479–83.

50. Benavente O R, White C L, Pearce L, *et al.* The Secondary Prevention of Small Subcortical Strokes (SPS3) study. *International Journal of Stroke.* 2011; **6**: 164–75.

51. Chimowitz M I, Lynn M J, Derdeyn C P, *et al.* Stenting versus aggressive medical therapy for intracranial arterial stenosis. *New England Journal of Medicine.* 2011; **365**:993–1003.

52. Wong K S L, Chen C, Fu J, *et al.* Clopidogrel plus aspirin versus aspirin alone for reducing embolisation in patients with acute symptomatic cerebral or carotid artery stenosis (CLAIR study): A randomised, open-label, blinded-endpoint trial. *Lancet Neurology.* 2010; **9**:489–97.

53. Wang Y, Wang Y, Zhao X, *et al.* Clopidogrel with aspirin in acute minor stroke or transient ischemic attack. *New England Journal of Medicine.* 2013; **369**:11–19.

54. Geeganage C M, Diener H-C, Algra A, *et al.* Dual or mono antiplatelet therapy for patients with acute ischemic stroke or transient ischemic attack: systematic review and meta-analysis of randomized controlled trials. *Stroke.* 2012; **43**:1058–66.

55. Markus H S, Droste D W, Kaps M, *et al.* Dual antiplatelet therapy with clopidogrel and aspirin in symptomatic carotid stenosis evaluated using Doppler embolic signal detection: the clopidogrel and aspirin for reduction of emboli in symptomatic carotid stenosis (CARESS) trial. *Circulation.* 2005; **111**: 2233–40.

56. Connolly S J, Pogue J, Hart R G, *et al.* Effect of clopidogrel added to aspirin in patients with atrial fibrillation. *New England Journal of Medicine.* 2009; **360**:2066–78.

57. Connolly S, Pogue J, Hart R, *et al.* Active writing group of the active investigators. Clopidogrel plus aspirin versus oral anticoagulation for atrial fibrillation in the atrial fibrillation clopidogrel trial with irbesartan for prevention of vascular events (Active W): A randomised controlled trial. *Lancet.* 2006; **367**:1903–12.

58. Nurden A T, Poujol C, Durrieu-Jais C, Nurden P. Platelet glycoprotein IIb/IIIa inhibitors: basic and clinical aspects. *Arteriosclerosis, Thrombosis, and Vascular Biology.* 1999; **19**:2835–40.

59. The Epic I. Use of a monoclonal antibody directed against the platelet glycoprotein IIb/IIIa receptor in high-risk coronary angioplasty. *New England Journal of Medicine.* 1994; **330**:956–61.

60. The EPILOG Investigators. Platelet glycoprotein IIb/IIIa receptor blockade and low-dose heparin during

percutaneous coronary revascularization. *New England Journal of Medicine.* 1997; **336**:1689–97.

61. Lincoff A M, Califf R M, Anderson K M, *et al.* Evidence for prevention of death and myocardial infarction with platelet membrane glycoprotein IIb/IIIa receptor blockade by abciximab (c7e3 Fab) among patients with unstable angina undergoing percutaneous coronary revascularization. *Journal of the American College of Cardiology.* 1997; **30**:149–56.

62. Qureshi A I. Adjunctive use of platelet glycoprotein IIb/IIIa inhibitors for carotid angioplasty and stent placement: Time to say good bye? *Journal of Endovascular Therapy.* 2003; **10**:42–4.

63. Velat G J, Burry M V, Eskioglu E, *et al.* The use of abciximab in the treatment of acute cerebral thromboembolic events during neuroendovascular procedures. *Surgical Neurology.* 2006; **65**:352–8.

64. Deshmukh V R, Fiorella D J, Albuquerque F C, *et al.* Intra-arterial thrombolysis for acute ischemic stroke: Preliminary experience with platelet glycoprotein IIb/IIIa inhibitors as adjunctive therapy. *Neurosurgery.* 2005; **56**.

65. Qureshi A I, Siddiqui A M, Hanel R A, *et al.* Safety of high-dose intravenous eptifibatide as an adjunct to internal carotid artery angioplasty and stent placement: A prospective registry. *Neurosurgery.* 2004; **54**.

66. Qureshi A I, Saad M, Zaidat O O, *et al.* Intracerebral hemorrhages associated with neurointerventional procedures using a combination of antithrombotic agents including abciximab. *Stroke.* 2002; **33**:1916–19.

67. Kellert L, Hametner C, Rohde S, *et al.* Endovascular stroke therapy tirofiban is associated with risk of fatal intracerebral hemorrhage and poor outcome. *Stroke.* 2013; **44**:1453–5.

68. Gotoh F, Tohgi H, Hirai S, *et al.* Cilostazol stroke prevention study: A placebo-controlled double-blind trial for secondary prevention of cerebral infarction. *Journal of Stroke and Cerebrovascular Diseases.* 2000; **9**:147–57.

69. Goto S. Cilostazol: Potential mechanism of action for antithrombotic effects accompanied by a low rate of bleeding. *Atherosclerosis Supplements.* 2005; **6**:3–11.

70. Gorter J. Major bleeding during anticoagulation after cerebral ischemia patterns and risk factors. *Neurology.* 1999; **53**:1319.

71. Smith E, Rosand J, Knudsen K, Hylek E, Greenberg S. Leukoaraiosis is associated with warfarin-related hemorrhage following ischemic stroke. *Neurology.* 2002; **59**:193–7.

72. Werring D, Coward L, Losseff N, Jäger H, Brown M. Cerebral microbleeds are common in ischemic stroke but rare in TIA. *Neurology.* 2005; **65**:1914–18.

73. Vernooij M, Van Der Lugt A, Ikram M, *et al.* Prevalence and risk factors of cerebral microbleeds: the Rotterdam Scan Study. *Neurology.* 2008; **70**:1208–14.

74. Greenberg S M, Eng J A, Ning M, Smith E E, Rosand J. Hemorrhage burden predicts recurrent intracerebral hemorrhage after lobar hemorrhage. *Stroke.* 2004; **35**:1415–20.

75. Jeon S-B, Kang D-W, Lee E-M, *et al.* Initial microbleeds at MR imaging can predict recurrent intracerebral hemorrhage. *Journal of Neurology.* 2007; **254**:508–12.

76. Vernooij M W, Haag M D, van der Lugt A, *et al.* Use of antithrombotic drugs and the presence of cerebral microbleeds: The Rotterdam scan study. *Archives of Neurology.* 2009.

77. Soo Y O, Yang S R, Lam W W, *et al.* Risk vs benefit of anti-thrombotic therapy in ischaemic stroke patients with cerebral microbleeds. *Journal of Neurology.* 2008; **255**:1679–86.

78. Wintzen A, De Jonge H, Loeliger E, Bots G. The risk of intracerebral hemorrhage during oral anticoagulant treatment: A population study. *Annals of Neurology.* 1984; **16**:553–8.

79. Greenberg S M. Cerebral amyloid angiopathy: prospects for clinical diagnosis and treatment. *Neurology.* 1998; **51**:690–4.

80. Rosand J, Hylek E M, O'Donnell H C, Greenberg S M. Warfarin-associated hemorrhage and cerebral amyloid angiopathy: a genetic and pathologic study. *Neurology.* 2000; **55**:947–51.

81. Wong K, Mok V, Lam W, *et al.* Aspirin-associated intracerebral hemorrhage: clinical and radiologic features. *Neurology.* 2000; **54**:2298–301.

82. Gregoire S M, Jäger H, Yousry T A, *et al.* Brain microbleeds as a potential risk factor for antiplatelet-related intracerebral haemorrhage: Hospital-based, case-control study. *Journal of Neurology, Neurosurgery & Psychiatry.* 2010; **81**:679–84.

83. Buresly K, Eisenberg M J, Zhang X, Pilote L. Bleeding complications associated with combinations of aspirin, thienopyridine derivatives, and warfarin in elderly patients following acute myocardial infarction. *Archives of Internal Medicine.* 2005; **165**:784.

84. Dale J, Myhre E, Storstein O, Stormorken H, Efskind L. Prevention of arterial thromboembolism with acetylsalicylic acid: A controlled clinical study in patients with aortic ball valves. *American Heart Journal.* 1977; **94**:101–11.

85. Hansen M L, Sorensen R, Clausen M T, *et al.* Risk of bleeding with single, dual, or triple therapy with warfarin, aspirin, and clopidogrel in patients with atrial fibrillation. *Archives of Internal Medicine.* 2010; **170**:1433.

181

86. Rodgers R P, Levin J. A critical reappraisal of the bleeding time. *Semin Thromb Hemost.* 1990; **16**:1–20.

87. Yardumian D A, Mackie I J, Machin S J. Laboratory investigation of platelet function: A review of methodology. *Journal of Clinical Pathology.* 1986; **39**:701–12.

88. Davidson J F, Colvin B T, Barrowcliffe T W, *et al.* The British Society for Haematology Hemostasis and Thrombosis Task-force. Guidelines on platelet-function testing. *Journal of Clinical Pathology.* 1988; **41**:1322–30.

89. Seidel H, Rahman M M, Scharf R E. Monitoring of antiplatelet therapy. Current limitations, challenges, and perspectives. *Hamostaseologie.* 2011; **31**:41–51.

90. Breet N J, van Werkum J W, Bouman H J, *et al.* Comparison of platelet function tests in predicting clinical outcome in patients undergoing coronary stent implantation. *Journal of the American Medical Association.* 2010; **303**:754–62.

91. Sibbing D, Schulz S, Braun S, *et al.* Antiplatelet effects of clopidogrel and bleeding in patients undergoing coronary stent placement. *Journal of Thrombosis and Haemostasis.* 2010; **8**:250–6.

92. Godino C, Mendolicchio L, Figini F, *et al.* Comparison of Verifynow-p2y. *Thrombosis Journal.* 2009; **7**:4.

93. Jakubowski J A, Li Y G, Small D S, *et al.* A comparison of the Verifynow p2y12 point-of-care device and light transmission aggregometry to monitor platelet function with prasugrel and clopidogrel: An integrated analysis. *Journal of Cardiovascular Pharmacology.* 2010; **56**:29–37.

94. Mangiacapra F, Patti G, Peace A, *et al.* Comparison of platelet reactivity and periprocedural outcomes in patients with versus without diabetes mellitus and treated with clopidogrel and percutaneous coronary intervention. *American Journal of Cardiology.* 2010; **106**:619–23.

95. Ozben S, Ozben B, Tanrikulu A M, Ozer F, Ozben T. Aspirin resistance in patients with acute ischemic stroke. *Journal of Neurology.* 2011; **258**:1979–86.

96. Paniccia R, Antonucci E, Gori A M, *et al.* Different methodologies for evaluating the effect of clopidogrel on platelet function in high-risk coronary artery disease patients. *Journal of Thrombosis and Haemostasis.* 2007; **5**:1839–47.

97. Paniccia R, Antonucci E, Maggini N, *et al.* Comparison of methods for monitoring residual platelet reactivity after clopidogrel by point-of-care tests on whole blood in high-risk patients. *Thrombosis & Haemostasis.* 2010; **104**:287.

98. Altman R, Scazziota A, De Lourdes Herrera M, Gonzalez C. Recombinant factor VIIa reverses the inhibitory effect of aspirin or aspirin plus clopidogrel on in vitro thrombin generation. *Journal of Thrombosis and Haemostasis.* 2006; **4**:2022–7.

99. Flordal P A, Sahlin S. Use of desmopressin to prevent bleeding complications in patients treated with aspirin. *British Journal of Surgery.* 1993; **80**:723–4.

100. Gratz I, Koehler J, Olsen D, *et al.* The effect of desmopressin acetate on postoperative hemorrhage in patients receiving aspirin therapy before coronary artery bypass operations. *Journal of Thoracic and Cardiovascular Surgery.* 1992; **104**:1417–22.

101. James R F, Palys V, Lomboy J R, Lamm Jr J R, Simon S D. The role of anticoagulants, antiplatelet agents, and their reversal strategies in the management of intracerebral hemorrhage. *Neurosurgical Focus.* 2013; **34**:E6.

102. Gayle J A, Kaye A D, Kaye A M, Shah R. Anticoagulants: Newer ones, mechanisms, and perioperative updates. *Anesthesiology Clinics.* 2010; **28**:667–79.

103. Horwitz P A, Berlin J A, Sauer W H, *et al.* Bleeding risk of platelet glycoprotein IIb/IIIa receptor antagonists in broad-based practice (results from the Society for Cardiac Angiography and Interventions Registry). *American Journal of Cardiology.* 2003; **91**:803–6.

104. Ducruet A F, Hickman Z L, Zacharia B E, *et al.* Impact of platelet transfusion on hematoma expansion in patients receiving antiplatelet agents before intracerebral hemorrhage. *Neurological Research.* 2010; **32**:706–10.

105. Nishijima D K, Zehtabchi S, Berrong J, Legome E. Utility of platelet transfusion in adult patients with traumatic intracranial hemorrhage and preinjury antiplatelet use: A systematic review. *Journal of Trauma and Acute Care Surgery.* 2012; **72**.

106. Batchelor J S, Grayson A. A meta-analysis to determine the effect on survival of platelet transfusions in patients with either spontaneous or traumatic antiplatelet medication-associated intracranial haemorrhage. *BMJ Open.* 2012; **2**.

107. de Gans K, de Haan R J, Majoie C B, *et al.* PATCH: Platelet Transfusion in Cerebral Haemorrhage: Study protocol for a multicentre, randomised, controlled trial. *BMC Neurology.* 2010; **10**:19.

108. Qureshi A I. Intracerebral hemorrhage specific intensity of care quality metrics. *Neurocritical Care.* 2011; **14**:291–317.

109. Baker R I, Coughlin P B, Gallus A S, *et al.* Warfarin reversal: Consensus guidelines on behalf of the Australasian Society of Thrombosis and Haemostasis. *Medical Journal of Australia.* 2004; **181**:492–7.

110. Pollack Jr. C V, Reilly P A, Eikelboom J, *et al.* Idamcizumab for dabigatran reversal. *New England Journal of Medicine.* 2015; **373**:511–20.

111. Kazui S, Minematsu K, Yamamoto H, Sawada T, Yamaguchi T. Predisposing factors to enlargement of spontaneous intracerebral hematoma. *Stroke*. 1997; **28**:2370–5.

112. Dandapani B K, Suzuki S, Kelley R E, Reyes-Iglesias Y, Duncan R C. Relation between blood pressure and outcome in intracerebral hemorrhage. *Stroke*. 1995; **26**:21–4.

113. Vemmos K N, Tsivgoulis G, Spengos K, *et al.* Association between 24-h blood pressure monitoring variables and brain oedema in patients with hyperacute stroke. *Journal of Hypertension*. 2003; **21**:2167–73.

114. Anderson C S, Huang Y, Wang J G, *et al.* Intensive Blood Pressure Reduction in Acute Cerebral Haemorrhage Trial (INTERACT): A randomised pilot trial. *Lancet Neurology*. 2008; 7:391–9.

115. Qureshi A I. Antihypertensive Treatment of Acute Cerebral Hemorrhage (ATACH). *Neurocritical Care*. 2007; **6**:56–66.

116. Butcher K S, Jeerakathil T, Hill M, *et al.* The intracerebral hemorrhage acutely decreasing arterial pressure trial. *Stroke*. 2013; **44**:620–6.

117. Ropper A H. Lateral displacement of the brain and level of consciousness in patients with an acute hemispheral mass. *New England Journal of Medicine*. 1986; **314**:953–8.

118. Vespa P M, O'Phelan K, Shah M, *et al.* Acute seizures after intracerebral hemorrhage: a factor in progressive midline shift and outcome. *Neurology*. 2003; **60**:1441–6.

119. Qureshi A I. Acute hypertensive response in patients with stroke pathophysiology and management. *Circulation*. 2008; **118**:176–87.

120. Lee S H, Kim B J, Bae H J, *et al.* Effects of glucose level on early and long-term mortality after intracerebral haemorrhage: The acute brain bleeding analysis study. *Diabetologia*. 2010; **53**:429–34.

121. Reith J, Jorgensen H S, Pedersen P M, *et al.* Body temperature in acute stroke: Relation to stroke severity, infarct size, mortality, and outcome. *Lancet*. 1996; **347**:422–5.

122. Chastre J, Wolff M, Fagon J-Y, *et al.* Comparison of 8 vs 15 days of antibiotic therapy for ventilator-associated pneumonia in adults: A randomized trial. *Journal of the American Medical Association*. 2003; **290**:2588–98.

123. Ogata T, Yasaka M, Wakugawa Y, *et al.* Deep venous thrombosis after acute intracerebral hemorrhage. *Journal of the Neurological Sciences*. 2008; **272**:83–6.

124. Boeer A, Voth E, Henze T H, Prange H W. Early heparin therapy in patients with spontaneous intracerebral haemorrhage. *Journal of Neurology, Neurosurgery & Psychiatry*. 1991; **54**:466–7.

125. Tetri S, Hakala J, Juvela S, *et al.* Safety of low-dose subcutaneous enoxaparin for the prevention of venous thromboembolism after primary intracerebral haemorrhage. *Thrombosis Research*. 2008; **123**:206–12.

126. Misra U K, Kalita J, Pandey S, Mandal S K, Srivastava M. A randomized placebo controlled trial of ranitidine versus sucralfate in patients with spontaneous intracerebral hemorrhage for prevention of gastric hemorrhage. *Journal of the Neurological Sciences*. 2005; **239**:5–10.

127. Eddleston J M, Pearson R C, Holland J, *et al.* Prospective endoscopic study of stress erosions and ulcers in critically ill adult patients treated with either sucralfate or placebo. *Critical Care Medicine*. 1994; **22**:1949–54.

128. Finestone H M, Greene-Finestone L S, Wilson E S, Teasell R W. Prolonged length of stay and reduced functional improvement rate in malnourished stroke rehabilitation patients. *Archives of Physical Medicine and Rehabilitation*. 1996; **77**:340–5.

129. Qureshi A I, Suarez J I, Parekh P D, Bhardwaj A. Prediction and timing of tracheostomy in patients with infratentorial lesions requiring mechanical ventilatory support. *Critical Care Medicine*. 2000; **28**:1383–7.

130. Griffiths J, Barber V S, Morgan L, Young J D. Systematic review and meta-analysis of studies of the timing of tracheostomy in adult patients undergoing artificial ventilation. *British Medical Journal*. 2005; **330**:1243.

131. Dennis M S, Lewis S C, Warlow C. Routine oral nutritional supplementation for stroke patients in hospital (food): A multicentre randomised controlled trial. *Lancet*. 2005; **365**:755–63.

132. Hemphill J C 3rd, White D B. Clinical nihilism in neuroemergencies. *Emergency Medicine Clinics of North America*. 2009; **27**:27–37.

Chapter

18

Intracranial–extracerebral hemorrhage: complication of anticoagulation

Muhib Alam Khan

Introduction

Intracranial–extracerebral hemorrhage while on anticoagulation treatment has been described since the introduction and wide use of oral anticoagulants. Location of extracerebral bleeds are subdural, subarachnoid, and epidural. Extracerebral hemorrhages are fairly common comprising 50% of all anticoagulation-related hemorrhages [1–3]. These hemorrhages have significant impact on patient outcomes in the long term. They have financial implications raising lifetime healthcare-related cost through mortality and associated morbidity [4]. This is a major cause of concern for health policy makers. Every effort needs to be made in order to minimize the incidence of these hemorrhages. Most of the anticoagulation-related extracerebral hemorrhages are subdural in nature (70–90%) with very few subarachnoid and rarely epidural hemorrhages [1–5].

Predictors

The intensity of anticoagulation is strongly correlated with the incidence of intracranial hemorrhages with INR >3 putting patients at higher risk [3]. Moreover, older age is a significant predictor of intracranial hemorrhage by virtue of higher anticoagulation and falls in this age group [1]. It has been observed that INR at the time of bleeding is substantially elevated laying emphasis on better anticoagulation monitoring in a systematic manner [6]. Although anticoagulation increases the incidence of intracranial–extracerebral hemorrhages, it significantly reduces the risk of ischemic strokes making it a necessary evil [7,8].

It is also noted that the addition of aspirin to anticoagulation increases the risk of intracranial hemorrhage [9]. Aspirin is added to warfarin in patients with mechanical heart valves with an understanding that it would allow use of a lower-target INR. However, this approach at times leads to increased bleeding risk. Therefore a cautious approach is recommended when selecting such a management plan.

Falls are fairly common in elderly patients. Since most of the patients on anticoagulation are in the elderly age group, this poses major intracranial bleeding issues [6]. Therefore risk for falls in elderly patients should be carefully evaluated before putting them on anticoagulation. However, the risk of falls is usually overestimated by physicians leading to denial of warfarin therapy to many of those who would benefit from it [10].

Prevention of intracranial hemorrhages is an important aspect of patient management. Several clinical trials have analyzed their data in order to identify risk factors for bleeding. This has led to the development of predictive models such as HAS-BLED, HEMORR$_2$HAGES, mOBRI, and RIETE registry [11–14]. These predictive models provide a guide to patient selection for anticoagulation but should not be relied on completely. These models have their limitations and individualized clinical judgment is still recommended [15].

Mortality

Extracerebral hemorrhages have better outcomes as compared to intracerebral hemorrhages when resulting from anticoagulation [2]. This is most likely due to the fact that these hemorrhages are amenable to surgical evacuation as compared to intracerebral hemorrhage. Mortality is also affected by the intensity of anticoagulation with INR >3.5 leading to a higher mortality [2].

Subdural hemorrhage

Acute subdural hemorrhages (SDH) are a frequent complication of anticoagulation and comprise about

Treatment-Related Stroke, ed. Alexander Tsiskaridze, Arne Lindgren and Adnan Qureshi. Published by Cambridge University Press. © Cambridge University Press 2016.

20% of all anticoagulation-related intracranial hemorrhages [16]. Oral anticoagulation is associated with a significant risk of intracranial bleeding, even after minor head trauma. As a result, traumatic brain injury patients with coagulopathy are often included in a high-risk group regardless of clinical presentation [17–19]. As mentioned earlier, the outcomes of acute subdural hemorrhages are better than those of intracerebral hemorrhages most likely due to them being amenable to surgical evacuation [16]. Population-based studies have shown that five-year incidence of chronic subdural hematoma is significantly increased in patients on anticoagulation [20]. As expected, elderly patients are at higher risk of developing chronic subdural hematomas due to higher incidence of both falls and increased likelihood of being on anticoagulation [21]. Trauma resulting from falls plays a major role in the development of subdural hemorrhage in these patients. However, elderly patients develop non-traumatic chronic subdural hematomas as well [22]. Anticoagulation is also related to the recurrence of chronic subdural hematomas and need for repeat surgical evaluation. This leads to poor functional outcomes and adverse impact on quality of life [23]. The mainstay of treatment is surgical evacuation. Coagulopathy is the major deterrent for convincing surgeons to take the patient to the operating theater. Therefore the initial management in the emergency room and the neurocritical care unit is to reverse anticoagulation. This approach helps prevent hemorrhage expansion and facilitates potential neurosurgical intervention [24]. Warfarin has been traditionally reversed through the use of fresh frozen plasma (FFP). An alternate and faster method is to use prothrombin complex concentrate. Reversal of anticoagulation is also achieved with recombinant factor VIIa (rFVIIa). However, rFVIIa has major thrombotic side effects as well as extremely high cost. It has been noted that the risk of major thrombotic events in anticoagulation-related intracranial hemorrhages is not more than those with spontaneous intracerebral hemorrhage [25,26]. Contrary to general belief the overall outcome of these patients does not seem to differ from historical cohorts with SDH without anticoagulation [27]. Premorbid anticoagulation may predispose patients to developing SDH but does not increase the risk of morbidity or mortality following surgical intervention [28].

Subarachnoid hemorrhage

The incidence of subarachnoid hemorrhage (SAH) related to anticoagulation is low and constitutes only 10% of all anticoagulation-related intracranial hemorrhages [29]. The etiology is equally distributed in spontaneous and traumatic subgroups [29]. Presence of aneurysms and concomitant anticoagulation does not increase the risk of bleeding and these patients can be comfortably anticoagulated provided that general principles of asymptomatic aneurysm management are followed [30]. Subarachnoid hemorrhage can result from intracranial arterial dissection as well. Since the conventional treatment of intracranial arterial dissections is anticoagulation, the presence of SAH with these dissections puts physicians in a management dilemma. It has been noted that patients with SAH as a result of intracranial arterial dissection have poor prognosis if treated with anticoagulation. Most of these dissections were associated with ruptured fusiform aneurysms [31].

Resumption

Resumption of anticoagulation therapy, particularly following surgical evacuation, poses a significant management dilemma. Definitive recommendations are lacking in the literature. Timing of restarting anticoagulation following surgical drainage remains a matter of debate. The recommendations for the resumption of full-dose anticoagulation in high-risk patients involve considering the anticipated bleeding risk and adequacy of postoperative hemostasis in individual patients. A protocol-based approach is not ideal, and care should be individualized based on a patient's reason for anticoagulation. Serial neuroimaging should be used in monitoring these patients [32].

New anticoagulants

Recently randomized clinical trials have been reported using a new generation of anticoagulants in head-to-head comparison with warfarin. The rate of subdural hematomas was lower for patients taking 110 mg of dabigatrin as compared to warfarin and 150 mg dose of dabigatran. No significant difference was found in the rates of subarachnoid hemorrhages [29]. Rivaroxaban has similar intracranial–extracerebral bleeding events as compared to warfarin [33]. These newer agents show potential for reducing the most dreaded complication of anticoagulation, which is intracranial bleeding. Comprehensive data is not available on all agents regarding the specific sites of intracranial bleeding but hopefully subgroup analyses will be reported soon informing us about the role in reducing intracranial–extracerebral bleeding events.

References

1. Fang M C, Chang Y, Hylek E M, *et al.* Advanced age, anticoagulation intensity, and risk for intracranial hemorrhage among patients taking warfarin for atrial fibrillation. *Ann Intern Med.* 2004; **141**(10):745–52.

2. Fang M C, Go A S, Chang Y, *et al.* Thirty-day mortality after ischemic stroke and intracranial hemorrhage in patients with atrial fibrillation on and off anticoagulants. *Stroke.* 2012; **43**(7):1795–9.

3. DiMarco J P, Flaker G, Waldo A L, *et al.* AFFIRM Investigators. Factors affecting bleeding risk during anticoagulant therapy in patients with atrial fibrillation: Observations from the Atrial Fibrillation Follow-up Investigation of Rhythm Management (AFFIRM) study. *Am Heart J.* 2005; **149**(4):650–6.

4. Ghate S R, Biskupiak J, Ye X, Kwong W J, Brixner D I. All-cause and bleeding-related health care costs in warfarin-treated patients with atrial fibrillation. *J Manag Care Pharm.* 2011; **17**(9):672–84.

5. Mattle H, Kohler S, Huber P, Rohner M, Steinsiepe K F. Anticoagulation-related intracranial extracerebral haemorrhage. *J Neurol Neurosurg Psychiatry.* 1989; **52**(7): 829–37.

6. Baechli H, Nordmann A, Bucher H C, Gratzl O. Demographics and prevalent risk factors of chronic subdural haematoma: results of a large single-center cohort study. *Neurosurg Rev.* 2004; **27**(4):263–6.

7. Mant J, Hobbs F D, Fletcher K, *et al.* BAFTA investigators. Midland Research Practices Network (MidReC). Warfarin versus aspirin for stroke prevention in an elderly community population with atrial fibrillation (the Birmingham Atrial Fibrillation Treatment of the Aged Study, BAFTA): A randomised controlled trial. *Lancet.* 2007; **370**(9586):493–503.

8. Gulløv A L, Koefoed B G, Petersen P. Bleeding during warfarin and aspirin therapy in patients with atrial fibrillation: the AFASAK 2 study. Atrial Fibrillation Aspirin and Anticoagulation. *Arch Intern Med.* 1999; **159**(12):1322–8.

9. Hart R G, Benavente O, Pearce L A. Increased risk of intracranial hemorrhage when aspirin is combined with warfarin: A meta-analysis and hypothesis. *Cerebrovasc Dis.* 1999; **9**(4):215–17.

10. Bond A J, Molnar F J, Li M, Mackey M, Man-Son-Hing M. The risk of hemorrhagic complications in hospital in-patients who fall while receiving antithrombotic therapy. *Thromb J.* 2005; **3**(1):1.

11. Airaksinen K E, Suurmunne H, Porela P, *et al.* Usefulness of outpatient bleeding risk index to predict bleeding complications in patients with long-term oral anticoagulation undergoing coronary stenting. *Am J Cardiol.* 2010; **106**(2):175–9. Epub 2010 Jun 9.

12. Ruíz-Giménez N, Suárez C, González R, *et al.* RIETE Investigators. Predictive variables for major bleeding events in patients presenting with documented acute venous thromboembolism. Findings from the RIETE Registry. *Thromb Haemost.* 2008; **100**(1):26–31.

13. Gage B F, Yan Y, Milligan P E, *et al.* Clinical classification schemes for predicting hemorrhage: Results from the National Registry of Atrial Fibrillation (NRAF). *Am Heart J.* 2006; **151**(3):713–19.

14. Lip G Y, Frison L, Halperin J L, Lane D A. Comparative validation of a novel risk score for predicting bleeding risk in anticoagulated patients with atrial fibrillation: The HAS-BLED (Hypertension, Abnormal Renal/Liver Function, Stroke, Bleeding History or Predisposition, Labile INR, Elderly, Drugs/Alcohol Concomitantly) score. *J Am Coll Cardiol.* 2011; **57**(2):173–80.

15. Loewen P, Dahri K. Risk of bleeding with oral anticoagulants: an updated systematic review and performance analysis of clinical prediction rules. *Ann Hematol.* 2011; **90**(10):1191–200.

16. Fang M C, Go A S, Chang Y, *et al.* Death and disability from warfarin-associated intracranial and extracranial hemorrhages. *Am J Med.* 2007; **120**(8):700–5.

17. Gomez P A, Lobato R D, Ortega J M, de la Cruz J. Mild head injury: Differences in prognosis among patients with a Glasgow Coma Scale score of 13 to 15 and analysis of factors associated with abnormal CT findings. *Br J Neurosurg.* 1996; **10**:453–60.

18. Servadei F, Teasdale G, Merry G. Defining acute mild head injury in adults: A proposal based on prognostic factors, diagnosis, and management. *J Neurotrauma.* 2001; **18**:657–64.

19. Vos P E, Battistin L, Birbamer G, *et al.* EFNS guideline on mild traumatic brain injury: Report of an EFNS task force. *Eur J Neurol.* 2002; **9**:207–19.

20. Rust T, Kiemer N, Erasmus A. Chronic subdural haematomas and anticoagulation or anti-thrombotic therapy. *J Clin Neurosci.* 2006; **13**(8):823–7.

21. Baechli H, Nordmann A, Bucher H C, Gratzl O. Demographics and prevalent risk factors of chronic subdural haematoma: results of a large single-center cohort study. *Neurosurg Rev.* 2004; **27**(4):263–6.

22. Lindvall P, Koskinen L O. Anticoagulants and antiplatelet agents and the risk of development and recurrence of chronic subdural haematomas. *J Clin Neurosci.* 2009; **16**(10):1287–90.

23. Forster M T, Mathé A K, Senft C, *et al.* The influence of preoperative anticoagulation on outcome and quality of life after surgical treatment of chronic subdural hematoma. *J Clin Neurosci.* 2010; **17**(8):975–9.

24. Hanley J P. Warfarin reversal. *J Clin Pathol.* 2004; **57**(11):1132–9.

25. Ducruet A F, Grobelny B T, Zacharia B E, *et al.* The surgical management of chronic subdural hematoma. *Neurosurg Rev.* 2012; **35**(2):155–69.

26. Robinson M T, Rabinstein A A, Meschia J F, Freeman W D. Safety of recombinant activated factor VII in patients with warfarin-associated hemorrhages of the central nervous system. *Stroke.* 2010; **41**(7): 1459–63.

27. Senft C, Schuster T, Forster M T, Seifert V, Gerlach R. Management and outcome of patients with acute traumatic subdural hematomas and pre-injury oral anticoagulation therapy. *Neurol Res.* 2009; **31**(10): 1012–18.

28. Panczykowski D M, Okonkwo D O. Premorbid oral antithrombotic therapy and risk for reaccumulation, reoperation, and mortality in acute subdural hematomas. *J Neurosurg.* 2011; **114**(1):47–52.

29. Hart R G, Diener H C, Yang S, *et al.* Intracranial hemorrhage in atrial fibrillation patients during anticoagulation with warfarin or dabigatran: the RE-LY trial. *Stroke.* 2012; **43**(6): 1511–17.

30. Tarlov N, Norbash A M, Nguyen T N. The safety of anticoagulation in patients with intracranial aneurysms. *J Neurointerv Surg.* 2012, Jun 7.

31. Metso T M, Metso A J, Helenius J, *et al.* Prognosis and safety of anticoagulation in intracranial artery dissections in adults. *Stroke.* 2007; **38**(6): 1837–42.

32. Byrnes M C, Irwin E, Roach R, *et al.* Therapeutic anticoagulation can be safely accomplished in selected patients with traumatic intracranial hemorrhage. *World J Emerg Surg.* 2012; **7**(1):25.

33. Patel M R, Mahaffey K W, Garg J, *et al.* The ROCKET Steering Committee for the ROCKET AF Investigators. Rivaroxaban versus warfarin in nonvalvular atrial fibrillation. *N Engl J Med.* 2011; **365**: 883–91.

Chapter 19

Iatrogenic intracerebral hemorrhage due to oral anticoagulation therapy: risk factors and diagnosis

Alexander Tsiskaridze

Introduction

Although oral anticoagulants are largely underprescribed [1], there has been increasing use of these agents for prevention of thromboembolism in recent years [2]. This is true for traditional agents such as vitamin K agonists (VKAs), coumadin (warfarin), acenocoumarol, or phenprocoumon as well as for recently developed novel oral anticoagulants (NOACs), including direct thrombin inhibitor – dabigatran – and direct FXa inhibitors – apixaban, rivaroxaban, and edoxaban – which are at least as effective as VKAs in the prevention of ischemic strokes in atrial fibrillation (AF) patients with a more favorable safety profile including lower rates of bleeding complications [3–11]. Despite this, in patients on oral anticoagulation therapy, even in those taking NOACs, bleeding remains a non-rare condition.

Table 19.1 HAS-BLED score.

Letter	Variable	Points
H	Hypertension	1
A	Abnormal renal and liver function (1 point each)	1 or 2
S	Stroke	1
B	Bleeding	1
L	Labile INRs	1
E	Elderly (age >65)	1
D	Drugs or alcohol (1 point each)	1 or 2
	Total	**9**

INR: international normalized ratio

Risk of bleeding in patients on oral anticoagulation therapy

The bleeding risk in AF patients receiving oral anticoagulation therapy (OAT) can be determined by HEMORR$_2$HAGES (hepatic or renal disease, ethanol abuse, malignancy, older age, reduced platelet count or function, rebleeding, hypertension, anemia, genetic factors, excessive fall risk, and stroke), HAS-BLED (hypertension, abnormal renal/liver function, stroke, bleeding history or predisposition, labile international normalized ratio, elderly, drugs/alcohol), and ATRIA (anticoagulation and risk factors in atrial fibrillation) risk scores [12–14]. The HAS-BLED score (Table 19.1) is user friendly and contains 7 items with a maximal score of 9. A score ≥3 corresponds to an increased risk of bleeding. The HEMORR$_2$HAGES score (Table 19.2), which consists of 13 items (sum ≥2 indicative of intermediate to high risk), requires additional information, including genetic polymorphisms, and therefore is somehow complicated for routine use. It may also underestimate the need for utilization of anticoagulation in elderly patients [15]. The most recently released ATRIA risk score (Table 19.3) is simple to use, consists of 5 items, with a maximum score of 10. Score ≥4 indicates moderate to high risk. However, the recent comparison of those three bleeding risk-estimation scores has demonstrated only modest performance in predicting the outcome of any clinically relevant bleeding, although the HAS-BLED score performed better than the HEMORR$_2$HAGES and ATRIA scores.

Treatment-Related Stroke, ed. Alexander Tsiskaridze, Arne Lindgren and Adnan Qureshi. Published by Cambridge University Press. © Cambridge University Press 2016.

Table 19.2 HEMORR$_2$HAGES score.

Variable	Points
Liver disease	1
Renal disease	1
Alcoholism	1
Cancer	1
Age >75 years	1
Platelets count <75,000/mm^3	1
Concomitant antiplatelets treatment	1
Previous bleeding	1
Uncontrolled arterial blood hypertension	1
Hemotocrit <30%	1
CYP2C9*2 or CYP2C9*3 presence	1
High risk of falls or cognitive impairment	1
Previous stroke	1
Total	13

Table 19.3 ATRIA score.

Variable	Points
Anemia	3
Severe renal disease^a	3
Age ≥75 years	2
Any prior hemorrhage diagnosis	1
Diagnosed hypertension	1
Total	10

^{a} Defined as estimated glomerular filtration rate <30 ml/minute or dialysis dependent.

Moreover, the HAS-BLED demonstrated significant predictive performance for intracranial bleeding [15].

Intracranial bleeding is the most feared and devastating complication of OAT. Almost 70% of intracranial bleeding represents intracerebral hemorrhage (ICH) [16,17]. The OAT-related ICH (OAT-ICH) is a major bleeding, resulting in a life-threatening condition, sometimes fatal. Estimates of its incidence vary between the published studies across time, due to different factors including increasing prevalence of AF in an aging population, increasing long-term usage of oral anticoagulants, heterogeneity of patient characteristics included, and treatment methods used. Previous studies report the occurrence of OAT-ICH on VKA treatment at a rate of 2 to 9 per 100,000 population/year with an incidence of seven- to ten-fold higher than the incidence of ICH in patients who do not receive OAT [18,19].

Among patients presenting with ICH, the proportion of OAT-ICH has increased considerably in the past years, approaching 12 to 15% in the general population, and even 25% in tertiary care centers [20–24].

On the individual patient's level, the absolute risk of ICH in a patient with AF on OAT is also difficult to determine because of the reasons mentioned above. The reported rates of OAT-ICH, irrespective of medication used (VKAs or NOACs) and design of the study conducted, vary widely ranging from 0.1% to as high as 2.5% per year [16,25]. Interestingly, the individual patient cumulative risk of bleeding is directly related to the length of OAT [26–28]. In one study, the frequency of major bleeding decreased from 3.0% during the first month of outpatient OAT therapy to 0.8%/month during the rest of the first year of therapy and to 0.3%/month thereafter [29].

In recent years, there has been a consistent trend towards overall decreasing the absolute risk with reported rates of warfarin-associated ICH up to 0.6% per year [30]. This tendency may be explained by better regulation of anticoagulation with more careful monitoring of the INR, lower anticoagulation intensities, and improved control of hypertension. It is also noteworthy that the reported annual rates of warfarin-associated ICH from major randomized control trials (RCTs) of AF [3–10,31–35] are lower compared to the rates of ICH of non-inception and inception observational studies [36–40]. Thus some recent observational cohort studies of patients on VKAs reported as high as 2.5% risk of OAT-ICH at one year [41,42]. Obviously, observational cohort studies better represent the "real world" patient population and give more proper estimates of the risk of serious adverse events including ICH compared to RCTs, which include highly selected populations with better adherence to study medications and careful follow-up. Therefore the results of RCTs may not be fully generalizable and could underestimate the risk of VKA-related ICH occurring in "everyday clinical practice" [43,44].

As to NOACs, the large RCTs on stroke prevention in patients with AF (3–10) have reported the absolute annual risk rates of OAT-ICH ranging from 0.2 to 0.5%. Surprisingly, in the "real world," dabigatran showed ICH annual risk rates of 0.1% for dabigatran 150 mg bid, 0.3% for dabigatran 110 mg bid, and 0.29% overall, according to data from the Danish and US registries [45,46]. This magnitude of risk rate difference between RCTs and the "real world" (lower in the latter) possibly reflects the differences between the "real world" and clinical trial populations in terms of baseline ICH risk or completeness of ICH ascertainment [47].

Etiology and pathogenesis

The OAT-ICH basically shares etiology with spontaneous ICH. In both conditions cerebral arteriopathies such as subcortical hypertensive small-vessel disease (lipohyalinosis and arteriolosclerosis) or cerebral amyloid angiopathy (CAA) (an age-related condition characterized by the progressive deposition of amyloid-β in the media and adventitia of small arteries, arterioles, and capillaries in the cerebral cortex) play the major role in development of intracerebral bleeding. Intense oral anticoagulation appears to exaggerate the underlying risk of spontaneous ICH [48]. Anticoagulation by itself may not be a sole cause of ICH if cerebral vessels are intact, but the presence of angiopathy resulting in stiffness and fragility of vessels is a causative or aggravating factor for such hemorrhage. Once hemorrhage occurs, impaired hemostasis may lead to prolongation of bleeding resulting in larger hematoma volume and its growth over time. The mechanism of the prolonged hematoma growth by means of secondary mechanical shearing/breakdown of neighboring vessels (already damaged by hypertensive small-vessel disease or CAA) that also start to bleed in "domino" fashion due to expansion of the initial hemorrhage, resembles a feed-forward aspect of the avalanche process. This "avalanche model" for hematoma expansion was proposed by Miller Fisher decades ago, based on his observation of multiple recently ruptured vessels at the periphery of serially sectioned hematomas [49]. Several recent observations have supported this model, including the visualization of a computed tomography angiography (CTA) "spot sign" as site of active bleeding (visualized as contrast extravasation) following venous contrast injection [50,51]. Multiple spot signs in a single hematoma have been frequently seen [50,52,53] (Figure 19.1), suggesting simultaneous bleeding from several surrounding vessels as would be expected in an avalanche of secondary shearing rather than a single persistently bleeding vessel [54]. A successful computational simulation of the "avalanche model" identifying the characteristics of hemorrhages generated by simulated rupture of adjacent vessels surrounding an initial site of bleeding has been proposed recently. The simulation demonstrated the direct effect of anticoagulation on increasing the number of macrobleed events, enlarging the final ICH volumes, accelerating the rates of expansion, and prolonging the duration of hematoma growth [55].

Risk factors

There are several risk factors and predictors of intracerebral bleeding in patients receiving OACs (Table 19.4). Those firmly established by multiple sources such as RCTs or observational studies are advanced age, Asian, Hispanic, and Afro-American ethnicity, intensive anticoagulation, markedly elevated systolic blood pressure, and history of previous stroke or transient ischemic attack (TIA).

Age

A case-control analysis of 121 patients with ICH taking warfarin showed that age of 80 years and older was a significant risk factor for both intracerebral hemorrhage and subdural hematoma [57]. Another case-control study carried out in an academic medical center of 170 case patients who developed intracranial hemorrhage during warfarin therapy and 1,020 matched controls who did not, showed increasing odds of intracranial hemorrhage with age but most sharply at 85 years of age or older [58]. The SPAF II study revealed OAT-ICH rates of 1.8% per year in patients older than 75 years compared with 0.5% per year among patients 75 years or younger taking warfarin [59]. In the RE-LY trial, age was the independent, significant predictor of ICH (relative risk, 1.1 per year; $P < 0.001$) [9]; the same was found in the ROCKET AF trial – age was an independent predictor of an increased risk of ICH (hazard ratio 1.34; 95%CI 1.10–1.64 per ten-year increase) [10].

Race

There is a large body of evidence that ethnic/racial difference may determine the risk of OAT-ICH. In an observational study evaluating Medicare patients hospitalized for AF, warfarin use was associated with a 44% higher relative risk of major bleeding in black patients compared to whites [60]. In another study analyzing the risk of OAT-ICH in a multiethnic

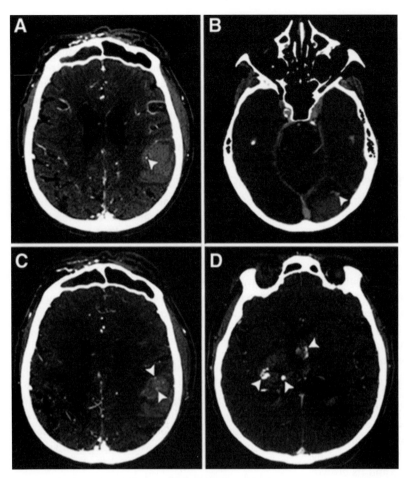

Figure 19.1 (A) and (B) Single spot signs on CTA. (C) and (D) Multiple spot signs on CTA. (Reproduced with permission of Brouwers H B, Goldstein J N, Romero J M, Rosand J. Clinical applications of the computed tomography angiography spot sign in acute intracerebral hemorrhage: A review. *Stroke*. 2012; 43: 3427–32)

cohort of AF patients hospitalized with AF (18,867 first-time hospitalizations in the six-year period), after adjusting for possible confounders, Hispanics and blacks had twice the risk for ICH as whites, whereas Asians were at four times the risk [61]. In the ROCKET AF trial population, the risk of ICH was significantly higher in Asians and blacks (hazard ratios, 2.02; 95% CI 1.39–2.94, and 3.25; 95% CI 1.43–7.41, respectively) as compared to whites [10].

Intensity of anticoagulation

Despite the fact that most (in terms of absolute numbers) ICHs associated with VKA treatment happen when patients are in the INR's therapeutic range of between 2 and 3 [24], the intensity of anticoagulation therapy is related to a greater risk of OAT-ICH. In the SPAF III study most warfarin-related ICH occurred at an INR greater than 3.0 [32]. A case-control study of 170 patients with ICH on warfarin showed that the risk of ICH increased with an INR of 3.5 to 3.9 [58].

A much larger well-designed study of more than 13,000 patients with AF showed no substantial increase in ICH rate in patients receiving warfarin until the INR reached 4.0 to 4.5 [62].

Hypertension

Hypertension is a well-established risk factor for ICH in general and a predictor for OAT-ICH in patients treated with VKAs. In a case-control study of 68 patients treated with warfarin, hypertension was independently associated with warfarin-associated ICH (odds ratio 2.69; 95% CI 1.04–6.97) [63]. A more recent retrospective study of 173 ICH patients with AF on warfarin therapy demonstrated a 3.3-fold increased risk of ICH in patients with hypertension compared to normotensive patients [61]. Another retrospective study of modifiable risk factors for warfarin-related intracerebral bleeding in 65 anticoagulated patients with ICH and 250 patients with spontaneous ICH revealed significantly higher mean

Table 19.4 Risk factors/predictors of OAT-ICH (adapted from Hart *et al.* [30] and Grysiewicz & Gorelick [56]).

Risk factors	Demographic at highest risk
Well established	
Age	>75 years of age
Race	Asian, Hispanic, and black
Intensity of anticoagulation	INR >4
Hypertension	Systolic blood pressure ≥160 mmHg
History of cerebrovascular disease	History of stroke or TIA
Probable	
Cerebral amyloid angiopathy	Presence of apoE epsilon 2 and 4 genotypes
Genetic polymorphisms of CYP45049	Presence of CYP2CP9*3 polymorphism
Concomitant antiplatelet use	INR above goal
Leukoaraiosis	Extensive leukoaraiosis
Cerebral microbleeds	Multiple microbleeds
Possible	
Reduced serum albumin	<4.5 g/dL
Reduced platelet count	<200×10^9/L

arterial pressure at presentation in patients receiving warfarin compared to those who did not (132 mmHg and 107 mmHg, respectively) [64]. In the most recent ROCKET AF study, increased diastolic blood pressure was independently and significantly associated with OAT-ICH (hazard ratio 1.17; 1.01–1.36 per 10 mmHg increase). Poorly controlled hypertension in patients on OAT imposes the highest risk of ICH when systolic blood pressure exceeds 159 mmHg [10,30] or in combination with other risk factors (e.g. INR >3 and cerebrovascular disease) [65].

History of cerebrovascular disease

In patients receiving OAT, a history of cerebrovascular disease (stroke or TIA) increases the risk of OAT-ICH occurrence. In a cohort of 565 patients starting outpatient therapy with warfarin upon discharge from a university hospital, a known history of stroke was associated with a 6.6-fold increased risk of ICH [29]. Afterwards, a case-control study revealed similar results showing a significant and independent association of previous stroke with warfarin-related ICH (odds ratio 2.3; 95% CI 1.4–3.7) [57]. These findings were confirmed by another large case-control study conducted in an academic medical center showing that patients with warfarin-related ICH were more likely than their matched controls to have a history of cerebrovascular disease (37% vs. 20%) [58]. More recently, in a prospective study of 783 AF patients for a total follow-up period of 2,567 patient/years, again, the risk of bleeding was significantly higher in patients with a history of ischemic stroke or TIA (odds ratio 2.5; 95% CI 1.3–4.8) [42].

Cerebral amyloid angiopathy

About 5 to 20% of cases of spontaneous ICH, mostly lobar, are attributed to CAA [66]. The presence of the apolipoprotein E (APOE) epsilon 2 and 4 genotypes, a genetic marker of CAA, may further increase the risk of ICH development in anticoagulated patients [67–71].

Genetic polymorphisms of cytochrome P45049

CYP2C9 is an important liver cytochrome P450 enzyme involved in the metabolism of VKAs [72]. Variant polymorphisms exist for CYP2C9 expression due to high polymorphism of the CYP2C9 gene. Thus CYP2CP9*2 and CYP2CP9*3 expression occurs in approximately 12 and 8%, respectively, of Caucasians, while their prevalence is much lower in Afro-Americans (1 to 3%) [73]. A retrospective cohort study conducted at anticoagulation clinics demonstrated the significantly increased risk of an overanticoagulation (hazard ratio 1.40; 95% CI 1.03–1.90) as well as a serious or life-threatening bleeding event (hazard ratio 2.39; 95% CI 1.18–4.86) in patients with CYP2C9*2 and CYP2C9*3 variant polymorphisms [74]. These polymorphisms of CYP2C9 expression may explain the difference in the risk of OAT-ICH between the different ethnicities. Concerning the novel anticoagulants, dabigartan is not metabolized by CYP450 unlike VKAs and other NOACs [75], and therefore may not comprise an additional risk of bleeding related to P45049 polymorphism. A recent analysis of the ENGAGE AF-TIMI 48 trial data

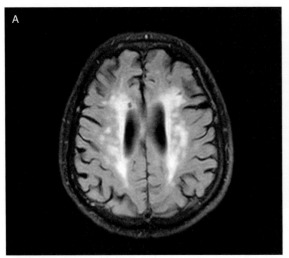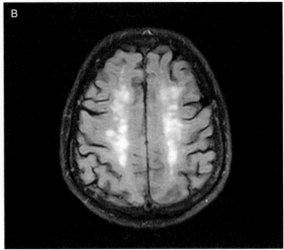

Figure 19.2 (A) and (B) Leukoaraiosis (cerebral white matter lesion) as seen on different brain T2-weighted MRI slices. (Courtesy of Dr M Okujava.)

demonstrated that sensitive and highly sensitive responders to warfarin, classified by CYP2C9 and VKORC1, have much higher rates of early bleeding than normal responders when treated with warfarin. This is not the case for edoxaban, which, compared with warfarin, reduced bleeding more so in sensitive and highly sensitive responders than in normal responders [76].

Concomitant antiplatelet use

About 20% of elderly AF patients receiving warfarin for stroke prophylaxis also take aspirin [58,77]. Adding aspirin to VKAs appears to increase the ICH risk. Thus in a retrospective study of a large hospital discharge cohort of 10,093 elderly patients receiving warfarin for atrial fibrillation, use of combined warfarin–antiplatelet treatment was associated with a three-fold increase in ICH (0.9% vs. 0.3%/year; relative risk 3.0, 95% CI 1.6–5.5) [77]. Meta-analysis of five randomized trials (some of them suffering from methodological shortcomings), in which aspirin was added to equal intensities of anti-coagulation by VKAs, revealed more than a 2.5-fold increased risk of ICH in patients receiving combination therapy (relative risk 2.6; 95% CI 1.3 to 5.4) [30]. In contrast, two case-control studies did not find concomitant aspirin use to be a predictor of ICH in patients receiving VKAs [58,63]. For atrial fibrillation patients, results of three randomized trials appear conflicting, but differences in study design and small numbers of ICHs preclude meaningful comparisons and definite conclusions [30]. Although the data are inconsistent, it is likely that concomitant use of aspirin and warfarin increases the risk of ICH. In younger patients with prosthetic cardiac valves or coronary artery disease who have inherently low ICH risks, absolute rates of ICH with combined warfarin–aspirin therapy are low. However, in older patients or in patients with target INRs >3.0, adding aspirin to VKAs may be associated with increased risk of ICH [30].

Leukoaraiosis

Leukoaraiosis or cerebral white matter lesion revealed by attenuation of the cerebral white matter on computed tomography (CT) or better on magnetic resonance imaging (MRI) (Figure 19.2), is a frequent finding in the elderly. It is associated with cerebral small-vessel disease and CAA and, not rarely, coincides with the presence of microbleeds. Since the pathological substrates of leukoaraiosis are heterogeneous in nature and severity (ranging from myelin loss, axon loss, and mild gliosis, to microinfarction, and dilation of perivascular spaces), it does not represent a specific marker of underlying bleeding-prone microangiopathy [78,79]. The presence of leukoaraiosis has been linked to the risk of warfarin-associated ICH [80,81], although a clinical application of this finding awaits the ability to standardize its detection and to ascertain its positive and negative predictive values.

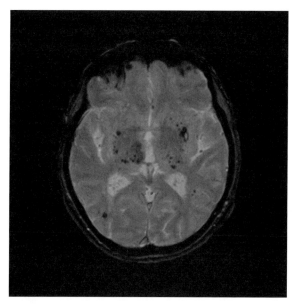

Figure 19.3 Predominately subcortical microbleeds on gradient recalled-echo T2*-weighted MRI. (Courtesy of Dr M Okujava.)

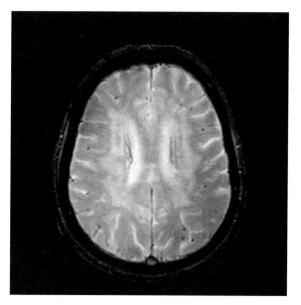

Figure 19.4 Lobar microbleeds on gradient recalled-echo T2*-weighted MRI. (Courtesy of Dr M Beraia.)

Cerebral microbleeds

Similarly to leukoaraiosis, cerebral microbleeds are neuroimaging markers of hypertensive cerebral small-vessel disease or CAA. The microbleeds are visualized on the gradient recalled-echo T2*-weighted MRI or susceptibility-weighted imaging (SWI) sequences as small, rounded, homogeneous, hypointense lesions, not seen with conventional spin echo sequences [82], and provide direct evidence of blood leakage from pathologically fragile small vessels [44]. Distribution of the microbleeds within the brain provides additional information on the underlying etiology; deep subcortical microbleeds correspond to hypertensive small-vessel disease (Figure 19.3), while strictly lobar microbleeds reflect CAA (Figure 19.4) [44].

The presence of cerebral microbleeds seems to increase the risk OAT-ICH. A case-control study of 24 patients with symptomatic warfarin-related ICH and 48 control subjects on warfarin therapy without history of ICH showed that the cases had significantly more microbleeds than the controls (79.2% vs. 22.9%). Moreover, the number of microbleeds was correlated with the presence of OAT-ICH (r =0.299, P <0.001) [83]. With regard to the location, microbleeds in the lobar area, basal ganglia, and cerebellum were significantly associated with warfarin-related ICH while those in the brainstem and thalamus were not [83]. In addition, a cohort study of 87 consecutive AF

patients with acute recurrent stroke on warfarin therapy revealed that the presence of cerebral microbleeds was associated with ICH independent of increased INR and hypertension (OR 7.383; 95% CI 1.052–51.830) [84]. A more recent systematic review of published and unpublished data from a cohort of 3,817 patients with ischemic stroke or TIA and a cohort of 1,460 patients with ICH showed an excess of cerebral microbleeds in warfarin users vs. non-users (OR 2.7; 95% CI 1.6–4.4) [85]. In pooled follow-up data for 768 antithrombotic users, presence of microbleeds at baseline was associated with a substantially increased risk of subsequent ICH (OR 12.1; 95% CI 3.4–42.5) [85]. Large, randomized, prospective clinical trials are needed to validate these findings. A large prospective European multicenter study aiming to establish the value of cerebral microbleeds detected on MRI as indicators of an increased risk of hemorrhagic complications is currently underway [44].

It has been recently reported that superficial siderosis, if disseminated, is associated with an increased risk of symptomatic lobar ICH in CAA [86]. Whether it comprises an additional risk of OAT-ICH is yet to be determined.

Reduced serum albumin and reduced platelet count

These possible prognostic factors for OAT-ICH, which are unique for the ROCKET AF population

195

(e.g., reduced serum albumin and reduced platelet count below $210\times10^9/L$), await external validation in other independent populations of anticoagulated AF patients [10,47].

Clinical presentation and diagnosis

Diagnosis of OAT-ICH is not difficult to establish. Like spontaneous ICH, it may present with focal neurological signs (e.g., hemiparesis, aphasia, ataxia) often accompanied by unusual headache, nausea and vomiting, confusion, stupor, or dizziness [16]. Sudden ("stroke-like") onset of such symptoms in a patient on OAT raises suspicion of intracerebral bleeding and warrants urgent transfer to the relevant medical facility and neuroimaging. Almost 40% of strokes in patients taking OAT are ICHs [16], and it is impossible to distinguish ICH from ischemic stroke on the basis of clinical presentation only. Widespread availability of CT in an acute setting makes it the primary diagnostic modality for ICH. ICHs (both spontaneous and OAT-associated) are immediately visible on CT scans; in OAT patients an almost unique fluid–blood interface can be seen within the first 12 hours as a result of uncongealed blood (visualized as a dark rim) in actively bleeding patients (Figure 19.5) [14]. However, gradient-recalled echo MRI is equally sensitive for diagnosing acute ICH [87]. An advantage of MRI over CT is its ability to detect microbleeds that are indicative of underlying vascular disease and a risk factor for recurrent lobar ICH [82,88].

Regarding other neuroimaging characteristics, according to data extracted from the CHANTS study, OAT-ICHs were larger than spontaneous ICHs with more frequent lobar location [89]. Another study also showed association of warfarin use with larger initial ICH volume, but this effect was merely observed for INR values >3.0 [90]. OAT-ICHs tend to be larger when they have a lobar location compared to deep cerebral [90]. With regard to hematoma shape, there is no difference between OAT-ICH and spontaneous ICH [91]. Warfarin-associated ICH is also characterized by less early edema than spontaneous ICH [92]. Additional characteristics of OAT complications are higher risk of intraventricular hemorrhage (IVH), higher IVH volume at presentation, IVH expansion in both lobar and deep OAT-ICH [93], and certain predilection of the bleeding to cerebellum [16,90,94,95].

There are two distinct temporal profiles of clinical course in OAT-ICH: those that present with rapidly

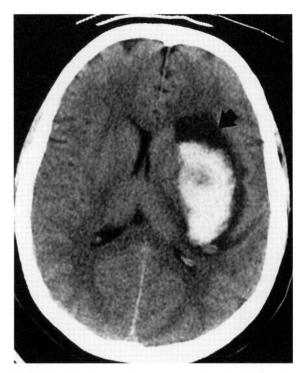

Figure 19.5 The dark rim of uncongealed blood surrounds hyperdense clot. (Reproduced with permission of Hart R G, Boop B S, Anderson D C. Oral anticoagulants and intracranial haemorrhage: Facts and hypotheses. *Stroke.* 1995; 26:1471–7)

evolving neurological deficits proceeding to stupor and coma with a high mortality; and those where the bleeding evolves slowly, for 24 hours or more (up to 50% of cases). This is in contrast to spontaneous ICH patients, in whom the duration of bleeding is usually brief (only 12% suffer from progressive bleeding in the first 24 hours) (16,22,96). Oral anticoagulant-associated ICHs often continue to expand after the diagnosis is made by neuroimaging studies since the median time of hematoma growth is 21.4 hours in OAT-ICH (range 4.6 to 61) vs. 8.4 hours in spontaneous ICH (range 2.4 to 31) [22]. Hematoma expansion, defined as >33% increase in ICH volume, is a major determinant of a poor prognosis and is seen in 54 to 56% of OAT-ICH vs. 16 to 26% of patients with spontaneous ICH. Predictors of hematoma expansion are time to neuroimaging (the earlier the presentation, the higher the risk of expansion), "spot sign" (reflecting continuing bleeding), OAT and INR >2, larger initial hemorrhage, heterogeneity of hematoma, larger intraventricular blood volume, and some blood biomarkers (increased IL-6, MMP-9, c-FN, and TNF, reduced platelet activity, reduced fibrinogen concentrations, and increased serum creatinine) [97]. The spot sign is highly specific for ICH growth [50,51]. Indeed, the recently developed "spot sign score," which is used to grade the number of spot signs and their maximum dimensions and attenuation, has been shown to be the strongest predictor of hematoma expansion [52].

Outcome

Mortality rates in patients with OAT-ICH range from 52 to 67%, and are higher than those observed in patients with spontaneous ICH [98]. A Swedish multicenter study reported the following case-fatality rates for OAT-ICH: 53.6% at 30 days, 63.6% at 6 months, and 77.5% at follow-up (mean 3.5 years). In the same study the 30-day case-fatality rate was as high as 96% among patients unconscious on admission and 80% among patients who became unconscious before active treatment was started [99].

Survivors of OAT-ICH also more frequently remain severely disabled compared with patients recovering from spontaneous ICH [22,100]. The only published data on variables responsible for outcome exclusively in patients with OAT-ICH revealed lower level of consciousness at presentation and larger initial ICH to be predictors of poor outcome including death and disability [101].

There are limited data on NOACs. In the RE-LY and ROCKET AF studies mortality did not differ between patients with NOAC therapy-related ICH and those with ICH during VKA treatment [9,10].

Treatment

Therapeutic strategy in OAT-ICH includes similar measures used for spontaneous ICH including general supportive care, prevention and treatment of complications, and neurosurgical intervention when indicated. Specific for OAT-ICH treatment implies prevention of hematoma expansion by immediate reversal of anticoagulation, applying the principle "time is brain."

References

1. Ogilvie I M, Newton N, Welner S A, Cowell W, Lip G Y H. Underuse of oral anticoagulants in atrial fibrillation: A systematic review. *Am J Med.* 2010; **123**:638–45.

2. Shroff G R, Solid C A, Herzog C A. Temporal trends in ischemic stroke and anticoagulation therapy among Medicare patients with atrial fibrillation: A 15-year perspective (1992–2007). *JAMA Intern Med.* 2013; **173**:159–60.

3. Connolly S J, Ezekowitz M D, Yusuf S, et al. Dabigatran versus warfarin in patients with atrial fibrillation. *N Engl J Med.* 2009; **361**:1139–51.

4. Patel M R, Mahaffey K W, Garg J, et al. Rivaroxaban versus warfarin in nonvalvular atrial fibrillation. *N Engl J Med.* 2011; **365**:883–91.

5. Granger C B, Alexander J H, McMurray J J V, et al. Apixaban versus warfarin in patients with atrial fibrillation. *N Engl J Med.* 2011; **365**:981–92.

6. Connolly S J, Eikelboom J, Joyner C, et al. Apixaban in patients with atrial fibrillation. *N Engl J Med.* 2011; **364**:806–17.

7. Giugliano R P, Ruff C T, Rost N S, et al. Cerebrovascular events in 21 105 patients with atrial fibrillation randomized to edoxaban versus warfarin: Effective Anticoagulation with Factor Xa Next Generation in Atrial Fibrillation-Thrombolysis in Myocardial Infarction 48. *Stroke.* 2014; **45**:2372–8.

8. Connolly S J, Wallentin L, Ezekowitz M D, et al. The long-term multicenter observational study of dabigatran treatment in patients with atrial fibrillation (RELY-ABLE) study. *Circulation.* 2013; **128**:237–43.

9. Hart R G, Diener H C, Yang S, et al. Intracranial hemorrhage in atrial fibrillation patients during anticoagulation with warfarin or dabigatran: The RE-LY trial. *Stroke.* 2012; **43**:1511–17.

10. Hankey G J, Stevens S R, Piccini J P, et al. Intracranial hemorrhage among patients with atrial fibrillation anticoagulated with warfarin or rivaroxaban: The rivaroxaban once daily, oral, direct factor Xa inhibition compared with vitamin K antagonism for prevention of stroke and embolism trial in atrial fibrillation. *Stroke.* 2014; **45**:1304–12.

11. Ruff C T, Giugliano R P, Braunwald E, et al. Comparison of the efficacy and safety of new oral anticoagulants with warfarin in patients with atrial fibrillation: a meta-analysis of randomised trials. *Lancet.* 2014; **383**:955–62.

12. Gage B F, Yan Y, Milligan P E, Waterman A D, et al. Clinical classification schemes for predicting hemorrhage: results from the National Registry of Atrial Fibrillation (NRAF). *Am Heart J.* 2006; **151**:713–19.

13. Pisters R, Lane D A, Nieuwlaat R, et al. A novel user-friendly score (HAS-BLED) to assess 1-year risk of major bleeding in patients with atrial fibrillation: The Euro Heart Survey. *Chest.* 2010; **138**:1093–100.

14. Fang M C, Go A S, Chang Y, et al. A new risk scheme to predict warfarin-associated hemorrhage: the ATRIA (Anticoagulation and Risk Factors in Atrial Fibrillation) study. *J Am Coll Cardiol.* 2011; **58**:395–401.

15. Apostolakis S, Lane D A, Guo Y, Buller H, Lip G Y. Performance of the HEMORR(2)HAGES, ATRIA, and

HAS-BLED bleeding risk-prediction scores in patients with atrial fibrillation undergoing anticoagulation: The AMADEUS (evaluating the use of SR34006 compared to warfarin or acenocoumarol in patients with atrial fibrillation) study. *J Am Coll Cardiol.* 2012; **60**:861–7.

16. Hart R G, Boop B S, Anderson D C. Oral anticoagulants and intracranial hemorrhage. Facts and hypotheses. *Stroke.* 1995; **26**:1471–7.

17. Fang M C, Go A S, Chang Y, Hylek E M, *et al.* Death and disability from warfarin-associated intracranial and extracranial hemorrhages. *Am J Med.* 2007; **120**:700–5.

18. Steiner T, Kaste M, Forsting M, *et al.* The European Stroke Initiative Writing Committee and the Writing Committee for the EUSI Executive Committee. Recommendations for the management of intracranial haemorrhage – part I: Spontaneous intracerebral haemorrhage. *Cerebrovasc Dis.* 2006; **22**:294–316.

19. Själander A, Engström G, Berntorp E, Svensson P. Risk of haemorrhagic stroke in patients with oral anticoagulation compared with the general population. *J Intern Med.* 2003; **254**:434–8.

20. Go A S, Hylek E M, Phillips K A, Chang Y, *et al.* Prevalence of diagnosed atrial fibrillation in adults: National implications for rhythm management and stroke prevention: the AnTicoagulation and Risk factors in Atrial Fibrillation (ATRIA) Study. *JAMA.* 2001; **285**:2370–5.

21. Franke C L, de Jonge J, van Swieten J C, Op de Coul A A, van Gijn J. Intracerebral hematomas during anticoagulant treatment. *Stroke.* 1990; **21**:726–30.

22. Flibotte J J, Hagan N, O'Donnell J, Greenberg S M, Rosand J. Warfarin, hematoma expansion, and outcome of intracerebral hemorrhage. *Neurology.* 2004; **63**:1059–64.

23. Sacco S, Marini C, Toni D, Olivieri L, Carolei A. Incidence and 10-year survival of intracerebral hemorrhage in a population-based registry. *Stroke.* 2009; **40**:394–9.

24. Horstmann S, Rizos T, Lauseker M, *et al.* Intracerebral hemorrhage during anticoagulation with vitamin K antagonists: a consecutive observational study. *J Neurol.* 2013; **260**:2046–51.

25. Lip G Y, Andreotti F, Fauchier L, *et al.* Bleeding risk assessment and management in atrial fibrillation patients: A position document from the European Heart Rhythm Association, endorsed by the European Society of Cardiology Working Group on Thrombosis. *Europace.* 2011; **13**:723–46.

26. Petitti D, Strom B, Melmon K. Duration of warfarin anticoagulation therapy and the probabilities or recurrent thromboembolism and hemorrhage. *Am J Med.* 1986; **81**:255–9.

27. Fihn S D, McDonnel M, Martin D, *et al.* Warfarin Optimized Outpatient Follow-up Study Group. Risk factors for complications of chronic anticoagulation: A multicenter study. *Ann Intern Med.* 1993; **118**:511–20.

28. Palareti G, Leali N, Coccheri S, *et al.* Bleeding complications of oral anticoagulant treatment: An inception-cohort, prospective collaborative study (ISCOAT). *Lancet.* 1996; **348**:423–8.

29. Landefeld C S, Goldman L. Major bleeding in outpatients treated with warfarin: Incidence and prediction by factors known at the start of outpatient therapy. *Am J Med.* 1989; **87**:144–52.

30. Hart R G, Tonarelli S B, Pearce L A. Avoiding central nervous system bleeding during antithrombotic therapy: Recent data and ideas. *Stroke.* 2005; **36**:1588–93.

31. Atrial Fibrillation Investigators. Risk factors for stroke and efficacy of antithrombotic therapy in atrial fibrillation. Analysis of pooled data from five randomized controlled trials. *Arch Intern Med.* 1994; **154**:1449–57.

32. SPAF-Investigators. Warfarin versus aspirin for prevention of thromboembolism in atrial fibrillation: Stroke prevention in atrial fibrillation II study. *Lancet.* 1994; **343**:687–91.

33. Olsson S B. Stroke prevention with the oral direct thrombin inhibitor ximelagatran compared with warfarin in patients with non-valvular atrial fibrillation (SPORTIF III): Randomised controlled trial. *Lancet.* 2003; **362**:1691–8.

34. Albers G W, Diener H C, Frison L, *et al.* Ximelagatran vs warfarin for stroke prevention in patients with nonvalvular atrial fibrillation: a randomized trial. *JAMA.* 2005; **293**:690–8.

35. Di Marco J P, Flaker G, Waldo A L, *et al.* Factors affecting bleeding risk during anticoagulant therapy in patients with atrial fibrillation: Observations from the Atrial Fibrillation Follow-up Investigation of Rhythm Management (AFFIRM) study. *Am Heart J.* 2005; **149**:650–6.

36. Landefeld C S, Goldman L. Major bleeding in outpatients treated with warfarin: Incidence and prediction by factors known at the start of outpatient therapy. *Am J Med.* 1989; **87**:144–52.

37. van der Meer F J, Rosendaal F R, Vandenbroucke J P, Briet E. Bleeding complications in oral anticoagulant therapy. An analysis of risk factors. *Arch Intern Med.* 1993; **153**:1557–62.

38. Steffensen F H, Kristensen K, Ejlersen E, Dahlerup J F, Sorensen H T. Major haemorrhagic complications during oral anticoagulant therapy in a Danish population-based cohort. *J Intern Med.* 1997; **242**:497–503.

39. Beyth R J, Quinn L M, Landefeld C S. Prospective evaluation of an index for predicting the risk of major bleeding in outpatients treated with warfarin. *Am J Med*. 1998; **105**:91–9.

40. Go A S, Hylek E M, Chang Y, *et al*. Anticoagulation therapy for stroke prevention in atrial fibrillation: How well do randomized trials translate into clinical practice? *JAMA*. 2003; **290**:2685–92.

41. Hylek E M, Evans-Molina C, Shea C, Henault L E, Regan S. Major hemorrhage and tolerability of warfarin in the first year of therapy among elderly patients with atrial fibrillation. *Circulation*. 2007; **115**:2689–96.

42. Poli D, Antonucci E, Grifoni E, *et al*. Bleeding risk during oral anticoagulation in atrial fibrillation patients older than 80 years. *J Am Coll Cardiol*. 2009; **54**:999–1002.

43. Vandenbroucke J P. Why do the results of randomised and observational studies differ? *BMJ*. 2011; **343**:d7020.

44. Charidimou A, Shakeshaft C, Werring D J. Cerebral microbleeds on magnetic resonance imaging and anticoagulant-associated intracerebral hemorrhage risk. *Front Neurol*. 2012; **19**:133.

45. Larsen T B, Rasmussen L H, Skjøth F, Due K M, *et al*. Efficacy and safety of dabigatran etexilate and warfarin in "real-world" patients with atrial fibrillation: A prospective nationwide cohort study. *J Am Coll Cardiol*. 2013; **61**:2264–73.

46. Southworth M R, Reichman M E, Unger E F. Dabigatran and postmarketing reports of bleeding. *N Engl J Med*. 2013; **368**:1272–4.

47. Hankey G J. Intracranial hemorrhage and novel anticoagulants for atrial fibrillation: What have we learned? *Curr Cardiol Rep*. 2014; **16**:480.

48. Wintzen A R, De Jonge H, Loeliger E A, Botts G T A M. The risk of intracerebral hemorrhage during oral anticoagulant treatment: A population study. *Ann Neurol*. 1984; **16**:533–8.

49. Fisher C M. Pathological observations in hypertensive cerebral hemorrhage. *J Neuropathol Exp Neurol*. 1971; **30**:536–50.

50. Brouwers H B, Goldstein J N, Romero J M, Rosand J. Clinical applications of the computed tomography angiography spot sign in acute intracerebral hemorrhage: A review. *Stroke*. 2012; **43**:3427–32.

51. Demchuk A M, Dowlatshahi D, Rodriguez-Luna D, *et al*. PREDICT/Sunnybrook ICH CTA study group. Prediction of hematoma growth and outcome in patients with intracerebral haemorrhage using the CT-angiography spot sign (PREDICT): A prospective observational study. *Lancet Neurol*. 2012; **11**:307–14.

52. Delgado Almandoz J E, Yoo A J, Stone M J, *et al*. Systematic characterization of the computed tomography angiography spot sign in primary intracerebral hemorrhage identifies patients at highest risk for hematoma expansion: The spot sign score. *Stroke*. 2009; **40**:2994–3000.

53. Brouwers H B, Biffi A, McNamara K A, *et al*. Apolipoprotein E genotype is associated with CT angiography spot sign in lobar intracerebral hemorrhage. *Stroke*. 2012; **43**:2120–5.

54. Brouwers H B, Greenberg S M. Hematoma expansion following acute intracerebral hemorrhage. *Cerebrovasc Dis*. 2013; **35**:195–201.

55. Greenberg C H, Frosch M P, Goldstein J N, Rosand J, Greenberg S M. Modeling intracerebral hemorrhage growth and response to anticoagulation. *PLoS One*. 2012; **7**:e48458.

56. Grysiewicz R, Gorelick P B. Incidence, mortality, and risk factors for oral anticoagulant-associated intracranial hemorrhage in patients with atrial fibrillation. *J Stroke Cerebrovasc Dis*. 2014; **23**:2479–88.

57. Hylek E M, Singer D E. Risk factors for intracranial hemorrhage in outpatients taking warfarin. *Ann Intern Med*. 1994; **120**:897–902.

58. Fang M C, Chang Y, Hylek E M, *et al*. Advanced age, anticoagulation intensity, and risk for intracranial hemorrhage among patients taking warfarin for atrial fibrillation. *Ann Intern Med*. 2004; **16**:745–52.

59. Stroke Prevention in Atrial Fibrillation (SPAF) II Study. Warfarin versus aspirin for prevention of thromboembolism in atrial fibrillation. *Lancet*. 1994; **343**:687–91.

60. Birman-Deych E, Radford M J, Nilasena D S, Gage B F. Use and effectiveness of warfarin in Medicare beneficiaries with atrial fibrillation. *Stroke*. 2006; **37**:1070–4.

61. Shen A Y, Yao J F, Brar S S, Jorgensen M B, Chen W. Racial/ethnic differences in the risk of intracranial hemorrhage among patients with atrial fibrillation. *J Am Coll Cardiol*. 2007; **50**:309–15.

62. Hylek E M, Go A S, Chang Y, Jensvold N G, *et al*. Effect of intensity of oral anticoagulation on stroke severity and mortality in atrial fibrillation. *N Engl J Med*. 2003; **349**:1019–26.

63. Berwaerts J, Webster J. Analysis of risk factors involved in oral-anticoagulant-related intracranial haemorrhages. *QJM*. 2000; **93**:513–21.

64. Fric-Shamji E C, Shamji M F, Cole J, Benoit B G. Modifiable risk factors for intracerebral hemorrhage: study of anticoagulated patients. *Can Fam Physician*. 2008; **54**:1138–9.

65. The Stroke Prevention In Reversible Ischemia Trial (SPIRIT) Study Group. A randomized trial of anticoagulants versus aspirin after cerebral ischemia of presumed arterial origin. *Ann Neurol*. 1997; **42**:857–65.

66. Revesz T, Holton J L, Lashley T, *et al.* Sporadic and familial cerebral amyloid angiopathies. *Brain Pathol.* 2002; **12**:343–57.

67. Greenberg S M, Rebeck G W, Vonsattel J P, Gomez-Isla T, Hyman B T. Apolipo-protein E epsilon 4 and cerebral hemorrhage associated with amyloid angiopathy. *Ann Neurol.* 1995; **38**:254–9.

68. Nicoll J A, Burnett C, Love S, *et al.* High frequency of apolipoprotein E epsilon 2 allele in hemorrhage due to cerebral amyloid angiopathy. *Ann Neurol.* 1997; **41**:716–21.

69. Biffi A, Sonni A, Anderson C D, *et al.* Variants at APOE influence risk of deep and lobar intracerebral hemorrhage. *Ann Neurol.* 2010; **68**:934–43.

70. Rosand J, Hylek E M, O'Donnell H C, Greenberg S M. Warfarin-associated hemorrhage and cerebral amyloid angiopathy: A genetic and pathologic study. *Neurology.* 2000; **55**:947.

71. Melo T P, Bogousslavsky J, Regli F, Janzer R. Fatal hemorrhage during anticoagulation of cardioembolic infarction: Role of cerebral amyloid angiopathy. *Eur Neurol.* 1993; **33**:9–12.

72. Flockhart D A, O'Kane D, Williams M S, *et al.* Pharmacogenetic testing of CYP2C9 and VKORC1 alleles for warfarin. *Genet Med.* 2008; **10**:139–50.

73. Stehle S, Kirchheiner J, Lazar A, Fuhr U. Pharmacogenetics of oral anticoagulants: A basis for dose individualization. *Clin Pharmacokinet.* 2008; **47**:565–94.

74. Higashi M K, Veenstra D L, Kondo L M, *et al.* Association between CYP2C9 genetic variants and anticoagulation-related outcomes during warfarin therapy. *JAMA.* 2002; **287**:1690–8.

75. Rybak I, Ehle M, Buckley L, Fanikos J. Efficacy and safety of novel anticoagulants compared with established agents. *Ther Adv Hematol.* 2011; **2**:175–95.

76. Mega J L, Walker J R, Ruff C T, *et al.* Genetics and the clinical response to warfarin and edoxaban: Findings from the randomised, double-blind ENGAGE AF-TIMI 48 trial. *Lancet.* 2015; **385**:2280–7.

77. Shireman T I, Howard P A, Kresowik T F, Ellerbeck E F. Combined anticoagulant-antiplatelet use and major bleeding events in elderly atrial fibrillation patients. *Stroke.* 2004; **35**:2362–7.

78. Gouw A A, Seewann A, Van Der Flier W M, *et al.* Heterogeneity of small vessel disease: A systematic review of MRI and histopathology correlations. *J Neurol Neurosurg Psychiatr.* 2010; **82**:126–35.

79. Schmidt R, Grazer A, Enzinger C, *et al.* MRI-detected white matter lesions: Do they really matter? *J Neural Transm.* 2011; **118**:673–81.

80. Gorter J W. Major bleeding during anticoagulation after cerebral ischemia: Patterns and risk factors. Stroke Prevention In Reversible Ischemia Trial (SPIRIT). European Atrial Fibrillation Trial (EAFT) study groups. *Neurology.* 1999; **53**:1319–27.

81. Smith E E, Rosand J, Knudsen K A, Hylek E M, Greenberg S M. Leukoaraiosis is associated with warfarin-related hemorrhage following ischemic stroke. *Neurology.* 2002; **59**:193–7.

82. Greenberg S M, Vernooij M W, Cordonnier C, *et al.* Cerebral microbleeds: A guide to detection and interpretation. *Lancet Neurol.* 2009; **8**:165–74.

83. Lee S H, Ryu W S, Roh J K. Cerebral microbleeds are a risk factor for warfarin-related intracerebral hemorrhage. *Neurology.* 2009; **72**:171–6.

84. Ueno H, Naka H, Ohshita T, *et al.* Association between cerebral microbleeds on T2*-weighted MR images and recurrent hemorrhagic stroke in patients treated with warfarin following ischemic stroke. *Am J Neuroradiol.* 2008; **29**:1483–6.

85. Lovelock C E, Cordonnier C, Naka H, *et al.* Edinburgh Stroke Study Group. Antithrombotic drug use, cerebral microbleeds, and intracerebral hemorrhage: a systematic review of published and unpublished studies. *Stroke.* 2010; **41**:1222–8.

86. Charidimou A, Peeters A P, Jäger R, *et al.* Cortical superficial siderosis and intracerebral hemorrhage risk in cerebral amyloid angiopathy. *Neurology.* 2013; **81**:1666–73.

87. Kidwell C S, Chalela J A, Saver J L, *et al.* Comparison of MRI and CT for detection of acute intracerebral hemorrhage. *JAMA.* 2004; **292**:1823–30.

88. Greenberg S M, Eng J A, Ning M, Smith E E, Rosand J. Hemorrhage burden predicts recurrent intracerebral hemorrhage after lobar hemorrhage. *Stroke.* 2004; **35**:1415–20.

89. Cucchiara B, Messe S, Sansing L, Kasner S, Lyden P; CHANT Investigators. Hematoma growth in oral anticoagulant related intracerebral hemorrhage. *Stroke.* 2008; **39**:2993–6.

90. Flaherty M L, Tao H, Haverbusch M, *et al.* Warfarin use leads to larger intracerebral hematomas. *Neurology.* 2008; **71**:1084–9.

91. Sheth K N, Cushing T A, Wendell L, *et al.* Comparison of hematoma shape and volume estimates in warfarin versus non-warfarin-related intracerebral hemorrhage. *Neurocrit Care.* 2010; **12**:30–4.

92. Levine J M, Snider R, Finkelstein D, *et al.* Early edema in warfarin-related intracerebral hemorrhage. *Neurocrit Care.* 2007; **7**:58–63.

93. Biffi A, Battey T W, Ayres A M, *et al.* Warfarin-related intraventricular hemorrhage: imaging and outcome. *Neurology.* 2011; **15**:1840–6.

94. Kase C S, Robinson R K, Stein R W, *et al.* Anticoagulant-related intracerebral hemorrhage. *Neurology.* 1985; **35**:943–8.

95. Toyoda K, Okada Y, Ibayashi S, *et al.* Antithrombotic therapy and predilection for cerebellar hemorrhage. *Cerebrovasc Dis.* 2007; **23**:109.

96. Brott T, Broderick J, Kothari R, *et al.* Early hemorrhage growth in patients with intracerebral hemorrhage. *Stroke.* 1997; **28**:1–5.

97. Balami J S, Buchan A M. Complications of intracerebral haemorrhage. *Lancet Neurol.* 2012; **11**:101–18.

98. Veltkamp R, Rizos T, Horstmann S. Intracerebral bleeding in patients on antithrombotic agents. *Semin Thromb Hemost.* 2013; **39**:963–71.

99. Sjöblom L, Hårdemark H G, Lindgren A, *et al.* Management and prognostic features of intracerebral hemorrhage during anticoagulant therapy: A Swedish multicenter study. *Stroke.* 2001; **32**:2567–74.

100. Rosand J, Eckman M H, Knudsen K A, Singer D E, Greenberg S M. The effect of warfarin and intensity of anticoagulation on outcome of intracerebral hemorrhage. *Arch Intern Med.* 2004; **164**:880–4.

101. Zubkov A Y, Mandrekar J N, Claassen D O, *et al.* Predictors of outcome in warfarin-related intracerebral hemorrhage. *Arch Neurol.* 2008; **65**:1320–5.

Stroke during pregnancy and the puerperium

Elisabetta Del Zotto and Alessandro Pezzini

Introduction

Stroke in young adults accounts for 5 to 10% of all stroke [1]. According to a recent study using the Nationwide Inpatient Sample there is an increasing trend in the prevalence of hospitalization rates for stroke among young adults [1]. The costs and the effect on long-term disability associated with stroke are of even greater consequence in this age group. Pregnancy and puerperium may partly contribute to an increased incidence of stroke in young women. Ischemic and hemorrhagic strokes associated with pregnancy and puerperium have long been recognized as uncommon complications, but when they occur, they represent a potentially devastating event for a young woman. Stroke is a significant cause of maternal mortality contributing to more than 12% of all maternal deaths [2] and this is disproportionately higher in black women, in older patients, and those with no prenatal care [3]. Trends in stroke during pregnancy and the postpartum period are a subject of special interest, since the World Health Organization proposed to consider stroke as a life-threatening (or "near-miss") obstetric complication [4].

Epidemiology

A recent study using the US Nationwide Inpatient Sample from 1994 to 1995 and from 2006 to 2007 showed a temporal increase of 54% in the proportion of pregnancy hospitalizations that were associated with a stroke, with a 47% increase for antenatal hospitalizations and 83% increase for postpartum hospitalizations, but no increase for delivery hospitalizations. According to these data at the end of the study period (2006 to 2007), the overall prevalence of pregnancy-related stroke hospitalizations was 0.71 per 1,000 delivery hospitalizations. Increases in the prevalence of heart disease and hypertensive disorders accounted for almost all the increase in postpartum stroke hospitalizations but not the antenatal stroke hospitalizations [5].

The reported incidence of stroke associated with pregnancy and the puerperium is widely variable. According to previous hospital-based and community-based reports, the incidence rates for strokes associated with pregnancy or the puerperium vary from 4.3 to 210 per 100,000 deliveries [6]. A reliable estimation requires very large population size; the wide variability reflects small sample sizes of most studies, inadequate consideration of referral bias, different study designs (e.g., not all were population based), and the incorporation of different subgroups of patients. Moreover, another limitation regards studies reported before CT scan became widely available. Therefore comparisons of available retrospective data are limited because authors used different methods to define and capture their populations and different definitions of strokes and stroke subtypes.

Data published since 1985 shows an incidence of ischemic stroke ranging from 4 to 41 per 100,000 pregnancies [6–14] while it ranges from 5 to 31 per 100,000 pregnancies for hemorrhagic stroke [6,7,10–12]. Data from the three population-based studies indicate a lower incidence, varying from 4 to 11 cases per 100,000 deliveries for ischemic stroke and, similarly, for hemorrhagic stroke ranging from 0 to 6 cases per 100,000 [6,8,10] (Table 20.1).

Recently, in the United States a large population study based on data from the Nationwide Inpatient Sample has found a rate of pregnancy-related stroke of 34.2 per 100,000 deliveries for the period from 2000 to 2001 [3]. Although in this study the incidence of stroke for women who were not pregnant was not computed, comparing data with those of other studies, the authors found a three-fold increased

Treatment-Related Stroke, ed. Alexander Tsiskaridze, Arne Lindgren and Adnan Qureshi. Published by Cambridge University Press. © Cambridge University Press 2016.

Table 20.1 Studies of pregnancy-related stroke since 1985.

Author, year	Methodology	Study period	Postpartum period	Deliveries No	Total stroke No	IS No	IS incidence (per deliveries)	HS No	HS incidence (per deliveries)	Notes
Wiebers and Whisnant, 1985 [8]	Retrospective population based study	1955–1979	NR	26,099[a]	1	1	NR	0	NR	[a] live births
Simolke et al. 1991 [51]	Retrospective single hospital-based study	1984–1990	NR	89,913	15	9[b]	1 in 10,000[b]	6	1 in 15,000	[b] including also cerebral venous thrombosis
Awada et al. 1995 [9]	Retrospective hospital based study	1983–1993	15 days	NR	12	9	NR	3	NR	
Sharshar et al. 1995 [6]	Retrospective and prospective multihospital-based study	1989–1992	2 weeks	348,295	31	15	4,3 per 100,000	16	4,6 per 100,000	
Kittner et al. 1996 [10]	Retrospective population based study	1988–1991	6 weeks	141,243	31	17[c]	11 per 100,000	14	9 per 100,000	[c] including cerebral venous thrombosis (1 patient)
Witlin et al. 1997 [11]	Retrospective single hospital-based study	1985–1995	4 weeks	79,301	24	5	NR	6	NR	
Jlagobin and Silver, 2000 [12]	Retrospective single hospital-based study	1980–1997	6 weeks	50,711	34	21[d]	41 per 100,000	13	26 per 100,000	[d] including cerebral venous thrombosis (8 patients)
Skidmore et al. 2001 [13]	Retrospective hospital based study	1992–1999	12 weeks	58,429	36	21	NR	11	NR	

Study	Design	Period	Follow-up	Deliveries						
Ros et al. 2001 [15]	Retrospective, records from birth register, Sweden	1987–1995	6 weeks	1,003,489	NR	NR	4 per 100,000	NR	3.8[e] per 100,000	[e] 2.4 per 100,000 for subarachnoid hemorrhage
Jeng et al. 2004 [14]	Retrospective single hospital-based study	1984–2002	6 weeks	49,796	49	16	32.1 per 100,000	19	38.2[f] per 100,000	[f] 6.0 per 100,000 for subarachnoid hemorrhage; 22.1 per 100 000 for cerebral venous thrombosis
Liang et al. 2006 [7]	Retrospective single hospital-based study	1992–2004	6 weeks	66,781	26	11[g]	16.5 per 100,000	21	25.4 per 100,000	[g] including cerebral venous thrombosis (3 patients)

Table 20.2 Relative risk of stroke according to timing of pregnancy and the puerperium.

	Cerebral infarction	Intracerebral hemorrhage	Subarachnoid hemorrhage
	RR (95% CI)	RR (95% CI)	RR (95% CI)
Kittner et al. 1996 [10]			
during pregnancy	0.7 (03–1.6)	2.5 (1.0–6.4)	nr
during 6 weeks after pregnancy	5.4 (2.9–10.0)	18.2 (8.7–38.1)	nr
Ros et al. 2001 [15]			
third trimester (>28 weeks to 3 days before delivery)	2.2 (0.8–4.8)	13 (0.3–41)	0.8 (0.2–2.5)
around delivery (2 days before to 1 day after delivery)	33.8 (10.5–84.0)	95.0 (42.1–194.8)	46.9 (19.3–98.4)
2 days to 6 weeks postpartum	8.3 (4.4–14.8)	11.7 (6.1–21.6)	1.8 (0.5–4.9)

nr: not reported.

incidence of stroke during pregnancy than outside pregnancy in women of childbearing age.

With regard to the timing of stroke associated with pregnancy, the third trimester and the six weeks after pregnancy are associated with the greatest risk of stroke, with a peak in the first postpartum week [6,10,13] (Table 20.2)

In a large Swedish cohort of over 650,000 women with over 1 million deliveries in an eight-year time period the greatest risk of ischemic and hemorrhagic stroke was around the delivery (two days before and one day after) with relative risk (RR) of 33.8, (95% confidence interval (CI) 10.5–84.0 for ischemic stroke); of 95.0 (95% CI 42.1–194.8) for intracerebral hemorrhage, and of 46.9 (95% CI 19.3–98.4) for subarachnoid hemorrhage), with an increased but declining risk over the subsequent six weeks for all strokes except subarachnoid hemorrhage [15]. The clustering of events in the third trimester and postpartum period implies a possible link between the physiological changes of pregnancy and stroke; in particular with delivery there is a rapid normalization in hemodynamic and coagulation profile that potentially may increase the risk in susceptible patients and may explain the increased risk found in several studies in the postpartum period.

Maternal physiological changes

Maternal physiological alterations occur during pregnancy as a consequence of the variations of the hormonal status, involving the hemostatic and hemodynamic systems. Whether this adaptation could affect the risk of stroke is still unclear and the relationship is likely complex.

Hemodynamic and connective tissue adaptations

In the first ten weeks of pregnancy a volume shifting develops due an increase in the level of aldosterone and rennin activity with an increase of total body water; this physiological adaptation remains stably increased until one to two weeks after delivery, after which it gradually returns to normal.

Increasing circulatory demands of the fetus and placenta combined with this hypervolemic state results in a rise of 30 to 50% of cardiac output, stroke volume, and heart rate. Half of this change occurs during the first eight weeks of pregnancy, reaching a peak at 25 to 30 weeks. During labor there is a dramatic change in cardiac output that increases progressively as labor advances by a mean value of 30%. Heart rate also increases consistently. Then, in the first days after delivery, there is a strong fall of stroke volume and heart rate, and cardiac output gradually decreases to 50% above prepregnancy level within two weeks after delivery and returns to normal by six to twelve weeks [16]. As a consequence of the decrease in systemic vascular resistance, blood pressure starts to lower around the seventh week, hits the lowest levels at 24 to 32 weeks, and then increases progressively to pre-pregnancy levels at term. Venous compliance increases throughout pregnancy, leading to decreased blood flow, increased stasis, and a

Table 20.3 Modifications of hemostatic system during pregnancy.

Procoagulant factors	
Fibrinogen, von Willebrand factor, Factors VII, VIII, IX, X, XII	↑
Factors V, XIII	↑↓
Factor II, XI	C
Coagulation inhibitors	
Protein S	↓
Protein C, antithrombin III	=
Fibrinolytic factors	
Tissue plasminogen activator	↓
Plasminogen activator inhibitor 1 and 2 (PAI-1, PAI-2), Thrombin activable fibrinolysis inhibitor (TAFI)	↑
Others	
Platelet count	↓
Prothrombin fragment 1+2, Thrombin-antithrombin complex, D-dimer, fibrinopeptide-A	↑

↑: increase; ↓: decrease; =: no significant change; ↑↓: early increase followed by decrease; C: controversial data.

tendency toward orthostatic pressure drops. A remodelling in arterial composition with a reduction in collagen and elastin contents and a loss of distensibility that partially normalizes near term has also been observed during pregnancy.

Hemostatic adaptations

Pregnancy is normally associated with significant changes in venous flow and in the molecular mediators of hemostasis, to the extent that the overall balance shifts towards a hypercoagulable state (Table 20.3) [17]. Procoagulant changes are more marked around term and in the immediate postpartum period, presumably related to the expulsion of the placenta and release of thromboplastic substances at the site of separation. Blood coagulation and fibrinolysis get back to those of the non-pregnant state approximately three weeks after delivery [17]. This resulting hypercoagulable state in association with a venous stasis condition may likely account for an increased risk of thromboembolic complications, in particular during the third trimester and the puerperium.

Diagnostic work-up of pregnancy-related stroke

There are few specific causes of pregnancy-related stroke; in most cases, stroke has the same etiologies commonly observed in a young non-pregnant woman. As a consequence, a complete stroke work-up should be completed as for non-pregnant women.

In a pregnant women, as in other patients, it is important to differentiate timely hemorrhagic from ischemic stroke, considering the different treatment implications and to determine as soon as possible the specific etiology, since some of these conditions may need specific management (i.e., eclampsia). To answer this question, brain imaging in the form of CT or MRI scan should be carried out as quickly as possible after symptom onset. However, neuroimaging as part of the work-up causes several concerns for the clinician about fetal exposure to radiation. The harmful effects of radiation depend on the stage of gestation at which the fetus is exposed, the total dose of radiation absorbed, and the rate at which the dose is absorbed. Potential risk of birth defects due to radiation are limited to the first few weeks, the embryogenesis period, when the patient may not be aware of the pregnancy. Radiation-protection precautions for the developing fetus should be used whenever the question of pregnancy arises. A CT perfusion study should be avoided, due to a significant increase of the X-ray exposure and to the necessity of administering intravenous contrast, unless the information is critical to guide therapy. The use of iodinated contrast material during pregnancy may pose some risk to the fetus. Cerebral angiography requires approximately the same amount of fetal exposure plus whatever results from fluoroscopy during catheter insertion before abdominal shielding begins, which can be limited by skilled hands. Digital angiography procedures decrease the X-ray exposure and the amount of administered iodinated agents.

There is no evidence of adverse fetal effects in humans to the magnetic field exposure for magnetic resonance imaging (MRI). It has been hypothesized that some risk for the fetus may arise due to exposure to very powerful magnetic fields, minimal increases in body temperature, and loud tapping noises of the coils [18]. Although a possible teratogenic effect has been found in some studies on animal models [19], MRI is the preferred imaging option in pregnancy. According to the American College of Radiology guidelines an MRI study during pregnancy is recommended when it provides information that cannot be achieved via safer means, when the data are needed to determine the care of the patient and/or fetus during the pregnancy, and when the referring physician does not feel that it is prudent to wait to obtain this data until after the pregnancy [19]. The American College of Obstetricians and Gynecologists and the National Radiological Protection Board have stated that there have been no adverse fetal effects reported, but advise against the use of MRI in the first trimester [18].

Regarding the use of gadolinium during MRI study, animal reproduction studies showed that gadolinium at high dose can have teratogenic effects [18]. Therefore the use of gadolinium should be avoided in a pregnant woman unless specifically indicated in a particular situation where the decision must be made after a well-documented and thoughtful risk–benefit analysis [19].

Pregnancy does not contraindicate to performance of transesophageal echocardiography [20].

Risk factors and specific causes of stroke in pregnancy

Although the risk of pregnancy-related stroke is found to be higher among women aged 35 years and older [3], an ischemic subtype has been associated with a younger maternal age [10], and a mean age under of 30 has been reported in patients with pregnancy-related stroke in hospital-based series.

Several medical conditions were associated with stroke in pregnancy, such as hypertension, diabetes, heart disease, sickle cell disease, anemia, thrombocytopenia, and thrombophilia. Among lifestyle factors, alcohol, smoking, and substance abuse were found to be significantly associated with stroke in pregnancy [3]. Pregnancy and delivery complications such as infection, transfusion, postpartum hemorrhage, and fluid and electrolyte imbalance were also linked to pregnancy-related stroke [3]. Multiple gestation and greater parity may also predispose to stroke.

Cesarean delivery has been shown to be associated with a 3 to 12-fold increased risk of peripartum and postpartum stroke [21,22]. However, a possible explanation for this association may be found in an increased number of cesarean deliveries among patients with previous stroke or with conditions that can increase the risk of stroke such as preeclampsia–eclampsia. Despite this, the association of postpartum stroke with cesarean delivery suggests that cesarean delivery may increase the risk of cerebrovascular events.

Amniotic fluid embolism

Amniotic fluid embolism is a rare complication with a variable presentation, ranging from mild degree of organ dysfunction to cardiovascular collapse, coagulopathy, and death [23]. The mortality rate varies from 61 to 86% and accounts for approximately 10% of all maternal deaths in the United States [23]. Most cases usually present at term during labor and should be suspected in any pregnant patient, specifically those with ruptured membranes, who develops sudden onset dyspnea with hypoxia, acute hypotension, and/or cardiac arrest followed by a profound coagulopathy. Seizures occur in 10 to 20% of cases. The clinical picture is rarely suggestive of a stroke, but focal deficits are possible. The pathophysiology of amniotic fluid embolism remains enigmatic. Ischemic stroke due to paradoxical cerebral amniotic fluid emboli does occur, but its true incidence is unknown.

Preeclampsia and eclampsia

Preeclampsia–eclampsia represents a major obstetric problem accounting for a substantial maternal and perinatal morbidity and mortality, especially in developing countries [24]. It consists of a multisystem disorder of unknown cause that occurs in the later stages of pregnancy and in the first six to eight weeks after delivery [25].

Preeclampsia is usually diagnosed in the presence of elevated gestational blood pressure accompanied by proteinuria. In the absence of proteinuria, preeclampsia should be considered when hypertension is associated with persistent cerebral symptoms, epigastric or right upper-quadrant pain with nausea or vomiting, or with thrombocytopenia and abnormal liver enzymes [24]. Although preeclampsia is usually asymptomatic, patients may complain of headaches, visual abnormalities, confusion, and impairment of consciousness. In addition, in some patients a manifestation of sudden onset focal neurological deficits may be consistent with a clinical diagnosis of stroke. Eclampsia is defined as the onset of convulsions or coma in women who have either gestational hypertension or preeclampsia. About 2 to 12% of patients with eclampsia develop HELLP syndrome, a life-threatening condition characterized by hemolytic anemia (H), elevated liver enzymes (EL), and low platelet count (LP) [24].

Preeclampsia affects approximately 6 to 8% of all pregnancies, whereas eclampsia has an incidence of 1/1,000 to 1/2,000 deliveries in the United States [24,25]. The proportion of patients with ischemic stroke related to preeclampsia–eclampsia during pregnancies varies from 18 to 47%, while for hemorrhagic stroke it ranges from 14 to 44% [6,10].

The pathophysiology underlying preeclampsia–eclampsia is not completely understood. An abnormal vascular response to placentation represents a typical characteristic, which is associated with increased vascular tone and sensitivity to mediators of vasoconstrictions; this results in hypertension, vasospasm, and organ hypoperfusion [26]. Endothelial cell dysfunction represents another common response including instability of vascular tone, enhanced platelet aggregation, and activation of the coagulation system leading to local thrombosis [26]. Loss of endothelial integrity may lead to hemorrhage and severe vasospasm, and thrombosis may lead to infarction. Therefore as a consequence of these manifestations, pathological changes may occur in the placenta, liver, brain, and kidney.

A CT scan is normal or shows multiple bilateral and almost symmetrical hypodensities involving the cerebral white matter and the adjacent cerebral cortex, often with posterior predominance, and the basal ganglia. Notwithstanding MR imaging is superior to CT in demonstrating the effects of preeclampsia and eclampsia on the brain. The MRI findings include cortical and/or subcortical hyperintensities and, even less commonly, in the brainstem and cerebellum on T2-weighted sequences there may or may not be associated enhancement. In rare cases, subarachnoid hemorrhage can also be present, usually located in the sulci over the cerebral convexities.

The management of preeclampsia is aimed at delivery of the fetus and placenta and drug therapy of hypertension. Magnesium sulfate is the first-line therapy for seizures, as it prevents vascular spasm, and this could also be used in prophylaxis in preeclamptic patients.

Peripartum cardiomyopathy

Peripartum cardiomyopathy is a rare dilating cardiomyopathy that develops in the last gestational month of pregnancy or in the first five months after delivery, with no identifiable cause for heart failure and in the absence of heart disease. A cardiomyopathy that develops during the first stage of pregnancy has also been reported; clinical presentation and maternal outcome are similar with peripartum cardiomyopathy suggesting that these two conditions may represent a continuum of a spectrum of the same disease [27]. The true incidence is widely variable according to geographical differences, being uncommon in Europe and more frequent in Africa. A reported incidence in the United States is of 1 in 3,000 to 1 in 4,000 live births [28,29].

Risk factors include advanced age (>30 years), obesity, black race, multiparity, twin pregnancies, preeclampsia, and severe hypertension during pregnancy [29]. However, a recent study did not support the association with multiparity, since almost 40% of cardiomyopathy developed in first pregnancy women and >50% with the first two pregnancies [27].

Many hypotheses have been suggested to explain the etiology of peripartum cardiomyopathy, including abnormal immune response to pregnancy, myocarditis, viral infection, maladaptive response to the hemodynamic stresses of pregnancy, stress-activated cytokines, and prolonged tocolysis [28].

The diagnosis remains a challenge because many normal women in the last month of a normal pregnancy experience dyspnea, fatigue, and pedal edema – symptoms identical to early congestive cardiac failure. A suspicion of heart failure should rise in the presence of symptoms and signs such as paroxysmal nocturnal dyspnea, chest pain, nocturnal cough, new regurgitant murmurs, pulmonary crackles, elevated jugular venous pressure, and hepatomegaly. Other late complications of pregnancy such as massive pulmonary embolism, amniotic fluid embolism (most often during labor and delivery), and severe toxemia may also simulate heart failure. Peripartum cardiomyopathy is a diagnosis of exclusion, distinguished by rapid onset, occurrence in the peripartum period, and significant improvement in up to 50% of affected women.

The estimated incidence of systemic and pulmonary embolization varies from 25 to 40% [30]. Ischemic stroke represents about 5% of cases and more rarely may result from cerebral hypoperfusion secondary to cardiac failure [30].

Prognosis of peripartum cardiomyopathy depends on recovery of systolic function and mortality is high. Approximately 20% of women with the disorder either die or survive only because they receive cardiac transplants; the majority recover partially or completely. Recurrences during subsequent pregnancies are common.

Postpartum cerebral angiopathy

Postpartum cerebral angiopathy is often grouped with other conditions unified under the term of reversible cerebral vasoconstriction syndrome (RCVS). It has been described using various labels, including postpartum angiopathy, postpartum angiitis, and puerperal vasospasm.

This condition is characterized by multifocal narrowing of cerebral arteries in the absence of inflammation, and is clinically associated with acute-onset, severe, recurrent headaches, with or without additional neurologic signs and symptoms. Although the pathophysiology of this condition is scarcely understood, a disturbance in the control of cerebral vascular tone seems to be a critical element, determining a prolonged but reversible vasoconstriction of the cerebral arteries. Though typically considered a benign disorder with favorable prognosis, recent data has highlighted the possibility of a malignant course with residual neurological symptoms or death, suggesting a close neurological monitoring with prompt brain imaging for patients with neurological symptoms in the postpartum period [31].

Though most patients have a history of uncomplicated pregnancy and normal labor and delivery, a recent study found that proteinuria was present in half of pregnant patients supporting the suggestion that there is an overlap between preeclampsia or eclampsia and postpartum angiopathy [31]. The authors also showed that an initial angiogram in symptomatic patients may be normal, especially if performed early in the clinical course of postpartum angiopathy, and the necessity to repeat angiography for diagnosis when clinical suspicion remains high [31].

A brain MRI in patients with postpartum angiopathy may show acute stroke (hemorrhagic or ischemic). On both magnetic resonance angiography (MRA) and CT angiography multifocal segmental narrowing of large and medium-size cerebral arteries may be present. Arterial abnormalities are better visualized with CT angiography and conventional invasive catheter angiography, both of which require the use of iodinated contrast material.

Choriocarcinoma

Choriocarcinoma develops from placental trophoblastic tissue, usually as a consequence of a molar pregnancy but also following a term delivery, abortion, and ectopic pregnancy. This malignant neoplasm has a tendency to early metastases, especially to the lungs, brain, liver, and vagina [32]. Brain metastasis complicates about 20% of choriocarcinomas. Patients may present with headache, focal neurological deficits, seizures, encephalopathy, signs of elevated intracranial pressure, and excessively elevated serum β human choriogonadotrophic hormone level. Due to high vascularization, choriocarcinoma is extremely prone to hemorrhage. In the brain, trophoblasts may invade blood vessels, just as they would in the uterus. Thrombosis may occur in the damaged vessels with single or multiple cerebral infarctions as a consequence, or an embolus may fail to lodge and pass distally, leading to transient ischemic attacks. Other vessels may develop neoplastic aneurysms or varicosities resulting in intraparenchymal or subarachnoid space bleeding [30].

Cerebral venous sinus thrombosis

The several changes in the coagulation system induced by pregnancy and the puerperium have been regarded as important factors contributing to the risk of cerebral venous thrombosis (CVT). Data from the National Hospital Discharge Survey with the limiting cerebrovascular events to the hospitalization showed an incidence of 8.9 CVT per 100,000 deliveries [33]. However, when antepartum and postpartum data were included, the incidence was 11.4 per 100,000 for CVT [34].

As for arterial ischemic stroke, the risk of pregnancy-related venous infarction is significantly higher in the puerperium. Jaigobin and Silver identified eight cases of CVT associated with pregnancy over a 17-year period and seven of these occurred postpartum [12]. A study in Taiwanese women reported 11 cases of pregnancy-related CVT, 73% of which occurred during the puerperium [14]. Most of these patients had a pre-existing hereditary coagulopathy.

Cerebral venous thrombosis is characterized by a variety of clinical manifestations depending on the site involved, which can be grouped in three major syndromes: isolated headache with or without features of the intracranial hypertension syndrome (vomiting, papilledema, and visual symptoms), focal syndrome (focal deficits, seizures, or both), and encephalopathy (multifocal signs, mental status changes, stupor, or coma). Subarachnoid hemorrhage, pulsatile tinnitus, and cranial nerve palsies are a less frequent presentation of CVT. The symptoms and signs can develop acutely in a stroke-like picture, but often had a subacute course or even a chronic presentation.

Risk factors associated with CVT during pregnancy and the puerperium include increasing maternal age, cesarean delivery, and the presence of several comorbid conditions such as hypertension, infections other than pneumonia and influenza, and excessive vomiting in pregnancy [21].

In their study based on data from the Healthcare Cost and Utilization Project, Lanska and Kryscio found no fatalities attributed to CVT [21]. The death rate from CVT is thought to be lower in pregnant than in non-pregnant women of comparable age [35]. When maternal deaths occur, they usually result from secondary intracranial hemorrhage [21].

Standard management of CVT during pregnancy includes anticoagulation. The use of these agents during pregnancy is discussed in the subsequent section of the present chapter. AHA/ASA guidelines for management of CVT recommend for women with a history of CVT, prophylaxis with low molecular weight heparin during future pregnancies and the postpartum period; moreover these patients may be reassured that future pregnancies are not contraindicated.

Treatment of ischemic stroke during pregnancy

Therapeutic decision for an ischemic stroke in pregnancy is conditioned by potentials of fetal toxicity, by concerns about the possibility of adverse outcomes both to the mother and the fetus, and the consideration of the term of pregnancy. On the other side it is influenced by the identification of underlying etiology and the related effectiveness of the treatment.

Prevention strategy: antiplatelet and anticoagulant treatments

Since a suitable comparison between treatment options for this group of patients through randomized controlled trials is lacking, the choice of agents for prophylactic strategies is largely based upon inferences from other studies, primarily on prevention of deep vein thrombosis and the use of anticoagulants in women with high-risk cardiac conditions. However, even in these situations there are no specific randomized controlled trials.

Therefore according to the American Heart Association (AHA) guidelines for pregnant women with ischemic stroke or TIA and high-risk thromboembolic conditions such as coagulopathy and mechanical heart valves, three possible therapeutic options can be used: (1) adjusted-dose unfractionated heparin (UFH) throughout pregnancy; (2) adjusted-dose low molecular weight heparins (LMWHs) throughout pregnancy; (3) either UFH or adjusted-dose LMWHs until week 13, then restarted from the middle of the third trimester until delivery and warfarin at other times [36]. For lower risk conditions, either UFH or LMWH therapy is recommended in the first trimester, followed by low-dose aspirin for the remainder of the pregnancy [36].

Particular women with a history of venous thromboembolism plus a known thrombophilia, particularly antithrombin-III deficiency, antiphospholipid antibody syndrome, prothrombin gene mutation or Factor V Leiden, may be treated with prophylactic-dose LMWH or UFH during pregnancy followed by postpartum anticoagulation with warfarin [36,37]. For women with antiphospholipid antibody syndrome and no history of venous thromboembolism, but recurrent pregnancy loss, prophylactic UFH or LMWH plus aspirin throughout pregnancy is recommended [36,37].

Antiplatelet therapy

The safety of treatment with aspirin during the first trimester of pregnancy is not clear. Prospective studies have not confirmed the teratogenic effect of aspirin in pregnant women reported in retrospective studies. Fetal and maternal bleeding, premature closure of the ductus arteriosus, prolongation of labor, and delay in the onset of labor are reported as possible complications of aspirin use in late pregnancy [30].

Whether aspirin use during the first trimester of pregnancy is associated with an increased risk of congenital malformations was evaluated in a meta-analysis of eight studies (seven observational and one randomized). This analysis found no evidence of an overall increase in rates of major congenital malformations, and suggested that aspirin is safe even when used early in pregnancy [38]. However, this meta-analysis showed that exposure to aspirin may be associated with an increased risk of gastroschisis, but the reliability of this result should be biased because of the limitations of the studies involved related to the use of other drugs, the selection of control subjects, and failure to definitively confirm the diagnosis in all patients. According to data reported in another meta-analysis of 14 randomized studies including a total of 12,416 women there is no evidence of fetal and maternal adverse effects of low-dose aspirin therapy (60 to 150 mg/d) administered during the second and the third trimester of pregnancy in women at risk for preeclampsia [39].

Therefore available evidence suggests that a safe use of aspirin during the first trimester of pregnancy remains controversial but low-dose aspirin (<150 mg/d) can be used safely during the second and third trimester.

Clopidogrel has not been found to cause significant feto-toxicity in animal studies at high doses but there are no adequate and well-controlled studies in pregnant women so far. Only a few cases reported pregnant women who had a successful outcome while taking clopidogrel. Thus there are insufficient data to judge about the safety of clopidogrel in this setting.

Although dipyridamole has not been found to cause significant fetal adverse effects, there are no adequate data regarding safety or effectiveness of dipyridamole in humans during pregnancy.

Anticoagulant therapy

Maternal complications About 2% of the pregnant women treated with UFH develop a major bleeding, which is consistent with the observed rate in non-pregnant women receiving UFH and warfarin therapy [37]. Given the possibility of a persistent anticoagulant effect (for up to 28 hours after the last injection of heparin), the use of heparin therapy prior to labor may complicate the delivery by increasing the risk of bleeding and contraindicates epidural analgesia [37]. Bleeding complications are rarely associated with LMWH use; in particular LWMH therapy is not associated with an increased risk of severe peripartum bleeding [40].

However, there is the possibility in about 3% of patients treated with UFH therapy and some patients receiving LMWH to develop heparin-induced thrombocytopenia (HIT), an acquired IgG-mediated immune condition, which is frequently complicated by extension of the pre-existing thrombotic phenomena or new arterial thrombosis. In pregnant women who develop HIT and require ongoing anticoagulant therapy, use of the heparinoid danaparoid sodium is recommended because it is an effective antithrombotic agent, does not cross the placenta, and has much less

cross-reactivity with UFH, and therefore less potential to produce recurrent HIT than LMWH [37].

Long-term heparin therapy has been associated with the development of osteoporosis and with an increased risk of osteoporotic fracture. In pregnancy the risk of fracture (2.2%) does not seem to be different from that observed in non-pregnant women; nevertheless a small randomized trial of pregnant women treated with UFH reported a higher incidence of osteoporotic fracture (15%), which may be due to the older age of the patients than patients of the other studies [40]. Moreover LMWHs are associated with a lower risk of osteoporosis than heparin [40].

Fetal complications UFH and LMWH do not cross the placenta [37]; thus these agents do not have teratogenic effects, but a bleeding at the utero-placental junction is possible. UFH/LMWH use is safe for the fetus. By contrast, warfarin crosses the placenta and can cause bleeding and malformation in the fetus. This agent is probably safe if administered during the first six weeks of gestation, but confers a risk of embryopathy if given between six weeks and twelve weeks of gestation [37]. Besides, warfarin causes an anticoagulant effect in the fetus, which is a concern, particularly at the time of delivery, when the combination with the trauma of delivery can lead to bleeding in the neonate. Heparin and LMWHs do not reach the maternal milk and can be safely given to nursing mothers. Reported evidence showed that warfarin therapy administered to a nursing mother does not induce an anticoagulant effect in the breast-fed infant.

Acute treatment: thrombolysis

To date experience with the use of thrombolytic agents in pregnancy and the puerperium is limited only to case reports and case series, including different thromboembolic conditions. Due to its large molecular size, recombinant human tissue plasminogen activator (rt-PA) does not cross the placental barrier. Studies on animal models have not shown teratogenic effects but fetal adverse effects remain largely unknown.

rt-PA is listed as a category C drug and pregnancy is considered a relative contraindication for administration, but there are multiple case reports of successful use in pregnant women. The major concerns regarding the use of thrombolytics during pregnancy include their possible effects on the placenta, possibly resulting in premature labor, placental abruption, or fetal demise; other concerns regard the possibility of hemorrhage during parturition or cesarean delivery, if the patient goes into labor within the context sensitive half-time (the time of the drug's effective physiologic and pharmacologic effects in the setting of the disease process being studied) after the administration of the thrombolytic.

Thrombolysis has been carried out in pregnant patients with pulmonary embolism, thrombosis of cardiac valve prosthesis, myocardial infarcts, and deep venous thrombosis. Thrombolysis for acute ischemic stroke in pregnancy has been described in only 13 patients [41–48]. In most cases, patients received thrombolysis during the first trimester, sometimes inadvertently. One of seven patients treated with systemic rt-PA died; the other six women were treated with catheter-based therapy (four intra-arterial rt-PA, one intra-arterial urokinase, and one local urokinase). Five patients did not have complications, while three had cerebral hemorrhage with clinical worsening in one case. Hemorrhagic complications also included intrauterine hematoma in one case and buttock hematoma in another one. Two women had an elective therapeutic abortion and one a spontaneous miscarriage. Moreover, thrombolysis in the postpartum period was also reported, within fifteen hours after a cesarean delivery in one case and after six days from delivery in another one, without complications for the patients [49,50] (Table 20.4).

However, because of the differences in etiologies, as well as in thrombolytic agents used and the method of administration, it is difficult to draw any major efficacy or safety conclusions. The suggestion from these data is that pregnant women generally can be safely treated with thrombolytics for acute ischemic stroke and can have reasonably good outcome in most cases, whereas fetal effects remain unclear. Therefore thrombolytic therapy should not be withheld for potentially disabling stroke during pregnancy, but in each clinical situation, since experience is limited, the ultimate choice of therapies must be based on careful assessment of the maternal and fetal risks and benefits.

Cerebral hemorrhage during pregnancy

The most common underlying disorders of a cerebral hemorrhage during pregnancy include preeclampsia–eclampsia, rupture of an aneurysm, and arteriovenous malformation (AVM). Choriocarcinoma is also a rare cause of intracerebral or subarachnoid hemorrhage to consider during pregnancy (Table 20.5).

The physiological maternal adaptations such as arterial intima and media changes, cardiac output increase, progressive increase in blood volume and pressure reaching a maximum at term, and significant compression of the aorta and inferior vena cava by the gravid uterus, which may cause redistribution of blood flow, may play a role in the rupture of aneurysms or AVM. However, whether pregnancy truly increases risk of bleeding is a topic of ongoing debate. Most cases of subarachnoid hemorrhage (SAH) are due to ruptured cerebral aneurysms, and typically present with thunderclap headache, vomiting, seizures, or reduced level of conscious. Presentation in pregnancy may be confused with eclampsia, and the diagnosis should be confirmed with neuroimaging or cerebrospinal fluid (CSF) analysis. Approximately 85% of cases of SAH can be associated with a saccular aneurysm and about 10% are related to non-aneurysmal perimesencephalic hemorrhage. More rarely SAH can be attributed to dural arteriovenous fistula, septic aneurysm, AVM, vascular lesions around the spinal cord, and arterial dissection.

The natural history of unruptured aneurysms during pregnancy possibly differs significantly from that of the general population. Over 50% of all ruptured arterial aneurysms in women under the age of 40 are pregnancy related [51]. Subarachnoid hemorrhage is estimated to complicate as many as 0.01 to 0.05% of all pregnancies with an estimated incidence of SAH from an intracranial aneurysm during pregnancy ranging from 2 to 7 per 100,000 deliveries [2,30,51].

The rupture risk potentially correlates with the hemodynamic changes that occur as pregnancy advances [2], becoming increasingly likely toward the 3rd trimester, peaking at 30 to 34 weeks [2]. Rupture risk also appears to increase with both maternal age and parity. Aneurysmal rupture is an important contributor to mortality and morbidity. Maternal mortality related to a ruptured aneurysm is high, with a reported rate ranging from 40 to 83%, and is the third most common cause of maternal deaths from non-obstetric causes [2].

The risk of rebleeding with a conservative approach varies from 33 to 50% with a maternal mortality rate of 70% [2].

The management of an intracranial aneurysm in a pregnant patient is controversial. Whether an unruptured aneurysm should be treated or

Table 20.4 Reported cases of the use of thrombolytic treatments in ischemic stroke during pregnancy and the puerperium.

Author, year	Thrombolytic treatment	Maternal age (years)	Gestational age	Maternal complications	Fetal outcome	Associated conditions
Dapprich, 2002 [42]	IV rt-PA	31	12 weeks	minor hemorrhagic inhibition of infarct area	good	protein S deficiency
Elford, 2002 [43]	IA rt-PA	28	1 week	hematoma in basal ganglia	good	ovarian hyperstimulation syndrome
Johnson, 2005 [44]	IA rt-PA	39	37 weeks	none	good	undetermined cause
Leonhardt, 2006 [41]	IV rt-PA	26	23 weeks	basal ganglia infarction	good	elevated IgG and IgM anti-cardiolipin antibodies
Murugappan, 2006 [46]	(a) IV rt-PA	37	12 weeks	intrauterine hematoma	MTP	mitral valve replacement
	(b) IV rt-PA	31	4 weeks	none	MTP	decreased protein S activity
	(c) IV rt-PA	29	6 weeks	death from dissection during angioplasty	died	aortic valve replacement
	(d) IA rt-PA	43	37 weeks	none	good	AT III, protein C and S deficiencies
	(e) IA UK	28	6 weeks	buttock hematoma	good	protein C and S deficiencies, PFO
	(f) local UK	25	first trimester	asymptomatic ICH	SA	bacterial endocarditis
Wiese, 2006 [45]	IV rt-PA	33	13 weeks	none	good	mitral valve replacement
Mendez, 2008 [49]	IA UK	37	15 hours after cesarean delivery	none		undetermined cause
Ronning, 2010 [50]	IA rt-PA	29	6 days after delivery	none		peripartum cardiomyopathy
Ly, 2012 [47]	IA rt-PA	24	11 weeks	recurrent stroke at 13 weeks	good	PFO, pulmonary AVM
Mantoan Ritter, 2014 [48]	IV rt-PA	32	36 weeks	none	good	undetermined cause

IV: intravenous; IA: intra-arterial; rt-PA: recombinant tissue plasminogen activator; UK: urokinase; ICH: intracerebral hemorrhage; MTP: medical termination of pregnancy; SA: spontaneous abortion; PFO: patent foramen ovale; AVM: arteriovenous malformations.

Table 20.5 Etiologies of stroke complicating pregnancy and the puerperium.

Author, year	Sharshar et al., 1995 [6]	Kittner et al., 1996 [10]	Jiagobin and Silver, 2000 [12]	Skidmore et al., 2001 [13]	Jeng et al., 2004 [14]	Liang et al., 2006 [7]
Ischemic stroke						
Total number	15	17	13	21	16	11
Large artery disease, N (%)	0	0	1 (8)	0	0	1 (9)
Cardiac disease, N (%)	0	1 (5.9)	4 (30.7)	5 (23.7)	9 (56)	4 (36)
Coagulopathy, N (%)	1 (6.6)	0	2 (15.3)	2 (9.6)	3 (19)	0
Other causes, N (%)	1 (6.6)[a]	6 (35.3)[c]	0	5 (23.7)[e]	1 (6)[f]	3 (27)[g]
Preeclampsia/eclampsia, N (%)	7 (47)	4 (23.5)	3[d]	3 (14.4)	1 (6)	2 (18)
Other causes pregnancy-related, N (%)	2 (13.2)[b]	0	0	0	0	1 (9)[h]
Undeterminated causes, N (%)	4 (26.6)	6 (35.3)	6 (46)	6 (28.6)	2 (13)	0
Notes	[a] vertebral artery dissection; [b] 1 postpartum cerebral angiopathy, 1 amniotic fluid embolism	[c] 2 primary CNS vasculopathy, 1 cerebral artery dissection, 1 CVT, 1 postherpetic vasculitis, 1 TTP	[d] preeclampsia–eclampsia was considered as a risk factor	[e] 1 cerebral vasculitis, 1 migrainous infarct, 1 mucormycosis, 1 hypotension, 1 TTP	[f] giant cerebral aneurysm	[g] CVT; [h] amniotic fluid embolism
Hemorrhagic stroke						
Total number	16	14	13	11	22	21
Type of cerebral hemorrhage						
Subarachnoid hemorrhage, N	0	0	7	1	3	5

Table 20.5 (cont.)

Author, year	Sharshar et al., 1995 [6]	Kittner et al., 1996 [10]	Jiagobin and Silver, 2000 [12]	Skidmore et al., 2001 [13]	Jeng et al., 2004 [14]	Liang et al., 2006 [7]
Intracerebral hemorrhage, N	16	14	6	10	19	16
Aneurysm, N (%)	2 (12.5)	0	3 (23)	1 (9)	3 (13.6)	2 (9)
Arteriovenous malformation, N (%)	2 (12.5)	3 (21.5)	5 (38.5)	4 (36.4)	5 (22.8)	4 (19)
Preeclampsia/eclampsia, N (%)	7 (44)	2 (14.5)	0	4 (36.4)	7 (31.8)	5 (24)
Other causes, N (%)	2 (12.5)[i]	4 (29)[j]	2 (15.5)[k]	0	2 (9)[l]	5 (24)[m]
Undetermined causes, N (%)	3 (18.5)	5 (35)	3 (23)	2 (18.2)	5 (22.8)	5 (24)
Notes	[i] 2 cavernous angioma	[j] 1 sarcoid vasculitis, 1 primary CNS vasculopathy, 2 cocaine use	[k] 2 DIC		[l] 2 coagulopathy	[m] 1 infective endocarditis, 4 coagulopathy

CVT: cerebral venous thrombosis; TTP: thrombotic thrombocytopenic purpura; DIC: disseminated intravascular coagulation.

observed and whether a ruptured aneurysm should be endovascularly coiled or microsurgically clipped is unclear. The International Subarachnoid Aneurysm Trial (ISAT) and the International Study on Unruptured Intracranial Aneurysms (ISUIA) did not specifically address this condition [55]. Unruptured aneurysms affecting a pregnant patient should only be treated if they are symptomatic or enlarging. Other authors suggest a more aggressive management than in non-pregnant women, since pregnancy increases the risk of aneurysm rupture [52]. Ruptured aneurysms in a pregnant patient should be treated as in the non-pregnant patient. Treatment of a ruptured aneurysm determines a lower fetal and maternal mortality [2]. When an aneurysmal subarachnoid hemorrhage occurs, treatment should consist of securing the aneurysm. Endovascular coiling is now the preferred treatment of choice [53,54] and the intervention should be effectuated as soon as possible to avoid recurrent hemorrhage prior to delivery. Successful treatment of the aneurysm allows the pregnancy to progress to term. However, concerns may be raised about the safety during pregnancy of endovascular coiling and some implications, often to be discussed with patients during counseling, include:

a) *Irradiation:* a first concern is regarding the prolonged radiation exposure implied with coil embolization. Laboratory data showed that the risks associated with even relatively prolonged embolizations are, however, orders of magnitude below that which naturally prevails [55].

b) *General management:* a second concern is related to fetal monitoring (and potential precipitous labor) in an unfamiliar environment such as an angiographic suite, potentially prolonged systemic anticoagulation and a continued risk of postembolization rupture by virtue of potentially incomplete coiling. Moreover, where complications occur (such as coil prolapse back into the parent artery) intravenous heparinization, along with antiplatelet agents, might be deemed necessary for more protracted periods still. Such requirements have potentially significant hemorrhagic implications in cases where labor spontaneously commences during or soon after embolization, or where an emergency cesarean section is indicated for fetal distress. However unlikely such scenarios may be, some pregnant women might feel drawn toward

clipping over coil embolization while preempting them during comprehensive counseling. Moreover, the increased experience and the diversification in procedures available will inevitably reduce the prevalence of inadequate endovascular obliteration.

When urgent obstetric issues, such as active labor, eclampsia, or fetal distress, occur, it is best to proceed to cesarean delivery followed by aneurysm treatment [52]. Most clinicians feel that a vaginal delivery is the safest option; however, cesarean section may be a better choice if the clinical state of the mother is severe (e.g., coma or brain stem damage), the aneurysm is diagnosed at the time of delivery, or the interval between the surgical treatment of the aneurysm and labor is less than 8 days [2,53]. Pregnancy does not seem to confer an increased hemorrhagic risk of previously asymptomatic AVMs. Bateman *et al.* found that the rate of hemorrhage attributable to cerebrovascular malformations was similar in pregnant and non-pregnant women, at 0.50 and 0.33 per 100,00 person-years, respectively [56], but the risk seems to increase on the day of delivery. Whether surgery is effective to reduce maternal or fetal mortality is still controversial and it would seem reasonable to postpone treatment of an asymptomatic AVM that has not bled until after delivery. After an initial hemorrhage the rate of new bleeding has been reported to be 25% [57]. In these patients the decision of interventional treatment is more difficult. Dias and Sekhar found the maternal mortality from hemorrhage of an AVM to be 28%, compared with only 10% in the general population, and fetal mortality 14% [2]. However, the current treatment for AVMs is primarily endovascular intervention, which has a relatively low risk of mortality and morbidity. A patient with a treated AVM in which the feeding vessels have all been occluded can undergo a normal labor and delivery. If definitive treatment is accomplished before delivery, there are no data about an advantage to cesarean section over vaginal delivery in maternal and fetal outcome, and obstetrical principles should determine the type of delivery. Cesarean section to avoid the risk of hypertension related to Valsalva maneuver in vaginal delivery has been suggested, but the risk of anesthesia has also to be considered. Epidural anesthesia would be recommended in a vaginal delivery to limit pushing in the second stage of labor and to shorten delivery. Although epidural anesthesia is generally regarded as safe, a few cases of intracranial or subarachnoid hemorrhage occurring following dural puncture have been described. The hypothesis is that a prolonged low CSF pressure can lead to an increase in trans-mural pressure across an arterial wall facilitating rupture of an aneurysm or AVM. For this reason, insertion of an epidural catheter in this context should be carried out by an experienced operator to reduce the risk of a dural tap.

Guidelines for medical management of ICH or SAH are lacking for pregnant patients. Caution during pregnancy must be used with agents utilized on a routine basis in non-pregnant patients, such as mannitol for elevated intracranial pressure, antiepi-leptics for prevention or management of seizures, and nimodipine for vasospasm. Mannitol crosses the placenta and accumulates in the fetus and may result in fetal hypoxia and acid–base shifts; antiepi-leptic drugs are associated with varying degrees of teratogenic risk, and nimodipine has been linked with teratogenicity in some animal experiments, but there is slender data in humans, and the risk is linked to the potential for iatrogenic hypotension and consequent fetal ischemia [58]. However, ultimately, the use of these drugs in critically ill pregnant patients may outweigh the potential risks. Careful monitoring of hemodynamic parameters in both the mother and fetus is a priority.

Assisted reproductive technology and arterial cerebral thromboembolic complications

Assisted reproductive technology (ART) includes all treatments or procedures that are related to the in-vitro handling of human oocytes and sperm or embryos for the purpose of establishing a pregnancy.

It has been assisted by an ever-increasing ART diffusion in the last decade. In 2002 over 110,000 ART procedures were performed in the United States, resulting in 45,751 infants or 1% of all US infants born that year [59].

The most common procedure performed to assist reproduction includes in-vitro fertilization–embryo transfer (IVF-ET). The process of IVF comprises the administration of exogenous hormones to achieve cycle control, stimulate the ovaries, and support implantation.

Thromboembolic complications, both arterial and venous, have usually been associated with the presence of ovarian hyperstimulation syndrome (OHSS), a well-recognized complication of ART [60]. Ovarian hyperstimulation syndrome occurs most often when the ovaries are stimulated with exogenous gonado-trophins and clomiphene for the purpose of acquiring oocytes for fertilization; notwithstanding, a sponta-neous form of OHSS has been described but represents a rare event. Ovarian hyperstimulation syndrome usually develops after the administration of human chorionic gonadotrophin (hCG) during stimulation and oocyte retrieval to enhance luteal function, and it lasts for 10 to 14 days [60]. The frequency of this syndrome ranges from 1 or 2% to 30% [60]. In the majority of cases the form is mild, self-limiting and needs no or few therapeutic measures. In OHSS, there is an enlarge-ment of the ovaries, associated with leaky capillaries and a "third-spacing" of fluid, resulting in symptoms from pleural, pericardial, or abdominal fluid accumulation. As a consequence of this extravasation of fluid, leukocy-tosis, hemoconcentration, and electrolyte imbalance occur. This syndrome is also associated with a state of hypercoagulability. In about 1% of cases the syndrome is severe and can result in thromboembolism, adult respiratory distress syndrome, pleural effusions, signifi-cant ascites, renal insufficiency, liver dysfunction, and even death.

To date, there are no guidelines regarding the need for thromboprophylaxis in patients who develop OHSS; generally, thromboprophylaxis is initiated in view of the severity and the hospitalization of the patient [60]. Chan and Dixon analyzed previously published reports on the association between ART or OHSS, and thromboembolic, both arterial and venous, complications were reviewed [61]. Seventy-one episodes of thromboembolic complications in 70 women were gathered. In all but one case, throm-bosis occurred after hCG was administered to induce ovulation; in all cases, clomiphene, exogenous follicle-stimulating hormone (FSH), gonadotrophin releasing hormone (GnRH), or GnRH agonists were administered to cause follicular formation. Pregnancy was attained in 69% (n = 49) of these cases. Twenty-six out of 71 events concerned arterial throm-bosis and about 60% involved cerebrovascular events. There were two fatalities in patients with arterial ischemic stroke. On average, the timing for arterial thrombosis was 10.5 days after embryo transfer in IVF pregnancies and 8.2 days after hGC administration for ovulation induction cycles, respectively, while for venous complications it was 40.0 days and 26.6, respectively. Another condition that seems to be involved in thrombotic complications in women undergoing ovarian stimulation is a pre-existing polycystic ovary condition, but this may be expected since patients with this condition often have fertility problems.

The mechanism of thrombosis in ART is not completely understood. Ovarian stimulation is likely a trigger factor for arterial and venous thrombotic phenomena since evidence from studies performed on women undergoing controlled ovarian stimulation showed changes in the hemostatic system with an increase in coagulation factors and a decrease in many markers promoting fibrinolysis; overall these changes suggest that a prothrombotic state could be present over the course of ovarian stimulation. This activation in both coagulation and fibrinolytic systems appears to be exaggerated with the development of OHSS, especially if arterial thrombotic complications arise [62].

The therapeutic approach has been general supportive measures, adequate fluid compensation, cortisone, and anticoagulants or aspirin. The appropriate length of therapy, based on the future risk of recurrence in patients who develop these complications, is currently unknown. Data could be extrapolated from studies in pregnant women, and patient counseling accordingly. Moreover, the recognition of OHSS may be the key in preventing the possible devastating development of thromboses and timely intervention critical in maternal and fetal prognosis. In line with this, a case of successful use of rt-PA in a cerebral arterial stroke resulting from severe OHSS in a young woman undergoing an ART procedure was reported [43]. Therapeutic abortion was also a frequent measure utilized in the overall management of these patients.

Although the true incidence of thrombotic complications resulting from ART cannot be determined, the increasing reporting of these cases in the literature suggests that these complications of ART are not rare. Moreover, it should be noted that with the increasing diffusion of ART in clinical practice, the frequency of these complications will likely also increase and much effort is needed to reduce the potential devastating consequence of thromboembolic complications related to this elective procedure.

References

1. George M G, Tong X, Kuklina E V, Labarthe D R. Trends in stroke hospitalizations and associated risk factors among children and young adults, 1995–2008. *Ann Neurol*. 2011; **70**:713–21.

2. Dias M, Sekhar L. Intracranial hemorrhage from aneurysms and arteriovenous malformations during pregnancy and the puerperium. *Neurosurgery*. 1990; **27**:855–65.

3. James A, Bushnell C D, Jaminson M G, Myers E R. Incidence and risk factors for stroke in pregnancy and puerperium. *Obstet Gynecol*. 2005; **106**:509–16.

4. Say L, Souza J P, Pattinson R C; WHO working group on Maternal Mortality and Morbidity classifications. Maternal near miss: Towards a standard tool for monitoring quality of maternal health care. *Best Pract Res Clin Obstet Gynaecol*. 2009; **23**:287–96.

5. Kuklina E V, Tong X, Bansil P, George M G, Callaghan W M. Trends in pregnancy hospitalizations that included a stroke in the United States from 1994 to 2007: Reasons for concern? *Stroke*. 2011; **42**:2564–70.

6. Sharshar T, Lamy C, Mas J L, The Stroke in Pregnancy Group. Incidence and causes of stroke associated with pregnancy and puerperium: a study in public hospitals of Ile de France. *Stroke*. 1995; **26**:930–6.

7. Liang C C, Chang S D, Lai S L, *et al*. Stroke complicating pregnancy and the puerperium. *Eur J Neurol*. 2006; **13**:1256–60.

8. Wiebers D O, Whisnant J P. The incidence of stroke among pregnant women in Rochester, Minn, 1955 through 1979. *JAMA*. 1985; **254**:3055–7.

9. Awada A, al Rajeh S, Duarte R, Russell N. Stroke and pregnancy. *Int J Gynaecol Obstet*. 1995; **48**:157–61.

10. Kittner S J, Stern B J, Feeser B R, *et al*. Pregnancy and the risk of stroke. *N Engl J Med*. 1996; **335**:768–74.

11. Witlin A G, Friedman S A, Egerman R S, Frangieh A Y, Sibai B M. Cerebrovascular disorders complicating pregnancy: beyond eclampsia. *Am J Obstet Gynecol*. 1997; **176**:1139–45.

12. Jaigobin C, Silver F L. Stroke and pregnancy. *Stroke*. 2000; **31**:2948–51.

13. Skidmore F M, Williams L S, Fradkin K D, Alonso R J, Biller J. Presentation, etiology and outcome of stroke in pregnancy and puerperium. *J Stroke Cerebrovasc Dis*. 2001; **10**:1–10.

14. Jeng J S, Tang S C, Yip P K. Incidence and etiologies of stroke during pregnancy and puerperium as evidenced in Taiwanese women. *Cerebrovasc Dis*. 2004; **18**:290–5.

15. Ros H S, Lichtestein P, Bellocco R, Petersson R, Cnattingius S. Increased risks of circulatory diseases in late pregnancy and puerperium. *Epidemiology*. 2001; **12**:456–60.

16. Hunter S, Robson S C. Adaptation of the maternal heart in pregnancy. *Brit Heart J*. 1992; **68**:540–3.

17. Bremme K A. Haemostatic changes in pregnancy. *Best Pract Res Clin Haematol*. 2003; **16**:153–68.

18. ACOG Committee on Obstetric Practice. ACOG Committee Opinion Number 299, September 2004.

Guidelines for diagnostic imaging during pregnancy. *Obstet Gynecol.* 2004; **104**:647–51.

19. Kanal E, Borgstede J P, Barkovich A J, *et al.* American College of Radiology. American College of Radiology White Paper on MR Safety. *Am J Roentgenol.* 2002; **178**:1335–47.

20. Stoddard M F, Longaker R A, Vuocolo L M, Dawkins P R. Trans-esophageal echocardiography in the pregnant patient. *Am Heart J.* 1992; **124**:785–7.

21. Lanska D J, Kryscio R J. Risk factors for peripartum and postpartum stroke and intracranial venous thrombosis. *Stroke.* 2000; **31**:1274–82.

22. Ros H S, Lichtenstein P, Bellocco R, Petersson G, Cnattingius S. Pulmonary embolism and stroke in relation to pregnancy: How can high-risk women be identified? *Am J Obstet Gynecol.* 2002; **186**:198–203.

23. Clark S L, Hankins G D, Dudley D A, Dildy G A, Porter T F. Amniotic fluid embolism: Analysis of the national registry. *Am J Obstet Gynecol.* 1995; **172**:1158–69.

24. Sibai B, Dekker G, Kupferminc M. Pre-eclampsia. *Lancet.* 2005; **365**:785–99.

25. Moodley J, Kalane G. A review of the management of eclampsia: practical issues. *Hypertens Pregnancy.* 2006; **25**:47–62.

26. Roberts J M, Cooper D W. Pathogenesis and genetics of pre-eclampsia. *Lancet.* 2001; **357**:53–6.

27. Elkayam U, Akhter M W, Singh H, *et al.* Pregnancy-associated cardiomyopathy: Clinical characteristics and a comparison between early and late presentation. *Circulation.* 2005; **111**:2050–5.

28. Abboud J, Murad Y, Chen-Scarabelli C, Saravolatz L, Scarabelli T. Peripartum cardiomyopathy: a comprehensive review. *Int J Cardiol.* 2007; **118**:295–303.

29. Pearson G D, Veille J C, Rahimtoola S, *et al.* Peripartum cardiomyopathy: National Heart, Lung, and Blood Institute and Office of Rare Diseases (National Institutes of Health) workshop recommendations and review. *JAMA.* 2000; **283**:1183–8.

30. Mas J L, Lamy C. Stroke in pregnancy and the puerperium. *J Neurol.* 1998; **245**:305–13.

31. Fugate J E, Ameriso S F, Ortiz G, *et al.* Variable presentations of postpartum angiopathy. *Stroke.* 2012; **43**:670–6.

32. Huang C Y, Chen C A, Hsieh C Y, Cheng W F. Intracerebral hemorrhage as initial presentation of gestational choriocarcinoma: A case report and literature review. *Int J Gynecol Cancer.* 2007; **17**:1166–71.

33. Lanska D J, Kryscio R J. Peripartum stroke and intracranial venous thrombosis in the National Hospital Discharge Survey. *Obstet Gynecol.* 1997; **89**:413–18.

34. Lanska D J, Kryscio R J. Stroke and intracranial venous thrombosis during pregnancy and puerperium. *Neurology.* 1998; **51**:1622–8.

35. Cantu C, Barinagarrementaria F. Cerebral venous thrombosis associated with pregnancy and the puerperium: a review of 67 cases. *Stroke.* 1993; **24**: 1880–4.

36. Furie K L, Kasner S E, Adams R J, *et al.* American Heart Association Stroke Council, Council on Cardiovascular Nursing, Council on Clinical Cardiology, and Interdisciplinary Council on Quality of Care and Outcomes Research. Guidelines for the prevention of stroke in patients with stroke or transient ischemic attack: a guideline for Healthcare Professionals from the American Heart Association/ American Stroke Association. *Stroke.* 2011; **42**:227–76.

37. Bates S, Greer I, Pabinger I, Sofaer S, Hirsch J. Venous thromboembolism, thrombophilia, antithrombotic therapy, and pregnancy. *Chest.* 2008; **133**:844S–886S.

38. Kozer E, Nikfar S, Costei A, *et al.* Aspirin consumption during the first trimester of pregnancy and congenital anomalies: a meta-analysis. *Am J Obstet Gynecol.* 2002; **187**:1623–30.

39. Coomarasamy A, Honest H, Papaioannou S, Gee H, Khan K S. Aspirin for prevention of preeclampsia in women with historical risk factors: a systematic review. *Obstet Gynecol.* 2003; **101**:1319–32.

40. Greer I A, Nelson-Piercy C. Low-molecular-weight heparins for thromboprophylaxis and treatment of venous thromboembolism in pregnancy: a systematic review of safety and efficacy. *Blood.* 2005; **106**:401–7.

41. Leonhardt G, Gaul C, Nietsch H H, Buerke M, Schleussner E. Thrombolytic therapy in pregnancy. *J Thromb Thrombolysis.* 2006; **21**:271–6.

42. Dapprich M, Boessenecker W. Fibrinolysis with alteplase in a pregnant woman with stroke. *Cerebrovasc Dis.* 2002; **13**:290.

43. Elford K, Leader A, Wee R, Stys P K. Stroke in ovarian hyperstimulation syndrome in early pregnancy treated with intra-arterial rt-PA. *Neurology.* 2002; **59**:1270–2.

44. Johnson D M, Kramer D C, Cohen E, *et al.* Thrombolytic therapy for acute stroke in late pregnancy with intra-arterial recombinant tissue plasminogen activator. *Stroke.* 2005; **36**:e53–e55.

45. Wiese K M, Talkad A, Mathews M, Wang D. Intravenous recombinant tissue plasminogen activator in a pregnant woman with cardioembolic stroke. *Stroke.* 2006; **37**:2168–9.

46. Murugappan A, Coplin W M, Al-Sadat A N, *et al.* Thrombolytic therapy of acute ischemic stroke during pregnancy. *Neurology.* 2006; **66**:768–70.

47. Li Y, Margraf J, Kluck B, Jenny D, Castaldo J. Thrombolytic therapy for ischemic stroke secondary to

paradoxical embolism in pregnancy: A case report and literature review. *Neurologist.* 2012; **18**:44–8.

48. Mantoan Ritter L, Schüler A, Gangopadhyay R, *et al.* Successful thrombolysis of stroke with intravenous alteplase in the third trimester of pregnancy. *J Neurol.* 2014; **261**:632–4.

49. Méndez J C, Masjuán J, García N, de Leciñana M. Successful intra-arterial thrombolysis for acute ischemic stroke in the immediate postpartum period: Case report. *Cardiovasc Intervent Radiol.* 2008; **31**:193–5.

50. Rønning O M, Dahl A, Bakke S J, Hussain A I, Deilkås E. Stroke in the puerperium treated with intra-arterial rt-PA. *J Neurol Neurosurg Psychiatry.* 2010; **81**:585–6.

51. Barrett J M, Van Hooydonk J E, Boehm F H. Pregnancy-related rupture of arterial aneurysms. *Obstet Gynecol Surv.* 1982; **37**:557–66.

52. Marshman L A, Aspoas A R, Rai M S, Chawda S J. The implications of ISAT and ISUIA for the management of cerebral aneurysms during pregnancy. *Neurosurg Rev.* 2007; **30**:177–80.

53. Meyers P M, Halbach V V, Malek A M, *et al.* Endovascular treatment of cerebral artery aneurysms during pregnancy: Report of three cases. *Am J Neuroradiol.* 2000; **21**:1306–11.

54. Piotin M, Filho C B A, Kothimbakam R, Moret J. Endovascular treatment of acutely ruptured intracranial aneurysm in pregnancy. *Am J Obstet Gynecol.* 2001; **185**:1261–2.

55. Marshman L A G, Aspoas A R, Rai M S. Endovascular treatment of ruptured intracranial aneurysms during pregnancy: Letter. *Arch Gynecol Obstet.* 2005; **272**:93.

56. Bateman B, Schumacher H, Bushnell C D, *et al.* Intracerebral hemorrhage in pregnancy. Frequency, risk factors, and outcome. *Neurology.* 2006; **67**:424–9.

57. Sawin P. Spontaneous subarachnoid hemorrhage in pregnancy and the puerperium. In Loftus C, ed. *Neurological Aspects of Pregnancy.* Park Ridge, IL: American Association of Neurological Surgeons; 1996: 85–99.

58. Roman H, Descargues G, Lopes M, *et al.* Subarachnoid hemorrhage due to cerebral aneurysmal rupture during pregnancy. *Acta Obstet Gynecol Scand.* 2004; **83**:330–4.

59. Wright V C, Schieve L A, Reynolds M A, Jeng G. Assisted reproductive technology surveillance in United States, 2002. *MMWR.* 2005; **54**:1–24.

60. Whelan J G, Vlahos N F. The ovarian hyperstimulation syndrome. *Fertil Steril.* 2000; **73**:893–6.

61. Chan W S, Dixon M E. The "ART" of thromboembolism: a review of assisted reproductive technology and thromboembolic complications. *Thromb Res.* 2008; **121**:713–26.

62. Kodama H, Fukuda J, Karube H, *et al.* Status of the coagulation and fibrinolytic systems in ovarian hyperstimulation syndrome. *Fertil Steril.* 1996; **66**:417–24.

Chapter 21

Cardioversion-related stroke

Morten L. Hansen and Steen Husted

Introduction

Cardioversion of atrial fibrillation to sinus rhythm carries a risk of procedure-related thromboembolic events. Treatment strategies with prolonged anticoagulation or shorter term anticoagulation with screening transesophageal echocardiography (TEE) can reduce the thromboembolic risk. In this chapter we discuss thromboembolism in relation to cardioversion; the aim of this work is to provide the necessary background information about how to minimize this risk by an optimal use of antithrombotic treatment strategies.

Left atrial thrombus

Embolism from preformed atrial thrombus

Embolization after cardioversion with the return of synchronous atrial contraction was initially thought to be caused by the dislodgement of left atrial thrombi preformed due to atrial fibrillation and present at the time of cardioversion [1]. However, normalization of mechanical atrial contraction often takes as long as a month after sinus rhythm has been restored and thrombi may also be dislodged later when atrial contraction in, for example, the left atrial appendix is stronger [2–6].

Embolism from de novo formed atrial thrombus

Cardioversion results in the development of temporal depression of left atrial and left appendage function, "atrial stunning," a condition that promotes the formation of new thrombi that later can become dislodged when atrial contraction is restored. After cardioversion, echocardiographic evidence of "smoke" or spontaneous echo contrast often develops or worsens in the atrium, which is associated with the formation of atrial thrombi [7]. Additionally, left atrial appendage emptying velocities decrease, in spite of the development of coordinated electrical activity after cardioversion. A number of TEE studies favor the assumption that thrombi develop in the atria after, and possibly as a consequence of, cardioversion [8–10].

Rationale for anticoagulation therapy in cardioversion

All patients with atrial fibrillation have an increased risk of embolization compared to those without. Studies have suggested that cardioversion of patients with atrial fibrillation represents a risk procedure with thromboembolic complications ranging from 1 to 7% during the first month after the procedure [11–15]. Most embolic events occur within ten days of cardioversion, and occur more often in patients who are not effectively anticoagulated [16,17]. There have been no randomized studies, but there are several reports of complications from studies in patients either not receiving anticoagulation or who have not been adequately anticoagulated [17]. In 1969, Bjerkelund and Orning demonstrated that anticoagulation could reduce the rate of embolic events [11]. Two hundred and twenty-eight patients received warfarin, with a subsequent embolic rate of 1.1%, while in 209 patients who received no anticoagulants 6.8% had thromboembolic complications.

Treatment before cardioversion

The efficacy of at least three weeks of therapeutic anticoagulation prior to cardioversion is thought to

Treatment-Related Stroke, ed. Alexander Tsiskaridze, Arne Lindgren and Adnan Qureshi. Published by Cambridge University Press. © Cambridge University Press 2016.

be sufficient for a possible existing left atrial thrombus to resolve. It is known that three weeks of anticoagulation is not sufficiently long for all thrombi to resolve, but anticoagulation for this period of time results in very few complications [18,19].

Treatment after cardioversion

Immediate postconversion anticoagulation The reason for at least one month of oral anticoagulant therapy after cardioversion comes from the observations that left atrial function may be "stunned" for up to four weeks and have a greater propensity for thrombus formation after cardioversion [6]. Furthermore, many patients have recurrent episodes of atrial fibrillation [20].

Long-term anticoagulation The rationale and indications for long-term anticoagulation after the period of postcardioversion anticoagulation are similar to those for the general population of patients with atrial fibrillation and are based on risk factors for thromboembolism [21].

Patients with atrial fibrillation of more than 48 hours duration

The latest 2010 guidelines, and the 2012 focused update from the European Society of Cardiology (ESC), recommend that patients who have been in atrial fibrillation for more than 48 hours, receive a month of therapeutic warfarin prior to cardioversion with a target international normalized ratio (INR) of 2.0 to 3.0 [21,22]. (For non-vitamin K antagonist oral anticoagulants please see below.) Patients undergoing cardioversion for atrial fibrillation of more than 48 hours duration represent a high-risk group and there are recommendations of an INR of 2.0 or greater to be documented for at least three consecutive weeks before cardioversion. The guidelines recommend that warfarin therapy should be continued for at least four weeks after cardioversion (target INR of 2.0 to 3.0) [23]. This recommendation only deals with protection from embolic events related to the pericardioversion period. The long-term recommendations for patients with recurrent AF who are at high risk for thromboembolism are similar to those in patients with atrial fibrillation. The guidelines also suggest an alternative approach using shorter term precardioversion anticoagulation with screening TEE. Although the TEE-guided approach may shorten the precardioversion

duration of anticoagulation, this does not change the requisite four weeks of anticoagulation after cardioversion [22].

Non-vitamin K antagonist oral anticoagulants (NOACs)

Dabigatran etexilate

The RE-LY trial compared etexilate 110 or 150 mg twice daily with warfarin in over 18,000 patients with non-valvular atrial fibrillation and found that the lower dose was similar to and the higher dose was superior to warfarin for the prevention of thromboembolism and stroke [24,25]. In a post hoc analysis of 1,983 cardioversions (85% electric) in 1,270 RE-LY participants, there was no significant difference in the rate of thromboembolism and stroke within 30 days in those who received dabigatran etexilate 110 or 150 mg twice daily or warfarin before cardioversion using the conventional or expedited TEE approach (0.8%, 0.3%, and 0.6%, respectively) [26,27]. Therefore the ESC guidelines state that dabigatran etexilate is a reasonable alternative for patients who require anticoagulation prior to and after cardioversion [22,28].

Apixaban

In the large ARISTOTLE trial [29], a total of 743 cardioversions were performed in 540 patients: 265 first cardioversions in patients assigned to apixaban and 275 in those assigned to warfarin [30]. There were no strokes or thrombembolisms in subjects undergoing cardioversion, and only one major bleeding event in each group. During the 30-day follow-up period, two patients in each group died. Consequently, the conclusion from the investigators was that stroke and bleeding risks for patients undergoing cardioversion with apixaban were low and similar to those observed with warfarin.

Rivaroxaban

In the ROCKET [31] trial patients were excluded if electrical cardioversion was planned. Therefore the X-VeRT [32] trial was conducted, the first prospective randomized trial of a NOAC in patients with AF undergoing elective cardioversion. A total of 1,504 patients with AF more than 48 hours or of unknown duration received rivaroxaban (20 mg once daily, 15 mg if creatinine clearance was between 30 and 49 mL/minute) or warfarin. In the rivaroxaban group, among 978 patients there were two strokes (0.51%) compared with two strokes among 492 warfarin-treated patients (1.02%) (relative risk [RR] 0.50, 95% confidence interval [CI] 0.15–1.73). There were no significant differences in terms of major bleeding events between the two treatment groups.

The aforementioned studies show that NOACs represent effective and safe alternatives to vitamin K antagonist (VKA) therapy in patients scheduled for cardioversion. Currently, two further randomized controlled studies are being performed comparing apixaban and edoxaban, respectively, with vitamin K antagonist therapy in patients undergoing cardioversion.

Role of TEE

The potential role of a TEE for evaluating stroke risk associated with cardioversion is based on exclusion of thrombus in the left atrium including the left atrial appendage, thereby providing an alternative to anticoagulation prior to cardioversion in patients with atrial fibrillation of longer than 48 hours duration. A screening TEE has been suggested as a useful tool for patients for whom there is a concern about risks with three weeks' delay of cardioversion. The recommendation of the TEE-based approach is based on the ACUTE trial comparing a TEE-guided strategy with a conventional strategy (including therapeutic [INR 2.0–3.0] anticoagulation for at least three weeks) prior to electrical cardioversion in 1,222 patients with atrial fibrillation of more than two days duration [22,33]. Within the eight weeks after study enrollment, there was no significant difference between the TEE and conventional treatment groups in the incidence of ischemic stroke, all embolic events, all-cause mortality, or cardiovascular death, but the point estimates for the risk ratio for all-cause mortality, ischemic stroke, and all embolic events were all worse with the TEE-guided approach. There were significantly fewer hemorrhagic events with the TEE strategy, but no significant difference in the incidence of major bleeding; in addition, the TEE strategy led to a shorter mean time to cardioversion (3 vs. 31 days) and a greater incidence of successful restoration of sinus rhythm (71% vs. 65% percent). Although the results of the ACUTE study raise concerns about possible worse outcomes in patients treated with this strategy, the TEE strategy may be considered as a reasonable alternative in some patients, such as those with a strong preference for early cardioversion, those with AF of less than three weeks' duration, and those at increased risk of hemorrhagic complications (because the duration of anticoagulation may be shortened).

Atrial fibrillation of less than 48 hours duration

The risk of embolization after cardioversion among patients with atrial fibrillation of less than 48 hours duration and no anticoagulant protection appears to be lower than that among patients with atrial fibrillation of longer extent than 48 hours. However, long-term anticoagulant therapy *after* cardioversion follows the same principles as for patients pretreated with anticoagulants.

A low risk of embolization was found in a study of 357 consecutive patients with atrial fibrillation of less than 48 hours duration, in whom conversion to sinus rhythm during the hospitalization occurred (spontaneously, or after pharmacological or electrical cardioversion) in 95% [34]. A clinical thromboembolic event occurred in three (0.8%), each of whom recovered spontaneously, and this rate is similar to what would have been expected with warfarin therapy prior to cardioversion. Similar findings have been reported in another study [17]. Although the risk of an embolic event appears to be low in these patients, TEE evidence of left atrial thrombus has been between 12 and 14% with AF duration of less than 72 hours [22,35,36]. These values, which did not differ in those with AF duration of ≤2 days and 2 to 3 days, are similar to the 12 to 13% incidence noted above in TEE studies of patients with new onset atrial fibrillation of more than two days' duration [37,38]. Thus despite the apparent low risk of embolization, the rationale for the use of pericardioversion heparin comes from these observations, and many experts administer either low molecular weight heparin (LMWH) or unfractionated heparin prior to cardioversion in patients with atrial fibrillation of short duration. Oral anticoagulant treatment is started simultaneously in these patients and continued in the postcardioversion period. ESC guidelines recommend at least four weeks of anticoagulation treatment after cardioversion irrespective of the CHADS$_2$ (or CHA$_2$DS$_2$-VASc) score, therapeutic heparin throughout the pericardioversion period, and extension of its use until therapeutic anticoagulation is achieved [22,39,40].

Immediate/emergency cardioversion

In patients with atrial fibrillation with hemodynamic instability immediate cardioversion may be required to prevent adverse clinical and hemodynamic consequences. Clinical indications for emergent cardioversion of atrial fibrillation are rare, but in the setting of hemodynamic instability due to rapid atrial fibrillation that is refractory to pharmacologic treatment, the need for restoration of sinus rhythm may take precedence over the need for protection from thromboembolism. Low molecular weight heparin or unfractionated heparin should be administered before cardioversion, oral anticoagulant therapy should be started at the same time, and heparin should be continued until the INR is at the therapeutic level (2.0–3.0). Duration of oral anticoagulant therapy after the standard four-week period will depend on the presence of risk factors for stroke [22].

Summary and recommendations

Conversion of atrial fibrillation to sinus rhythm is associated with a small, but important, incidence of clinical thromboembolism, particularly stroke, that may be due to either pre-existing or de novo thrombus formation. The risk of thromboembolism after cardioversion can be diminished by the use of at least three weeks of therapeutic anticoagulation prior to and extending for four weeks after cardioversion. A TEE strategy is a reasonable alternative to a conventional approach in some patients, but after cardioversion at least four weeks of anticoagulation is mandatory. In patients with estimated atrial fibrillation of duration less than 48 hours the risk is considered low and the current practice is to, after careful evaluation including TEE, cardiovert patients without weeks of prior anticoagulation – but before conversion, treatment with LMWH should be initiated and then continued until treatment with VKA is in the therapeutic range after the cardioversion. One alternative in this situation may be to start rivaroxaban before cardioversion and continue this treatment also after the cardioversion.

References

1. Watson T, Shantsila E, Lip G Y. Mechanisms of thrombogenesis in atrial fibrillation: Virchow's triad revisited. *Lancet.* 2009; **373**(9658):155–66.

2. Manning W J, *et al.* Impaired left atrial mechanical function after cardioversion: Relation to the duration of atrial fibrillation. *J Am Coll Cardiol.* 1994; **23**(7): 1535–40.

3. O'Neill P G, *et al.* Return of atrial mechanical function following electrical conversion of atrial dysrhythmias. *Am Heart J.* 1990; **120**(2):353–9.

4. Shapiro E P, *et al.* Transient atrial dysfunction after conversion of chronic atrial fibrillation to sinus rhythm. *Am J Cardiol.* 1988; **62**(17):1202–7.

5. Ikram H, Nixon PG, Arcan T. Left atrial function after electrical conversion to sinus rhythm. *Br Heart J.* 1968; **30**(1):80–3.

6. Manning W J, *et al.* Pulsed Doppler evaluation of atrial mechanical function after electrical cardioversion of atrial fibrillation. *J Am Coll Cardiol.* 1989; **13**(3): 617–23.

7. Grimm R A, *et al.* Impact of electrical cardioversion for atrial fibrillation on left atrial appendage function and spontaneous echo contrast: Characterization by simultaneous transesophageal echocardiography. *J Am Coll Cardiol.* 1993; **22**(5): 1359–66.

8. Black I W, *et al.* Exclusion of atrial thrombus by transesophageal echocardiography does not preclude embolism after cardioversion of atrial fibrillation. A multicenter study. *Circulation.* 1994; **89**(6):2509–13.

9. Black I W, *et al.* Evaluation of transesophageal echocardiography before cardioversion of atrial fibrillation and flutter in nonanticoagulated patients. *Am Heart J.* 1993; **126**(2):375–81.

10. Missault L, *et al.* Embolic stroke after unanticoagulated cardioversion despite prior exclusion of atrial thrombi by transoesophageal echocardiography. *Eur Heart J.* 1994; **15**(9):1279–80.

11. Bjerkelund C J, Orning O M. The efficacy of anticoagulant therapy in preventing embolism related to D.C. electrical conversion of atrial fibrillation. *Am J Cardiol.* 1969; **23**(2):208–16.

12. Lown B. Electrical reversion of cardiac arrhythmias. *Br Heart J.* 1967; **29**(4):469–89.

13. Oram S, Davies J P. Further experience of electrical conversion of atrial fibrillation to sinus rhythm: Analysis of 100 patients. *Lancet.* 1964; **1**(7346): 1294–8.

14. Resnekov L, McDonald L. Complications in 220 patients with cardiac dysrhythmias treated by phased direct current shock, and indications for electroconversion. *Br Heart J.* 1967; **29**(6):926–36.

15. McCarthy C, Varghese P J, Barritt D W. Prognosis of atrial arrhythmias treated by electrical counter shock therapy. A three-year follow-up. *Br Heart J.* 1969; **31**(4):496–500.

16. Berger M, Schweitzer P. Timing of thromboembolic events after electrical cardioversion of atrial fibrillation or flutter: A retrospective analysis. *Am J Cardiol.* 1998; **82**(12):1545–7.

17. Gallagher M M, *et al.* Embolic complications of direct current cardioversion of atrial arrhythmias: Association with low intensity of anticoagulation at the time of cardioversion. *J Am Coll Cardiol.* 2002; **40**(5): 926–33.

18. Arnold A Z, *et al.* Role of prophylactic anticoagulation for direct current cardioversion in patients with atrial fibrillation or atrial flutter. *J Am Coll Cardiol.* 1992; **19**(4):851–5.

19. Collins L J, *et al.* Cardioversion of nonrheumatic atrial fibrillation. Reduced thromboembolic complications with 4 weeks of precardioversion anticoagulation are related to atrial thrombus resolution. *Circulation.* 1995; **92**(2):160–3.

20. Israel C W, *et al.* Long-term risk of recurrent atrial fibrillation as documented by an implantable monitoring device: implications for optimal patient care. *J Am Coll Cardiol.* 2004; **43**(1):47–52.

21. Camm A J, *et al.* focused update of the ESC Guidelines for the management of atrial fibrillation: an update of the 2010 ESC Guidelines for the management of atrial fibrillation. Developed with the special contribution of the European Heart Rhythm Association. *Eur Heart J.* 2012; **33**(21):2719–47.

22. Camm A J, *et al.* Guidelines for the management of atrial fibrillation: The Task Force for the Management of Atrial Fibrillation of the European Society of Cardiology (ESC). *Eur Heart J.* 2010; **31**(19):2369–429.

23. www.uptodate.com/contents/warfarin-drug-information?source=see_link. [Accessed September 27, 2015].

24. Connolly S J, *et al.* Dabigatran versus warfarin in patients with atrial fibrillation. *N Engl J Med.* 2009; **361**(12):1139–51.

25. www.uptodate.com/contents/warfarin-drug-information?source=see_link. [Accessed September 27, 2015].

26. Nagarakanti R, *et al.* Dabigatran versus warfarin in patients with atrial fibrillation: an analysis of patients undergoing cardioversion. *Circulation.* 2011; **123**(2): 131–6.

27. www.uptodate.com/contents/warfarin-drug-information?source=see_link. [Accessed on September 27, 2015].

28. www.uptodate.com/contents/warfarin-drug-information?source=see_link. [Accessed September 27, 2015].

29. Granger C B, *et al.* Apixaban versus warfarin in patients with atrial fibrillation. *N Engl J Med.* 2011; **365**:981–92.

30. Flaker G, *et al.* Efficacy and safety of apixaban in patients after cardioversion for atrial fibrillation: Insights from the ARISTOTLE trial (apixaban for reduction in stroke and other thromboembolic events in atrial fibrillation). *Journal of the American College of Cardiology.* 2014; **63**:1082–7.

31. Patel M R, *et al.* Rivaroxaban versus warfarin in nonvalvular atrial fibrillation. *N Engl J Med.* 2011; **365**:883–91.

32. Cappato R, *et al.* Rivaroxaban vs. vitamin K antagonists for cardioversion in atrial fibrillation. *European Heart Journal.* 2014; **35**:3346–55.

33. www.uptodate.com/contents/warfarin-drug-information?source=see_link. [Accessed September 27, 2015].

34. Weigner M J, *et al.* Risk for clinical thromboembolism associated with conversion to sinus rhythm in patients with atrial fibrillation lasting less than 48 hours. *Ann Intern Med.* 1997; **126**:615–20.

35. Stoddard M F, *et al.* Transesophageal echocardiographic guidance of cardioversion in patients with atrial fibrillation. *Am Heart J.* 1995; **129**(6):1204–15.

36. Stoddard M F, *et al.* Left atrial appendage thrombus is not uncommon in patients with acute atrial fibrillation and a recent embolic event: A transesophageal echocardiographic study. *J Am Coll Cardiol.* 1995; **25**(2):452–9.

37. Klein A L, *et al.* Use of transesophageal echocardiography to guide cardioversion in patients with atrial fibrillation. *N Engl J Med.* 2001; **344**(19): 1411–20.

38. Weigner M J, *et al.* Early cardioversion of atrial fibrillation facilitated by transesophageal echocardiography: Short-term safety and impact on maintenance of sinus rhythm at 1 year. *Am J Med.* 2001; **110**(9):694–702.

39. Camm A J, *et al.* Guidelines for the management of atrial fibrillation: The Task Force for the Management of Atrial Fibrillation of the European Society of Cardiology (ESC). *Europace.* 2010; **12**(10):1360–420.

40. www.uptodate.com/contents/warfarin-drug-information?source=see_link. [Accessed September 27, 2015].

Chapter 22

Medication-induced stroke

Fazeel M. Siddiqui and Adnan I. Qureshi

Background

Oral and intravenous medications are uncommon but known precipitants of stroke. The resulting stroke can be either ischemic or intracerebral hemorrhage (ICH) [1]. The overall incidence of medication-induced stroke (MIS) is unknown [1]. Diagnosis is challenging, especially in elderly patients when a single drug cannot be considered a causative agent in the presence of multiple other cardiovascular risk factors. The cause–effect relationship is more complicated in polypharmacy regimens when multiple drugs can be implicated as the cause of stroke. Drugs such as oral contraceptive pills (OCPs) and hormone replacement therapies (HRTs) have conflicting evidence to support their causative role in stroke [1]. The association of ICH with anticoagulant therapy is the most well known. There is a rise in the incidence of anticoagulation-related ICH due to the increasing use of warfarin for the treatment of atrial fibrillation (AF) [2]. Over the counter sympathomimetics such as phenylpropranol-amine, ephedrine, and pseudoephedrine (part of cold preparations) have also been known to cause stroke mainly by inducing vasospasm or vasculopathy [3].

Classification of medication-induced stroke

Medications cause stroke by a variety of pathophysiological mechanisms that can result in both ischemic stroke and ICH. Medications can be broadly classified according to their proposed mechanism of stroke [1,4] (Table 22.1).

Medication-induced thromboembolism

Several drugs have been implicated in causing ischemic stroke by thromboembolism (Table 22.2).

Table 22.1 Classification of medication-induced stroke [1,4].

Stroke secondary to medication-induced thromboembolism

Stroke secondary to medication-induced vasospasm (RCVS)

Stroke secondary to medication-induced vasculitis

Stroke secondary to medication-induced coagulation dysfunction

Stroke secondary to medication-induced platelet dysfunction/thrombocytopenia

Stroke secondary to medication-induced thrombolysis

Stroke secondary to other/unknown mechanisms

RCVS: reversible cerebral vasoconstriction syndrome.

The major culprits include HRT, OCPs, and some chemotherapeutic agents. Drugs can cause thromboembolism by activating platelets, vascular damage, clotting dysfunction, altering blood viscosity (by increased production of blood cells/proteins), and lysis of pre-existing clots.

Oral contraceptive pills

There is a long-standing association of stroke with the use of OCPs. Despite several studies, this relationship remains controversial. Oral contraceptive pills can cause stroke secondary to two major mechanisms: arterial thrombo-occlusive disease and cerebral venous thrombosis (CVT) [5,6]. High plasma estrogen can cause endothelial and intimal proliferation leading to thrombotic occlusions. Oral contraceptive pills themselves do not cause arterial disease, but they act synergistically with other risk factors that damage vessel walls including smoking, hypertension, and atherosclerosis [7]. Oral contraceptive pills also have prothrombotic effects that may lead to CVT [7].

Treatment-Related Stroke, ed. Alexander Tsiskaridze, Arne Lindgren and Adnan Qureshi. Published by Cambridge University Press. © Cambridge University Press 2016.

Table 22.2 Medications causing thromboembolism.

Medications	Proposed mechanism
OCPs/HRT	Vascular damage Prothrombotic state
Testosterone/anabolic steroids	Increased platelet aggregation Polycythemia/increased blood viscosity
Heparin/heparin derivatives	Autoimmune/increased platelet activation/aggregation
Chemotherapeutic agents	Direct vascular damage Prothrombotic state Increased platelet aggregation Increased blood viscosity
Erythropoiesis stimulating agents	Polycythemia/increased viscosity
Antifibrinolytic agents	Prothrombotic state
Non-steroidal anti-inflammatory agents	Direct vascular damage Increased platelet aggregation Hypertension
Miscellaneous agents	
Intravenous immunoglobulins	Increased viscosity Prothrombotic state
All-trans retinoic acid	Accelerated atherosclerosis
Anti-retroviral medication	

OCP: Oral contraceptive pills; HRT: hormone replacement therapy.

Higher dose estrogen formulations have higher risk of reported stroke and lower doses have higher failure rates [8]. Higher doses are considered unsafe in patients over 35 years of age, and in those women with history of ischemic stroke, hyperlipidemia, or migraine headaches [1,9]. Due to early reports of major cardiovascular events associated with OCPs, major changes have been made in formulations over the past 30 to 40 years. New-generation OCPs contain a lower amount of estrogen along with progestins that have stronger progestogenic activity and reduced androgenic effects [5]. Studies have shown that the decreased amount of estrogen and third-generation progesterone (desogestrel, norgestimate, or gestodene) have lower risk of arterial ischemic strokes

[10]. Chan *et al.* performed a meta-analysis to investigate the risk of ischemic stroke or ICH with OCP use [11]. Four cohort and 16 case-control studies were included. This study did not stratify patients based upon their use of different generations of OCPs. The pooled odds ratio (OR) from the cohort studies demonstrated no increased stroke risk with OCP use; however, the pooled OR from the case-control studies showed a significant association (2.13; 95% confidence interval [CI], 1.59–2.86; P <0.001). The risk of stroke with OCP use, however, was significant only with thrombotic stroke (2.74; 95% CI 2.24–3.35; P = 0.009) and not with ICH. Another meta-analysis performed by Plu-Bureau *et al.* concluded that the new generation of OCPs carries a lower risk of stroke compared with first-generation OCPs. There was no risk of ICH. This study also did not find any evidence to support that non-oral hormonal contraceptives are safer than oral OCPs [5].

Use of OCPs in women with migraine with aura carries a higher risk of stroke. The risk increases further in women with the triad of migraine with aura, OCP use, and cigarette smoking [12].

Cerebral venous thrombosis is a rare cause of stroke (0.5 to 1% of all strokes) [13]. The relationship of OCP and CVT is well established, supported by various case series and meta-analyses [14–18]. The risk increases in the presence of other prothrombotic conditions (familial or acquired) [16]. In contrast to arterial strokes, there is potentially more risk of CVT with third-generation OCPs (that include a newer generation of progestins: drospirenone and cyproterone acetate) and with the use of non-oral contraceptive medication [6,19].

Hormone replacement therapy

Hormone replacement therapy (HRT) gained popularity in the late 1980s and early 1990s as a potential solution of postmenopausal syndrome (PMS) with the possibility of providing some cardiovascular benefits. However, after the publication of the results of the Women's Health Initiative (WHI) trial in 2002, HRT use dropped significantly [20,21]. This multicenter double-blind, placebo-controlled, randomized clinical trial (RCT) recruited 16,608 women aged 50 through 79 years with an average follow-up of 5.6 years. There was an absolute risk of an additional 12 strokes per 10,000 person-years. The association was seen with ischemic stroke and not with ICH. The risk was prevalent in all age groups and all categories of baseline stroke risk including hypertension, prior history of cardiovascular disease, and use of hormones, statins, or aspirin [21,22]. However, HRT use may still be considered for a shorter duration of time, considering its symptomatic benefit in severe PMS [20].

Testosterone/anabolic steroids

There is no association between endogenous levels of testosterone and risk of ischemic stroke [23]. In fact, higher testosterone concentrations may weakly protect against cardiovascular diseases in elderly men [24]. However, misuse of testosterone for performance enhancement has been implicated as a potential risk factor for ischemic stroke in young adults. Anabolic testosterone use can cause increased platelet aggregation that may result in acute thrombosis leading to ischemic stroke and other cardiovascular diseases [25]. High-dose testosterone can also cause polycythemia that can lead to stroke by increasing blood viscosity [26].

Heparin-induced thrombocytopenia

Heparin's utility in the treatment and prevention of thromboembolic diseases is well known. Heparin-induced thrombocytopenia (HIT) type 2 is an auto-immune-mediated, rare but life-threatening disorder associated with prolonged use of heparin (>4 days) [27,28]. It leads to formation of antibodies that react with heparin and platelet factor 4 (PF4) complexes. PF4 is a heparin-binding protein contained in platelet alpha-granules [29]. These complexes further interact with platelets leading to their activation and eventual thrombotic complications [30]. The incidence of ischemic stroke in HIT is low but well recognized [31,32]. Immediate recognition and early therapy with argatroban may decrease the risk of new or recurrent strokes in HIT patients [32].

Chemotherapeutic agents

Chemotherapeutic agents can cause stroke mainly by causing hypercoagulability or direct vascular damage. However, various other mechanisms have been described that can potentially lead to stroke (Table 22.2). In a retrospective review of 10,963 patients, the incidence of postchemotherapy ischemic stroke was 0.137% and the frequency of chemotherapy cycles complicated by ischemic stroke was 0.035% [33]. Adenocarcinoma was the most common type of cancer and platinum-based compounds were the most common chemotherapeutic agents. Prognosis was generally poor [33]. Overall, the rate of chemotherapy-related stroke is low (<1%) in different case series published to date [33–36].

Erythropoiesis stimulating agents

Erythropoietin is an endogenously produced glycoprotein that controls the production of red blood cells. Exogenously produced erythropoietin by recombinant DNA technology has been used for the treatment of anemia in patients with chronic kidney disease (CKD) and that are undergoing cancer chemotherapy. However, there is an increased risk of cardiovascular events including stroke when erythropoietin is used to normalize hemoglobin in the blood. This risk is not attributable to any baseline characteristics or to the postrandomization blood pressure, hemoglobin, platelet count, or dose of treatment [37,38]. Based upon these findings, the US Food and Drug Administration (FDA) established a risk evaluation and mitigation strategy (REMS) to ensure safe use of ESAs. In 2011, the FDA issued a safety communication recommending a more conservative dosing of erythropoiesis stimulating agents (ESAs) in chronic kidney diseases because of the increased risks of cardiovascular events, stroke, thrombosis, and death [39,40].

Interestingly, erythropoietin has been tested as a neuroprotective agent in stroke, independent of its role in erythropoiesis. It binds specifically to neuronal erythropoietin receptors and may help in neuroplasticity by its anti-apoptotic, anti-oxidant, anti-inflammatory, and neurotrophic actions [41]. However, a recent double-blind, placebo-controlled, RCT could not show this benefit in the human population [41].

Antifibrinolytic agents

Antifibrinolytic agents (AFAs) are classified into lysine analogs (aminocaproic acid and tranexamic acid) and the serine protease inhibitors (aprotinin). Traditionally these compounds have been used during major surgeries and trauma to minimize blood loss. Aprotinin was withdrawn from the market when it was shown to be independently associated with increased mortality, cardiovascular events, cerebrovascular events including stroke, and renal events when compared with lysine analogs in patients undergoing cardiac surgery [42,43]. Lysine analogs such as tranexamic acid are, however, considered safe and have been widely utilized to minimize bleeding especially in the setting of trauma [44]. Oral or parenteral AFAs have also been used in reducing rebleeding in subarachnoid hemorrhage (SAH) patients. A meta-analysis of nine trials concluded that AFAs may reduce the risk of rebleeding in SAH but this benefit is offset by an increased risk of cerebral ischemia [45]. Oral tranexamic acid has also been utilized in patients with excessive menorrhagia and melasma. It carries a small risk of stroke, especially in women on OCPs and oral all-trans retinoic acid, mainly by augmenting their procoagulant effects [46,47].

Intravenous immunoglobulin

The use of intravenous immunoglobulin (IVIG) is well established in a variety of immune-mediated disorders including primary immunodeficiencies, idiopathic thrombocytopenic purpura, Guillain–Barré syndrome, chronic inflammatory demyelinating polyneuropathy, myesthenia gravis, dermatomyositis, and Kawasaki syndrome. The risk of stroke is very small and is possibly related to rapid changes in serum viscosity, although many other theories have also been proposed [48]. Rapid infusion of high doses may be associated with increased stroke risk, although strokes have been reported in patients with standard doses and conventional infusion rates [48–50]. No association has been found between specific brands of IVIG and increased stroke risk. The risk of stroke is more common with elderly patients and those with multiple stroke-risk factors [51].

Non-steroidal anti-inflammatory drugs

Non-steroidal anti-inflammatory drugs (NSAIDs) are the most prescribed medications for pain relief. Several studies have shown a higher risk of cardiovascular and cerebrovascular ischemic events associated with extended use of high-dose NSAIDs. This risk was present with the use of both cyclo-oxygenase-2 enzyme (COX-2) selective NSAIDs as well as COX-2 non-selective NSAIDs. The risk of ischemic stroke is higher with certain COX-2 selective NSAIDs based upon several studies published in the past decade [52–56]. A similar risk exists for ICH (discussed later in the chapter). The possible mechanisms may include increased thrombotic effect of platelets, direct vascular damage, increased blood pressure, and effect

on the kidneys and salt retention [53]. In 2004, the FDA issued a public health advisory concerning use of specific NSAIDs (rofecoxib, valdecoxib, celecoxib, and naproxen) and increased risk of ischemic stroke [57]. Rofecoxib and valdecoxib were later withdrawn from the market and a black-box warning was issued for the other drugs [58].

Antiretroviral medications

Several reports have suggested an increased risk of stroke, particularly ischemic stroke, in patients suffering from human immunodeficiency virus (HIV) [59–61]. It was initially thought that this higher risk of ischemic stroke was related to HIV-related meningitis and protein S deficiency. However, further studies showed that protein S deficiency is a relatively common occurrence in HIV-infected patients and is not related to the increased risk of stroke [62,63]. These findings lead to a closer scrutiny of antiretroviral medications. Studies have shown that antiretroviral drugs can cause hypercholesterolemia and hypertriglyceridemia, insulin resistance, and lipodystrophy that may further lead to premature atherosclerosis [59]. Several large studies were performed to evaluate this relationship with conflicting results. Vaughn et al. analyzed a cohort of 5,667 HIV-infected individuals in Los Angeles County. The use of protease inhibitors was associated with increased risk of cardiovascular diseases including stroke (hazard ratio (HR) 6.22; 95% CI 3.13–12.39; p-value <0.001) [64]. However, other studies could not find a strong causative relationship between antiretroviral therapies and ischemic stroke incidence [65–68]. At best, caution should be advised in patients with baseline risk factors for stroke and use of antiretroviral medications especially protease inhibitors and non-nucleoside reverse transcriptase inhibitors that can cause accelerated metabolic syndrome and hence increased risk of ischemic stroke [69,70].

Medication-induced vasospasm

The association of oral sympathomimetics with stroke is well known. These medications can cause both systemic as well as intracranial vasoconstriction that can be transient or prolonged. Systemic vasoconstriction leads to hypertension and resultant ICH and intracranial vasoconstriction can lead to ischemic stroke [1]. Table 22.3 describes different medications that have been implicated in causing cerebral vasospasm-related strokes.

Table 22.3 Medications causing vasospasm/RCVS [71,125].

Medication class	Examples	Treatment strategies
Stimulants	Amphetamines	Removal of offending drug.
Cough suppressants	Phenylpropanolamine, pseudoephedrine, ephedrine	Symptomatic treatment for headache or seizures.
Serotonergic medications	SSRI, triptans	Calcium-channel blockers (nimodipine, nicardipine, verapamil).
Ergot derivatives	Ergotamine tartrate, methergine, bromocriptine, lisuride	Avoid steroids.
Immunosuppressant agents	Cyclophosphamide, interferon-a, tacrolimus	Intra-arterial nimodipine, nicardipine, or milrinone in severe cases.
Blood products	Erythropoietin, IVIG, red blood cell transfusion	
Hormonal supplements	OCPs, hormonal ovarian stimulation for intrauterine insemination	
Miscellaneous agents	Binge drinking, ginseng, indomethacin, licorice, nicotine patches	

RCVS: reversible cerebral vasoconstriction syndrome; SSRI: selective serotonin-reuptake inhibitors; IVIG: intravenous immunoglobulins; OCP: oral contraceptive pills.

Reversible cerebral vasoconstriction syndrome (RCVS) that involves prolonged and mostly reversible vasoconstriction of the intracranial vasculature has been described. Patients present with thunderclap headaches and may develop ischemic strokes in the arterial territories involved. The incidence of ischemic stroke in RCVS may range from 4 to 54% based upon various studies, followed by SAH (34%) and ICH (20%) [71]. Medications that can induce RCVS include vasoactive medications such as sympathomimetics, ergot derivatives, serotonergic drugs, and some immunosuppressant medications [71] (Table 22.3).

Medication-induced vasculitis

Vasculitis is the inflammation of small, medium, or large arteries that can affect the CNS vasculature. Although most of the drug-related vascular changes on angiography are possibly RCVS, there are reports of biopsy proven medication-induced vasculitis [72,73]. CNS vasculitis can lead to a variety of stroke subtypes including ischemic stroke, ICH, or SAH, and sometimes a combination of all [72]. Vasculitis may be self-limiting or rapidly progressive leading to clinical deterioration and permanent neurological deficits and death. The pathophysiological process may be hypersensitivity or abnormal immune response to the inciting drug. In most cases, removal of the causative agent may lead to improvement in symptoms [73]. The most definitive evidence of drug-induced vasculitis came from a series of 14 patients who abused amphetamines, and showed a clinical and histological evidence of multisystem necrotizing vasculitis [74]. Allopurinol can cause a hypersensitivity reaction leading to systemic vasculitis including cerebral vasculitis [75,76].

Medication-induced coagulation dysfunction

According to the Greater Cincinnati/Northern Kentucky Stroke Study (GCNKSS), the annual incidence of anticoagulant-associated ICH per 100,000 increased from 0.8 (95% CI 0.3–1.3) in 1988 to 1.9 (95% CI 1.1–2.7) in 1993/1994 and 4.4 (95% CI 3.2–5.5) in

Table 22.4 Medications causing coagulation dysfunction.

Class	Examples	Affected clotting factors	Treatment strategies
Vitamin K antagonists	Warfarin	Inhibition of vitamin K-dependent clotting factors II, VII, IX, and X [80]	Stop the medication 4-factor PCC and vitamin K (preferred) [134], FFP and rfVIIa [126]
Parenteral anticoagulants	UFH	AT-dependent inactivation of thrombin and factor Xa [127]	Stop the medication Protamine dose 0.5–0.75 mg/100 U if UFH stopped in 30–60 min; 0.375–0.5 mg/100 U if UFH stopped in 60–120 min; 0.25–0.375 mg/100 U if UFH stopped in >120 min [126]
	LMWH (enoxaparin)	Predominant factor Xa inhibitor Mild thrombin inhibitor [127]	Stop the medication Protamine dose 1 mg/100 anti-Xa units of LMWH [126]
	Fondaparinux	Selective indirect factor Xa inhibitor [128]	Stop the medication rfVIIa [129]
Direct thrombin inhibitors	Dabigatran etexilate	Direct inhibition of thrombin [80]	Stop the medication Praxbind (idarucizumab) [135] PCC, FFP, rfVIIa Hemodialysis [130] Desmopressin or antifibrolytic agents [129]
Factor Xa inhibitors	Rivaroxaban, apixaban	Direct inhibition of factor Xa [80]	Stop the medication PCC, FFP, rfVIIa [126]

UFH: unfractionated heparin; LMWH: low molecular weight heparin; AT: antithrombin; PCC: prothrombin complex concentrate; rfVIIa: recombinant activated factor VII.

1999 (P <0.001 for trend) [77]. Anticoagulant-associated ICH now causes nearly 20% of all ICH [2]. There is a higher risk of life-threatening ICH with all oral and parenteral anticoagulant medications. This risk is lower with newer anticoagulant medications such as direct thrombin inhibitors and factor Xa inhibitors. Table 22.4 describes medications that can affect the coagulation system and eventually result in stroke.

Oral anticoagulant therapy

Warfarin, a vitamin K antagonist, has been the primary anticoagulant therapy for decades. It has been used for the prevention of stroke in AF, treatment of deep venous thrombosis and pulmonary embolism, CVT, and other familial and acquired prothrombotic disorders [78–80]. Despite its therapeutic benefits, it has a narrow therapeutic index. For example, a subtherapeutic international normalized ratio (INR) of 1.5 to 1.9 reduces its preventive

efficacy in regards to ischemic stroke by a factor of 2 to 3.6 in AF patients compared with the recommended INR values (2.0 to 3.0) [81]. The risk of ICH with therapeutic INR is small (0.3 to 0.5% per 100 patient-years), but it increases to 2.7% at INR values 4 to 4.5 and to 9.4% when INR exceeds 4.5 [81]. This risk also increases with age, concomitant use of antiplatelet agents or heparin, previous ischemic stroke, cerebral amyloid angiopathy, and drug interactions [1,82]. Warfarin-associated hemorrhages are life-threatening and associated with high mortality and disability [83]. In the past few years, a new generation of oral anticoagulants has emerged that boasts lesser risk of ICH. The major players in this category include direct thrombin inhibitors such as dabigatran etexilate, and factor Xa inhibitors such as rivaroxaban [80]. Despite lower risk of ICH, the major drawback with these newer anticoagulants is the lack of antidote in cases of hemorrhage requiring rapid reversal [80]. The FDA recently approved

Praxbind (idarucizamab), an antibody fragment, to reverse the anticoagulant effects of dabigatran [135].

Heparin and its derivatives

Heparin is a parenterally administered compound that augments the action of antithrombin III and inhibits the tissue factor pathway resulting in prolonged partial thromboplastin time (PTT) [84,85]. Enoxaparin is a similar compound that is obtained by alkaline degradation of heparin benzyl ester. It is approximately one-third the molecular size of standard heparin and hence traditionally known as low molecular weight heparin [84]. As with the case of oral anticoagulants, risk of ICH increases with intensity of anticoagulation (PTT >80 to 90 seconds), age, and history of ischemic stroke [1]. Enoxaparin is renally eliminated, and hence there is a higher risk of ICH in patients with kidney disease [1].

Medication-induced platelet dysfunction

Although many medications cause platelet dysfunction, the most notable are antiplatelet agents. There are numerous agents that can either decrease the production of platelets or affect their function (Tables 22.5 and 22.6). Platelet dysfunction has been associated with all types of intracranial hemorrhages including microhemorrhages [86], spontaneous ICH [87], and intraventricular hemorrhages [88]. In this section, we will discuss medications that predominantly cause platelet dysfunction.

Antiplatelet agents

Antiplatelet therapy use is highly prevalent among patients presenting with ischemic stroke. Commonly used antiplatelet agents include aspirin, clopidogrel, and dipyridamole in combination with aspirin. Patients on antiplatelet therapy are at increased risk for ICH [89]. Patients presenting with spontaneous ICH are more commonly using antiplatelet therapy than anticoagulant therapy [90]. Antiplatelet agents also increase the chances of hematoma expansion and subsequent death and disability [90–104]. Many studies have been performed to evaluate the effect of premorbid antiplatelet therapy on clinical outcome and hematoma growth with conflicting results. A recently conducted meta-analysis established a relationship between prior antiplatelet therapy and higher in-hospital mortality in patients with spontaneous ICH

Table 22.5 Medications causing platelet dysfunction [131,132].

Medications	Proposed mechanism
Antiplatelet agents	
Aspirin, ibuprofen, naproxen	COX-I inhibitors
Thienopyridines (clopidogrel and prasugrel)	ADP-induced platelet aggregation inhibitors
Dipyridamole, long-acting dipyridamole/aspirin, cilostazol	Phosphodiesterase inhibitors
Abciximab, tirofiban, and eptifibatide	GpIIb/IIIa receptor inhibitors
Beta-Lactam antibiotics	
Penicillin, ampicillin, cephalothin, carbenicillin	ADP-induced platelet aggregation inhibition Interference with platelet–vWF interactions
Nitrates	Inhibit platelet aggregation
Antihypertensive medications	
Beta-blockers	Interference with platelet membranes
Calcium channel blockers	Inhibit serotonin-induced platelet aggregation
Hydralazine, furosemide	Inhibition of prostaglandin pathways
Antidepressant medications	
Selective serotonin-reuptake inhibitors	Decrease serotonin uptake from the blood by platelets
Tricyclic antidepressants	Interference with platelet membranes
Chemotherapeutic agents	
Vincristine, vinblastine	Phosphodiesterase inhibitors

COX: cyclo-oxygenase; ADP: adenosine diphosphate; vWF: von Willebrand factor.

[87]. Patients on antiplatelet therapy have a higher incidence of cerebral microbleeds that may convert to larger hematomas with continued use. This risk is lower with the use of anticoagulant medications [105].

Theoretically, platelet infusion therapy can help in reversing the effect of antiplatelet drugs and

Table 22.6 Medications causing immune-mediated thrombocytopenia [133].

Medications
Antiplatelet agents
GpIIb/IIIa receptor inhibitors (abciximab, tirofiban, and eptifibatide), NSAIDs
Antibiotics/antivirals
Penicillins, cephalosporins, sulfonamides, acyclovir, interferon, rifampin, vancomycin
Anticonvulsant agents
Valproic acid, phenytoin, carbamazepine
Antihistamine medications
Cimetidine
Antiarrhythmic agents
Procainamide, quinidine, digoxin
Anti-inflammatory agents
Gold salts, sulfasalazine
Antihypertensive medications
Hydrochlorothiazide, chlorthalidone
Alcohol

NSAIDs: nonsteroidal anti-inflammatory drugs.

help control hematoma growth and resultant mortality and morbidity [88,94,106,107]. Platelet Transfusion in Cerebral Hemorrhage (PATCH) is an ongoing randomized controlled trial that is investigating whether platelet transfusion improves outcome in ICH patients who are on antiplatelet treatment [108].

Parenteral glycoprotein IIb/IIIa inhibitors

The glycoprotein IIb/IIIa complex is an integrin found on the platelet surface [84]. It binds to fibrinogen and helps in platelet aggregation. Abciximab is an intravenous glycoprotein IIb/IIIa inhibitor that is used as an adjunct to percutaneous coronary intervention performed for the prevention of cardiac ischemic complications [84]. In a meta-analysis of 14 randomized trials of intravenous platelet glycoprotein IIb/IIIa receptor inhibitors, Memon *et al.* compared the incidence of ICH among 15,850 patients receiving glycoprotein IIb/IIIa inhibitors with that among 12,039 patients receiving placebo. The authors found that the incidence of ICH with heparin plus any IIb/IIIa inhibitor was similar to placebo with heparin (0.12% vs. 0.09%, OR 1.3, 95% CI 0.6 to 3.1, P = 0.59). The incidence of ICH with glycoprotein IIb/IIIa drugs alone was similar to that with heparin alone (0.07% vs. 0.06%, OR 1.2, 95% CI 0.1 to 16, P = 1.0). They concluded that intravenous glycoprotein IIb/IIIa receptor inhibitors alone or in combination with heparin do not cause a statistically significant excess of ICH compared with heparin alone [84,109].

In patients undergoing percutaneous intervention for cerebrovascular diseases, glycoprotein IIb/IIIa inhibitors have been associated with rapidly expanding fatal ICH [110,111]. There was a higher risk of fatal ICH in patients who received abciximab for the treatment of acute ischemic stroke within five hours from symptom onset. Approximately 5.5% of abciximab-treated and 0.5% of placebo-treated patients had symptomatic or fatal ICH (P = 0.002) within five days of enrollment [112]. This risk was even higher in wake-up strokes with similar baseline characteristics (13.6%) [113].

Medication-induced thrombolysis

Medication-induced thrombolysis (MIT) has been widely used for treatment of ischemic stroke, myocardial infarction, life-threatening pulmonary embolism, and major peripheral artery embolism [114]. The major complication of MIT is bleeding, including ICH. The risk of ICH increases with history of prior ICH or recent large ischemic stroke, age, concomitant use of antiplatelet agents or anticoagulants, hyperglycemia, hypertension, and delayed revascularization after initial ischemic stroke [1,115]. Frequency of ICH ranges from 2.1 to 9.4% in different trials [116]. Thrombolysis-related ICH is associated with poor outcome and severe neurological dysfunction [116].

MIS secondary to other/unknown mechanisms

Several studies and meta-analyses have suggested an association between increased risk of stroke and use of atypical antipsychotics, especially risperidone in dementia patients. Different mechanisms were proposed including orthostatic hypotension causing watershed infarctions, excessive sedation resulting in dehydration and hemoconcentration, and hyperprolactinemia causing increased aggregation of platelets. However, careful reanalysis showed that this relationship may be because of poor allotment of patients with higher stroke risk factors in the risperidone group [117]. At best, the risk of stroke is low and more common in patients with older age, cognitive impairment, and vascular illness [118].

Oral bisphosphonates are the mainstay of treatment for osteoporosis. Studies have shown a possible causative relationship between bisphosphonates and AF. So far no study has shown a higher incidence of stroke in patients on oral bisphosphonates [119]. However, there may be an increased risk of stroke in cancer patients on intravenous bisphosphonates [120]. Certain oral hypoglycemic agents have shown increased risk of stroke. Rosiglitazone increases the risk of myocardial infarction, stroke, and death – possibly by increasing serum triglycerides and LDL-cholesterol levels [121,122]. Similarly, muraglitazar increases the risk of myocardial infarction, or stroke due to unknown reasons [122].

Management and prevention

In most cases, general management of medication-induced ischemic stroke and ICH is similar to ischemic stroke and spontaneous ICH caused by traditional risk factors [1]. Comprehensive management guidelines are present for both ischemic stroke and spontaneous ICH and are beyond the scope of this chapter [123,124].

Early recognition and removal of the culprit drug is crucial in preventing further damage. The role of intravenous thrombolysis in medication-induced ischemic stroke is not clear but has been successfully used in certain cases. Cerebral venous thrombosis secondary to OCP use may require long-term anticoagulation [13]. Heparin-induced thrombocytopenia-related ischemic stroke may benefit from argatroban infusion [32]. Most of the previously known medication-induced vasculitidis are now known to be RCVS. Glucocorticoids are shown to be an independent predictor of bad outcome and should be avoided in RCVS-related strokes. Calcium-channel blockers such as nimodipine and nicardipine have shown some benefit and can be used cautiously with strict blood pressure monitoring [71]. In rare cases of true

vasculitis, disease process is self-limiting after removal of the inciting agent. However, in some cases long-term immunosuppression is needed.

Intracerebral hemorrhage secondary to drugs causing platelet dysfunction/thrombocytopenia may require platelet transfusion although its role is not clear in patients with normal platelet count [123]. Anticoagulation-related ICH requires the use of a specific antidote, if available, along with use of FFP, activated clotting factors, and other urgent remedies (Table 22.4).

The most effective way to prevent MIS is to avoid, or use the lowest effective doses of, those drugs that are associated with strokes, especially in high-risk populations.

Conclusion

Medication-induced stroke is not uncommon. General management of MIS may differ from strokes associated with the usual risk factors. Prompt recognition and discontinuation of medication may prevent further ischemic or hemorrhagic events and neurological deficits.

References

1. Tisdale J E, Miller D A. American Society of Health-System Pharmacists. *Drug-induced Diseases: Prevention, Detection, and Management.* Bethesda, MD: American Society of Health-System Pharmacists; 2005.

2. Flaherty M L. Anticoagulant-associated intracerebral hemorrhage. *Seminars in Neurology.* 2010; **30**:565–72.

3. Cantu C, Arauz A, Murillo-Bonilla L M, Lopez M, Barinagarrementeria F. Stroke associated with sympathomimetics contained in over-the-counter cough and cold drugs. *Stroke.* 2003; **34**:1667–72.

4. Jain K K. *Drug-induced Neurological Disorders.* Cambridge, MA: Hogrefe Pub; 2012.

5. Plu-Bureau G, Hugon-Rodin J, Maitrot-Mantelet L, Canonico M. Hormonal contraceptives and arterial disease: An epidemiological update. *Best Practice & Research. Clinical Endocrinology & Metabolism.* 2013; **27**:35–45.

6. Plu-Bureau G, Maitrot-Mantelet L, Hugon-Rodin J, Canonico M. Hormonal contraceptives and venous thromboembolism: An epidemiological update. *Best Practice & Research. Clinical Endocrinology & Metabolism.* 2013; **27**:25–34.

7. Godsland I F, Winkler U, Lidegaard O, Crook D. Occlusive vascular diseases in oral contraceptive users. Epidemiology, pathology and mechanisms. *Drugs.* 2000; **60**:721–869.

8. Meade T W, Greenberg G, Thompson S G. Progestogens and cardiovascular reactions associated with oral contraceptives and a comparison of the safety of 50- and 30-microgram oestrogen preparations. *British Medical Journal.* 1980; **280**:1157–61.

9. Lidegaard O. Oral contraceptives, pregnancy and the risk of cerebral thromboembolism: The influence of diabetes, hypertension, migraine and previous thrombotic disease. *British Journal of Obstetrics and Gynaecology.* 1995; **102**:153–9.

10. Lidegaard O, Kreiner S. Contraceptives and cerebral thrombosis: A five-year national case-control study. *Contraception.* 2002; **65**:197–205.

11. Chan W S, Ray J, Wai E K, *et al.* Risk of stroke in women exposed to low-dose oral contraceptives: A critical evaluation of the evidence. *Archives of Internal Medicine.* 2004; **164**:741–7.

12. Schurks M, Rist P M, Bigal M E, *et al.* Migraine and cardiovascular disease: Systematic review and meta-analysis. *British Medical Journal.* 2009; **339**:b3914.

13. Saposnik G, Barinagarrementeria F, Brown R D, Jr., *et al.* Diagnosis and management of cerebral venous thrombosis: A statement for healthcare professionals from the American Heart Association/American Stroke Association. *Stroke.* 2011; **42**:1158–92.

14. Saadatnia M, Naghavi N, Fatehi F, Zare M, Tajmirriahi M. Oral contraceptive misuse as a risk factor for cerebral venous and sinus thrombosis. *Journal of Research in Medical Sciences.* 2012; **17**:344–7.

15. Ashjazadeh N, Borhani Haghighi A, Poursadeghfard M, Azin H. Cerebral venous-sinus thrombosis: A case series analysis. *Iranian Journal of Medical Sciences.* 2011; **36**:178–82.

16. Martinelli I, Sacchi E, Landi G, *et al.* High risk of cerebral-vein thrombosis in carriers of a prothrombin-gene mutation and in users of oral contraceptives. *New England Journal of Medicine.* 1998; **338**:1793–7.

17. de Bruijn S F, Stam J, Koopman M M, Vandenbroucke J P. The Cerebral Venous Sinus Thrombosis Study Group. Case-control study of risk of cerebral sinus thrombosis in oral contraceptive users and in [correction of who are] carriers of hereditary prothrombotic conditions. *British Medical Journal.* 1998; **316**:589–92.

18. Dentali F, Crowther M, Ageno W. Thrombophilic abnormalities, oral contraceptives, and risk of cerebral vein thrombosis: A meta-analysis. *Blood.* 2006; **107**:2766–73.

19. Dunne C, Malyuk D, Firoz T. Cerebral venous sinus thrombosis in a woman using the etonogestrel-ethinyl estradiol vaginal contraceptive ring: A case report. *Journal of Obstetrics and Gynaecology Canada.* 2010; **32**:270–3.

20. Shetty K D, Vogt W B, Bhattacharya J. Hormone replacement therapy and cardiovascular health in the United States. *Medical Care.* 2009; **47**:600–6.

21. Rossouw J E, Anderson G L, Prentice R L, *et al.* Risks and benefits of estrogen plus progestin in healthy postmenopausal women: Principal results from the women's health initiative randomized controlled trial. *Journal of the American Medical Association.* 2002; **288**:321–33.

22. Wassertheil-Smoller S, Hendrix S L, Limacher M, *et al.* Effect of estrogen plus progestin on stroke in postmenopausal women: The women's health initiative: A randomized trial. *Journal of the American Medical Association.* 2003; **289**:2673–84.

23. Ruige J B, Mahmoud A M, De Bacquer D, Kaufman J M. Endogenous testosterone and cardiovascular disease in healthy men: A meta-analysis. *Heart.* 2011; **97**:870–5.

24. Yeap B B, Hyde Z, Almeida O P, *et al.* Lower testosterone levels predict incident stroke and transient ischemic attack in older men. *Journal of Clinical Endocrinology and Metabolism.* 2009; **94**:2353–9.

25. Ferenchick G, Schwartz D, Ball M, Schwartz K. Androgenic-anabolic steroid abuse and platelet aggregation: A pilot study in weight lifters. *American Journal of the Medical Sciences.* 1992; **303**:78–82.

26. Stergiopoulos K, Brennan J J, Mathews R, Setaro J F, Kort S. Anabolic steroids, acute myocardial infarction and polycythemia: A case report and review of the literature. *Vascular Health and Risk Management.* 2008; **4**:1475–80.

27. Warkentin T E, Greinacher A, Koster A, Lincoff A M. Treatment and prevention of heparin-induced thrombocytopenia: American College of Chest Physicians evidence-based clinical practice guidelines (8th edition). *Chest.* 2008; **133**:340S-380S.

28. Linkins L A, Dans A L, Moores L K, *et al.* Treatment and prevention of heparin-induced thrombocytopenia: Antithrombotic therapy and prevention of thrombosis, 9th ed: American College of Chest Physicians evidence-based clinical practice guidelines. *Chest.* 2012; **141**:e495S-530S.

29. Visentin G P, Ford S E, Scott J P, Aster R H. Antibodies from patients with heparin-induced thrombocytopenia/thrombosis are specific for platelet factor 4 complexed with heparin or bound to endothelial cells. *Journal of Clinical Investigation.* 1994; **93**:81–8.

30. Newman P M, Chong B H. Heparin-induced thrombocytopenia: New evidence for the dynamic binding of purified anti-pf4-heparin antibodies to platelets and the resultant platelet activation. *Blood.* 2000; **96**:182–7.

31. Giossi A, Del Zotto E, Volonghi I, *et al.* Thromboembolic complications of heparin-induced thrombocytopenia. *Blood Coagulation & Fibrinolysis.* 2012; **23**:559–62.

32. LaMonte M P, Brown P M, Hursting M J. Stroke in patients with heparin-induced thrombocytopenia and the effect of argatroban therapy. *Critical Care Medicine.* 2004; **32**:976–80.

33. Li S H, Chen W H, Tang Y, *et al.* Incidence of ischemic stroke post-chemotherapy: A retrospective review of 10,963 patients. *Clinical Neurology and Neurosurgery.* 2006; **108**:150–6.

34. Czaykowski P M, Moore M J, Tannock I F. High risk of vascular events in patients with urothelial transitional cell carcinoma treated with cisplatin based chemotherapy. *Journal of Urology.* 1998; **160**:2021–4.

35. Wall J G, Weiss R B, Norton L, *et al.* Arterial thrombosis associated with adjuvant chemotherapy for breast carcinoma: A cancer and leukemia group B study. *American Journal of Medicine.* 1989; **87**:501–4.

36. Bachaud J M, David J M, Shubinski R E, *et al.* Predictive factors of a complete response to and adverse effects of a cddp-5fu combination as primary therapy for head and neck squamous carcinomas. *Journal of Laryngology and Otology.* 1993; **107**:924–30.

37. Skali H, Parving H H, Parfrey P S, *et al.* Stroke in patients with type 2 diabetes mellitus, chronic kidney disease, and anemia treated with darbepoetin alfa: The trial to reduce cardiovascular events with aranesp therapy (treat) experience. *Circulation.* 2011; **124**:2903–8.

38. Pfeffer M A, Burdmann E A, Chen C Y, *et al.* A trial of darbepoetin alfa in type 2 diabetes and chronic kidney disease. *New England Journal of Medicine.* 2009; **361**:2019–32.

39. FDA Drug Safety Communication. Erythropoiesis-stimulating agents (ESAS): Procrit, epogen and aranesp. 2010.

40. FDA Drug Safety Communication. Modified dosing recommendations to improve the safe use of erythropoiesis-stimulating agents (ESAS) in chronic kidney disease. 2011.

41. Ehrenreich H, Weissenborn K, Prange H, *et al.* Recombinant human erythropoietin in the treatment of acute ischemic stroke. *Stroke.* 2009; **40**:e647–656.

42. Fergusson D A, Hebert P C, Mazer C D, *et al.* A comparison of aprotinin and lysine analogues in high-risk cardiac surgery. *New England Journal of Medicine.* 2008; **358**:2319–31.

43. Mangano D T, Tudor I C, Dietzel C. The risk associated with aprotinin in cardiac surgery. *New England Journal of Medicine.* 2006; **354**:353–65.

44. Roberts I, Perel P, Prieto-Merino D, *et al.* Effect of tranexamic acid on mortality in patients with traumatic bleeding: Prespecified analysis of data from randomised controlled trial. *British Medical Journal.* 2012; **345**:e5839.

45. Roos Y B, Rinkel G J, Vermeulen M, Algra A, van Gijn J. Antifibrinolytic therapy for aneurysmal subarachnoid haemorrhage. *Cochrane Database of Systematic Reviews.* 2003: CD001245.

46. Idbaih A, Crassard I, Vahedi K, Guichard J P, Woimant F. Thrombotic cocktail in stroke. *Neurology.* 2005; **64**:334.

47. Brown J E, Olujohungbe A, Chang J, *et al.* All-trans retinoic acid (ATRA) and tranexamic acid: A potentially fatal combination in acute promyelocytic leukaemia. *British Journal of Haematology.* 2000; **110**:1010–12.

48. Caress J B, Cartwright M S, Donofrio P D, Peacock J E, Jr. The clinical features of 16 cases of stroke associated with administration of IVIG. *Neurology.* 2003; **60**:1822–4.

49. Katz U, Shoenfeld Y. Review: Intravenous immunoglobulin therapy and thromboembolic complications. *Lupus.* 2005; **14**:802–8.

50. Orbach H, Katz U, Sherer Y, Shoenfeld Y. Intravenous immunoglobulin: Adverse effects and safe administration. *Clinical Reviews in Allergy & Immunology.* 2005; **29**:173–84.

51. Caress J B, Hobson-Webb L, Passmore L V, Finkbiner A P, Cartwright M S. Case-control study of thromboembolic events associated with IV immunoglobulin. *Journal of Neurology.* 2009; **256**:339–42.

52. Haag M D, Bos M J, Hofman A, *et al.* Cyclooxygenase selectivity of nonsteroidal anti-inflammatory drugs and risk of stroke. *Archives of Internal Medicine.* 2008; **168**:1219–24.

53. Roumie C L, Mitchel E F, Jr., Kaltenbach L, *et al.* Nonaspirin NSAIDS, cyclooxygenase 2 inhibitors, and the risk for stroke. *Stroke.* 2008; **39**:2037–45.

54. Andersohn F, Schade R, Suissa S, Garbe E. Cyclooxygenase-2 selective nonsteroidal anti-inflammatory drugs and the risk of ischemic stroke: A nested case-control study. *Stroke.* 2006; **37**:1725–30.

55. Fosbol E L, Olsen A M, Olesen J B, *et al.* Use of nonsteroidal anti-inflammatory drugs among healthy people and specific cerebrovascular safety. *International Journal of Stroke.* 2012; **9**:943–5.

56. Chang C H, Shau W Y, Kuo C W, Chen S T, Lai M S. Increased risk of stroke associated with nonsteroidal anti-inflammatory drugs: A nationwide case-crossover study. *Stroke.* 2010; **41**:1884–90.

57. Bennett J S, Daugherty A, Herrington D, *et al.* The use of nonsteroidal anti-inflammatory drugs (NSAIDS): A science advisory from the American Heart Association. *Circulation.* 2005; **111**:1713–16.

58. Antman E M, Bennett J S, Daugherty A, *et al.* Use of nonsteroidal antiinflammatory drugs: An update for clinicians: A scientific statement from the American Heart Association. *Circulation.* 2007; **115**:1634–42.

59. Sklar P, Masur H. HIV infection and cardiovascular disease: Is there really a link? *New England Journal of Medicine.* 2003; **349**:2065–7.

60. Engstrom J W, Lowenstein D H, Bredesen D E. Cerebral infarctions and transient neurologic deficits associated with acquired immunodeficiency syndrome. *American Journal of Medicine.* 1989; **86**:528–32.

61. Qureshi A I, Janssen R S, Karon J M, *et al.* Human immunodeficiency virus infection and stroke in young patients. *Archives of Neurology.* 1997; **54**:1150–3.

62. Mochan A, Modi M, Modi G. Protein S deficiency in HIV associated ischaemic stroke: An epiphenomenon of HIV infection. *Journal of Neurology, Neurosurgery, and Psychiatry.* 2005; **76**:1455–6.

63. Qureshi A I. HIV infection and stroke: If not protein S deficiency then what explains the relationship? *Journal of Neurology, Neurosurgery, and Psychiatry.* 2005; **76**:1331.

64. Vaughn G, Detels R. Protease inhibitors and cardiovascular disease: Analysis of the Los Angeles County Adult Spectrum of Disease cohort. *AIDS Care.* 2007; **19**:492–9.

65. Monsuez J J, Goujon C, Wyplosz B, *et al.* Cerebrovascular diseases in HIV-infected patients. *Current HIV Research.* 2009; **7**:475–80.

66. Corral I, Quereda C, Moreno A, *et al.* Cerebrovascular ischemic events in HIV-1-infected patients receiving highly active antiretroviral therapy: Incidence and risk factors. *Cerebrovascular Diseases.* 2009; **27**:559–63.

67. Ortiz G, Koch S, Romano J G, Forteza A M, Rabinstein A A. Mechanisms of ischemic stroke in HIV-infected patients. *Neurology.* 2007; **68**:1257–61.

68. Mangili A, Gerrior J, Tang A M, *et al.* Risk of cardiovascular disease in a cohort of HIV-infected adults: A study using carotid intima-media thickness and coronary artery calcium score. *Clinical Infectious Diseases.* 2006; **43**:1482–9.

69. Sen S, Rabinstein A A, Elkind M S, Powers W J. Recent developments regarding human immunodeficiency virus infection and stroke. *Cerebrovascular Diseases.* 2012; **33**:209–18.

70. Dobbs M R, Berger J R. Stroke in HIV infection and AIDS. *Expert Review of Cardiovascular Therapy.* 2009; **7**:1263–71.

71. Chen S P, Fuh J L, Wang S J. Reversible cerebral vasoconstriction syndrome: Current and future perspectives. *Expert Review of Neurotherapeutics.* 2011; **11**:1265–76.

72. Salvarani C, Brown R D, Jr., Hunder G G. Adult primary central nervous system vasculitis. *Lancet.* 2012; **380**:767–77.

73. Calabrese L H, Duna G F. Drug-induced vasculitis. *Current Opinion in Rheumatology.* 1996; **8**:34–40.

74. Citron B P, Halpern M, McCarron M, *et al.* Necrotizing angiitis associated with drug abuse. *New England Journal of Medicine.* 1970; **283**:1003–11.

75. Lim D, Rademaker M, Asztely F, Ratnaweera M, Coltman G. Cerebral vasculitis and multi-focal neurological deficits due to allopurinol-induced hypersensitivity syndrome. *Australasian Journal of Dermatology.* 2013.

76. Rothwell P M, Grant R. Cerebral vasculitis following allopurinol treatment. *Postgraduate Medical Journal.* 1996; **72**:119–20.

77. Flaherty M L, Kissela B, Woo D, *et al.* The increasing incidence of anticoagulant-associated intracerebral hemorrhage. *Neurology.* 2007; **68**:116–21.

78. Whitlock R P, Sun J C, Fremes S E, Rubens F D, Teoh K H. Antithrombotic and thrombolytic therapy for valvular disease: Antithrombotic therapy and prevention of thrombosis, 9th ed: American College of Chest Physicians evidence-based clinical practice guidelines. *Chest.* 2012; **141**:e576S–600S.

79. You J J, Singer D E, Howard P A, *et al.* Antithrombotic therapy for atrial fibrillation: Antithrombotic therapy and prevention of thrombosis, 9th ed: American College of Chest Physicians evidence-based clinical practice guidelines. *Chest.* 2012; **141**:e531S–575S.

80. Ageno W, Gallus A S, Wittkowsky A, *et al.* Oral anticoagulant therapy: Antithrombotic therapy and prevention of thrombosis, 9th ed: American College of Chest Physicians evidence-based clinical practice guidelines. *Chest.* 2012; **141**:e44S–88S.

81. Hylek E M, Skates S J, Sheehan M A, Singer D E. An analysis of the lowest effective intensity of prophylactic anticoagulation for patients with nonrheumatic atrial fibrillation. *New England Journal of Medicine.* 1996; **335**:540–6.

82. Hart R G, Boop B S, Anderson D C. Oral anticoagulants and intracranial hemorrhage. Facts and hypotheses. *Stroke.* 1995; **26**:1471–7.

83. Fang M C, Go A S, Chang Y, *et al.* Death and disability from warfarin-associated intracranial and extracranial hemorrhages. *American Journal of Medicine.* 2007; **120**:700–5.

84. Quinones-Hinojosa A, Gulati M, Singh V, Lawton M T. Spontaneous intracerebral hemorrhage due to coagulation disorders. *Neurosurgical Focus.* 2003; **15**:E3.

85. Hampton K K, Preston F E. ABC of clinical haematology. Bleeding disorders, thrombosis, and

anticoagulation. *British Medical Journal.* 1997; **314**:1026–9.

86. Vernooij M W, Haag M D, van der Lugt A, *et al.* Use of antithrombotic drugs and the presence of cerebral microbleeds: The Rotterdam scan study. *Archives of Neurology.* 2009; **66**:714–20.

87. Thompson B B, Bejot Y, Caso V, *et al.* Prior antiplatelet therapy and outcome following intracerebral hemorrhage: A systematic review. *Neurology.* 2010; **75**:1333–42.

88. Naidech A M, Bendok B R, Garg R K, *et al.* Reduced platelet activity is associated with more intraventricular hemorrhage. *Neurosurgery.* 2009; **65**:684–8.

89. He J, Whelton P K, Vu B, Klag M J. Aspirin and risk of hemorrhagic stroke: A meta-analysis of randomized controlled trials. *Journal of the American Medical Association.* 1998; **280**:1930–5.

90. Foerch C, Sitzer M, Steinmetz H, Neumann-Haefelin T. Pretreatment with antiplatelet agents is not independently associated with unfavorable outcome in intracerebral hemorrhage. *Stroke.* 2006; **37**:2165–7.

91. Toyoda K, Okada Y, Minematsu K, *et al.* Antiplatelet therapy contributes to acute deterioration of intracerebral hemorrhage. *Neurology.* 2005; **65**:1000–4.

92. Toyoda K, Yasaka M, Nagata K, *et al.* Antithrombotic therapy influences location, enlargement, and mortality from intracerebral hemorrhage. The bleeding with antithrombotic therapy (BAT) retrospective study. *Cerebrovascular Diseases.* 2009; **27**:151–9.

93. Saloheimo P, Ahonen M, Juvela S, *et al.* Regular aspirin-use preceding the onset of primary intracerebral hemorrhage is an independent predictor for death. *Stroke.* 2006; **37**:129–33.

94. Creutzfeldt C J, Weinstein J R, Longstreth W T, Jr., *et al.* Prior antiplatelet therapy, platelet infusion therapy, and outcome after intracerebral hemorrhage. *Journal of Stroke & Cerebrovascular Diseases.* 2009; **18**:221–8.

95. Caso V, Paciaroni M, Venti M, *et al.* Effect of on-admission antiplatelet treatment on patients with cerebral hemorrhage. *Cerebrovascular Diseases.* 2007; **24**:215–18.

96. Roquer J, Rodriguez Campello A, Gomis M, *et al.* Previous antiplatelet therapy is an independent predictor of 30-day mortality after spontaneous supratentorial intracerebral hemorrhage. *Journal of Neurology.* 2005; **252**:412–16.

97. Lacut K, Le Gal G, Seizeur R, *et al.* Antiplatelet drug use preceding the onset of intracerebral hemorrhage is associated with increased mortality. *Fundamental & Clinical Pharmacology.* 2007; **21**:327–33.

98. Hanger H C, Fletcher V J, Wilkinson T J, *et al.* Effect of aspirin and warfarin on early survival after intracerebral haemorrhage. *Journal of Neurology.* 2008; **255**:347–52.

99. Sansing L H, Messe S R, Cucchiara B L, *et al.* Prior antiplatelet use does not affect hemorrhage growth or outcome after ICH. *Neurology.* 2009; **72**:1397–402.

100. Moussouttas M, Malhotra R, Fernandez L, *et al.* Role of antiplatelet agents in hematoma expansion during the acute period of intracerebral hemorrhage. *Neurocritical Care.* 2010; **12**:24–9.

101. Stead L G, Jain A, Bellolio M F, *et al.* Effect of anticoagulant and antiplatelet therapy in patients with spontaneous intra-cerebral hemorrhage: Does medication use predict worse outcome? *Clinical Neurology & Neurosurgery.* 2010; **112**:275–81.

102. Ishibashi A, Yokokura Y, Adachi H. Is antiplatelet therapy for the prevention of ischemic stroke associated with the prognosis of intracerebral hemorrhage? *Kurume Medical Journal.* 2008; **55**:71–5.

103. Nicolini A, Ghirarduzzi A, Iorio A, *et al.* Intracranial bleeding: Epidemiology and relationships with antithrombotic treatment in 241 cerebral hemorrhages in Reggio Emilia. *Haematologica.* 2002; **87**:948–56.

104. Baldi G, Altomonte F, Altomonte M, *et al.* Intracranial haemorrhage in patients on antithrombotics: Clinical presentation and determinants of outcome in a prospective multicentric study in Italian emergency departments. *Cerebrovascular Diseases.* 2006; **22**:286–93.

105. Lovelock C E, Cordonnier C, Naka H, *et al.* Antithrombotic drug use, cerebral microbleeds, and intracerebral hemorrhage: A systematic review of published and unpublished studies. *Stroke.* 2010; **41**:1222–8.

106. Naidech A M, Bernstein R A, Levasseur K, *et al.* Platelet activity and outcome after intracerebral hemorrhage. *Annals of Neurology.* 2009; **65**:352–6.

107. Naidech A M, Jovanovic B, Liebling S, *et al.* Reduced platelet activity is associated with early clot growth and worse 3-month outcome after intracerebral hemorrhage. *Stroke.* 2009; **40**:2398–401.

108. de Gans K, de Haan R J, Majoie C B, *et al.* PATCH: Platelet Transfusion in Cerebral Haemorrhage: Study protocol for a multicentre, randomised, controlled trial. *BMC Neurology.* 2010; **10**:19.

109. Memon M A, Blankenship J C, Wood G C, Frey C M, Menapace F J. Incidence of intracranial hemorrhage complicating treatment with glycoprotein IIb/IIIa receptor inhibitors: A pooled analysis of major clinical trials. *American Journal of Medicine.* 2000; **109**:213–17.

110. Qureshi A I, Suri M F, Ali Z, *et al*. Carotid angioplasty and stent placement: A prospective analysis of perioperative complications and impact of intravenously administered abciximab. *Neurosurgery*. 2002; **50**:466–73.

111. Qureshi A I, Saad M, Zaidat O O, *et al*. Intracerebral hemorrhages associated with neurointerventional procedures using a combination of antithrombotic agents including abciximab. *Stroke*. 2002; **33**:1916–19.

112. Adams H P, Jr., Effron M B, Torner J, *et al*. Emergency administration of abciximab for treatment of patients with acute ischemic stroke: Results of an international phase III trial: Abciximab in emergency treatment of stroke trial (ABESTT-II). *Stroke*. 2008; **39**:87–99.

113. Adams H P, Jr., Leira E C, Torner J C, *et al*. Treating patients with "wake-up" stroke: The experience of the ABESTT-II trial. *Stroke*. 2008; **39**:3277–82.

114. Hirsh J, Guyatt G, Albers G W, Harrington R, Schunemann H J, American College of Chest Physicians. Antithrombotic and thrombolytic therapy: American College of Chest Physicians evidence-based clinical practice guidelines (8th edition). *Chest*. 2008; **133**:110S-112S.

115. The National Institute of Neurological Disorders and Stroke RT-PA Stroke Study Group. Tissue plasminogen activator for acute ischemic stroke. *New England Journal of Medicine*. 1995; **333**:1581–7.

116. Strbian D, Sairanen T, Meretoja A, *et al*. Patient outcomes from symptomatic intracerebral hemorrhage after stroke thrombolysis. *Neurology*. 2011; **77**:341–8.

117. Herrmann N, Lanctot K L. Do atypical antipsychotics cause stroke? *CNS Drugs*. 2005; **19**:91–103.

118. Sacchetti E, Turrina C, Valsecchi P. Cerebrovascular accidents in elderly people treated with antipsychotic drugs: A systematic review. *Drug Safety*. 2010; **33**:273–88.

119. Christensen S, Mehnert F, Chapurlat R D, Baron J A, Sorensen H T. Oral bisphosphonates and risk of ischemic stroke: A case-control study. *Osteoporosis International*. 2011; **22**:1773–9.

120. Wilkinson G S, Baillargeon J, Kuo Y F, Freeman J L, Goodwin J S. Atrial fibrillation and stroke associated with intravenous bisphosphonate therapy in older patients with cancer. *Journal of Clinical Oncology*. 2010; **28**:4898–905.

121. Gallagher A M, Smeeth L, Seabroke S, Leufkens H G, van Staa T P. Risk of death and cardiovascular outcomes with thiazolidinediones: A study with the general practice research database and secondary care data. *PloS One*. 2011; **6**:e28157.

122. Panicker G K, Karnad D R, Salvi V, Kothari S. Cardiovascular risk of oral antidiabetic drugs: Current evidence and regulatory requirements for new drugs. *J Assoc Physicians India*. 2012; **60**:56–61.

123. Morgenstern L B, Hemphill J C, 3rd, Anderson C, *et al*. Guidelines for the management of spontaneous intracerebral hemorrhage: A guideline for healthcare professionals from the American Heart Association/American Stroke Association. *Stroke*. 2010; **41**:2108–29.

124. Jauch E C, Saver J L, Adams H P, Jr. *et al*. Guidelines for the early management of patients with acute ischemic stroke: A guideline for healthcare professionals from the American Heart Association/American Stroke Association. *Stroke*. 2013; **44**:870–947.

125. Ducros A, Bousser M G. Reversible cerebral vasoconstriction syndrome. *Practical Neurology*. 2009; **9**:256–67.

126. Mittal M K, Rabinstein A A. Anticoagulation-related intracranial hemorrhages. *Current Atherosclerosis Reports*. 2012; **14**:351–9.

127. Hirsh J, Anand S S, Halperin J L, Fuster V. Mechanism of action and pharmacology of unfractionated heparin. *Arteriosclerosis, Thrombosis, and Vascular Biology*. 2001; **21**:1094–6.

128. Choay J, Petitou M, Lormeau JC, *et al*. Structure-activity relationship in heparin: A synthetic pentasaccharide with high affinity for antithrombin III and eliciting high anti-factor Xa activity. *Biochemical and Biophysical Research Communications*. 1983; **116**:492–9.

129. Crowther M A, Warkentin T E. Bleeding risk and the management of bleeding complications in patients undergoing anticoagulant therapy: Focus on new anticoagulant agents. *Blood*. 2008; **111**:4871–9.

130. Watanabe M, Siddiqui F M, Qureshi A I. Incidence and management of ischemic stroke and intracerebral hemorrhage in patients on dabigatran etexilate treatment. *Neurocritical Care*. 2012; **16**:203–9.

131. Baz R, Mekhail T. Disorders of platelet function and number. 2010.

132. Konkle B A. Acquired disorders of platelet function. *ASH Education Program Book*. 2011; 391–6.

133. Kenney B, Stack G. Drug-induced thrombocytopenia. *Archives of Pathology and Laboratory Medicine*. 2009; **133**:309–14.

134. Steiner T, Poli S, Griebe M, *et al*. Fresh frozen plasma versus prothrombin complex concentrate in patients with intracranial haemorrhage (INCH): a randomized trial. *Lancet*. 2016; **15**:566–73.

135. Pollack C V, Reilly P A, Eikelboom J, *et al*. Idarucizamab for dabigatran reversal. *New England Journal of Medicine*. 2015; **373**:511–20.

Chapter

23

Cerebral venous thrombosis

José M. Ferro and Patrícia Canhão

Introduction

In the general population, the risk of cerebral venous thrombosis (CVT) is low. However, it is considerably increased in pregnancy and the puerperium, in patients with prothrombotic clinical conditions such as cancer and the antiphospholipid syndrome, if drugs with a prothrombotic effect are prescribed (e.g., hormone replacement therapy, steroids, L-asparaginase) or if the patient has a non-diagnosed inherited prothombotic condition (e.g., deficiencies in protein S, C, and antithrombin or factor V Leiden and prothrombin G20210A mutations). Oncologic patients, who already have a prothrombotic state, must sometimes be treated with drugs with prothrombotic effects or undergo surgical procedures, which also increase the risk of venous thrombosis. In some brain and neck surgical interventions, veins have to be sacrificed. Because of the high variability of the cerebral venous circulation and its anastomosis, ligation for instance of an internal jugular vein can be either asymptomatic or produce an intracranial hypertension syndrome.

This chapter addresses CVT in relation to pharmacological treatment (Table 23.1); to interventional procedures; and finally gives an overview of treatment-related CVT in the large International Study of Cerebral Vein and Dural Sinus Thrombosis.

Cerebral venous thrombosis and pharmacological treatment

Hormone therapy

Combined oral contraceptives

Combined oral contraceptives (OCs) are known to confer a risk of CVT to otherwise healthy women and are

Table 23.1 Pharmacological therapies associated with cerebral vein and dural sinus thrombosis.

Hormone therapy

Combined oral contraceptives

Combined contraceptive vaginal rings

Glucocorticoids

Anabolic steroids

Drugs in cancer therapeutic regimens

Chemotherapy (L-asparaginase; cyclophosphamide, methotrexate, 5-fluorouracil; cisplatin; cyclosporine)

Hormonal therapy (tamoxifen, medroxyprogesterone acetate, chlormadinone)

Angiogenesis inhibitors (thalidomide, lenalidomide, bevacizumab, temozolomide)

Others (interleukin-2 and granulocyte-macrophage-colony stimulating factor; all-trans retinoic acid)

Hemostatic treatments

Epsilon-aminocaproic acid

Tranexamic acid

Factor VII concentrate

Heparin-induced thrombocytopenia

Heparin

Heparinoid pentosan sulfate

Enoxaparin

IV immunoglobulin therapy

Miscellaneous

Epoetin alfa therapy

Clozapine

Dihydroergotamine

Treatment-Related Stroke, ed. Alexander Tsiskaridze, Arne Lindgren and Adnan Qureshi. Published by Cambridge University Press. © Cambridge University Press 2016.

the most frequent risk factor for CVT in women. In the International Study in Cerebral Vein and Dural Sinus Thrombosis (ISCVT) study, the proportion of OC users was 54% in women less than 50 years old. Among OC users, the thrombotic risk is higher among carriers of hereditary thrombophilias (e.g., factor V Leiden, the prothrombin gene mutation, and deficiencies of protein S, protein C, and antithrombin) [1,2].

In OC users, activation of coagulation likely results from an imbalance between increased levels of coagulation and decreased inhibition of coagulation. Plasma levels of almost all coagulation factors increase. Plasma is resistant to the anticoagulant action of activated protein C, and decreased levels of protein S are frequently found.

Oral contraceptives containing third-generation progestins (desogestrel and norgestimate) may be associated with a greater risk of venous thrombosis when compared with earlier progestins (levonorgestrel-containing OCs). From the PharMetrics dataset, Jick *et al.* [3] assessed the risk of CVT in women using desogestrel-, norgestimate-, or levonorgestrel-containing OCs. They also assessed the risk among users of the contraceptive patch. In this study with over 1 million users of the four study drugs regimens, the CVT incidence rate ratios (IRRs) were 4.0 (95% CI 0.7–42.4) for desogestrel-containing OCs vs. levonorgestrel-containing OCs, and 2.4 (95% CI 0.5–24.0) for norgestimate-containing OCs vs. levonorgestrel-containing OCs. The IRR for the patch could not be calculated because no case of CVT occurred among current users of the contraceptive patch.

Third-generation and second-generation progestins have different effects on the anticoagulant pathway. Acquired resistance to activated protein C may be one mechanism by which the third generation OCs could predispose to venous thromboembolism. In addition, it has been suggested that second-generation progestins are more effective than third-generation progestins in counteracting the thrombotic effects of estrogen.

Combined contraceptive vaginal rings are used as an alternative to oral contraceptives with a purported advantage of allowing lower general hormonal doses, and thus potentially confer a lower venous thromboembolism risk. However, there are some cases of CVT reported in women using contraceptive vaginal rings suggesting an increased risk associated with their use [4]. There is also one report of CVT associated with emergency (day after) contraception.

Apart from contraceptive use, there are several conditions where estrogens or progestagens have been associated with CVT. The most reported is the use in postmenopausal women as hormone replacement therapy. In the ISCVT, 27 out of 57 CVT women aged more than 50 years reported the use of HRT.

There are some reports of CVT related to hormonal treatment for infertility and these are generally associated with the ovarian hyperstimulation syndrome [5]. One case has been reported on developing a CVT while receiving long-term estrogen therapy for approximately 15 years after feminizing genitoplasty [6]. Another woman developed a central CVT following intake of progestin-only pill (norethindrone acetate) for dysfunctional uterine bleeding secondary to polycystic ovary syndrome [7].

Glucocorticoids

Corticosteroids have been associated with CVT in several situations. Most of the patients who developed CVT while treated with corticosteroids presented other predisposing conditions for the thrombotic event, such as cancer or inflammatory diseases, or were submitted to some precipitant procedures, such as lumbar puncture [8], venous catheter insertion, surgery, or concomitant treatment with antineoplastic drugs. Corticosteroids may predispose to thrombosis by causing an increase in the levels of activated clotting factors by decreasing their clearance rate, and also by inhibiting the fibrinolytic activity of the blood.

Anabolic steroids

Anabolic steroids are used as therapy for hypoplastic anemias due to leukemia or kidney failure, and aplastic anemia. Three cases of dural sinus thrombosis have been reported in patients with aplastic anemia on treatment with anabolic steroids, such as metenolone acetate and oxymetholone [9–11].

Treatment with danazol, also known as 17alpha-ethinyl testosterone, was associated with the occurrence of CVT in one patient treated for immune hemolytic anemia [12] and in another case for endometriosis [13]. One patient with CVT had aplastic anemia and paroxysmal nocturnal hemoglobinuria, and had received danazol but also other prothrombotic drugs such as methylprednisolone, cyclosporine-A, and pregnenolone [14].

Finally, a few cases of CVT have been reported of androgen-induced cerebral venous sinus thrombosis in young body-builder men [15,16].

Hormonal therapy in cancer has been mentioned as one of the factors contributing to CVT in those patients (see below).

Drugs in cancer therapeutic regimens

Several chemotherapeutic agents used in the treatment of patients with malignancy have been associated with cerebral venous thrombosis. The attribution of thrombosis to chemotherapy in many published cases is speculative, because adequate prospective studies that include investigation for other thrombotic causes are not available. The best known associations with thrombosis are L-asparaginase, which is typically used in the induction therapy of acute lymphocytic leukemia, and combination hormonal therapy and chemotherapy for breast cancer.

L-asparaginase

Of 548 patients with acute lymphoblastic leukemia (ALL) treated at Dana–Farber Cancer Institute diagnosed between 1991 and 2008, sinus venous thrombosis occurred in 1.6% of patients [17]. Appearance of headaches, seizures, focal signs, or decrease of consciousness in patients with ALL treated with L-asparaginase should prompt physicians to exclude several potential causes of CNS dysfunction, such as meningeal infiltration, CNS infection or hemorrhage, and dural sinus occlusion. Brain imaging with magnetic resonance and veno-MRI, or alternatively veno-CT, would be required to establish the diagnosis of CVT. Early and vigilant recognition of CVT and anticoagulation may prevent further neurological damage.

L-asparaginase decreases both procoagulant and anticoagulant protein synthesis in the liver, leading to a possible alteration in the balance of the opposing forces of the hemostatic mechanism. There is some evidence that the prothrombotic state may be determined by a decrease of antithrombin levels. Qualitatively abnormal von Willebrand factor (vWf) has been found in several patients at the time of L-asparaginase-induced thrombosis. L-asparaginase may lead to a transient increase in unusually large plasma vWf multimers, which have enhanced platelet-agglutinating properties. Furthermore, induction chemotherapy in ALL also sometimes includes other agents such as corticosteroids that may increase the risk of a prothrombotic state.

Tamoxifen and chemotherapy of breast cancer

Tamoxifen is an antiestrogen that has weak estrogenic effects, which may contribute to its prothrombotic activity. It induces reduction of antithrombin and protein C. Several studies have shown an increased incidence of thromboembolic events in women with breast cancer treated with chemotherapy, tamoxifen, or both. The incidence of thromboembolic disease appears to be related to the stage of the disease, the chemotherapeutic regimen given, and whether tamoxifen is given concurrently or following the termination of chemotherapy. The risk is higher in patients with metastatic disease, which is probably due to the increased tumor burden. Several cases of thrombosis located in the dural sinuses have been described, as discussed below. Additional risk factors in those patients may include postmenopausal status, presence of an indwelling central venous catheter, and concurrent coagulation activation.

The mechanisms of the thrombogenic effects of chemotherapy in patients with breast cancer are not well understood. A decrease in protein C and protein S levels may be present during cyclophosphamide, methotrexate, and 5-fluorouracil (CMF) chemotherapy. Usually, the thrombotic events occurred while patients were receiving chemotherapy [18].

A number of studies, including large breast cancer prevention trials [19], demonstrated that tamoxifen use is associated with an increased rate of venous thromboembolic events and that there is a significant additional procoagulant effect when tamoxifen is added to chemotherapy [20]. Several reports have related tamoxifen to CVT in the absence of other risk factors [21]. A case of dural sinus thrombosis during medication with medroxyprogesterone acetate, which is a progestational agent, in a patient with metastasic lung carcinoma from breast carcinoma was also reported [22].

Angiogenesis inhibitors

Many new antineoplastic agents with antiangiogenic properties appear to be associated with an increased risk for thrombosis. There are a few reports of CVT occurring in patients treated with the following antiangiogenic agents: (1) thalidomide [23] and lenalidomide [24] in patients with multiple myeloma; (2) bevacizumab in two patients, one with colon cancer [25] and one with glioma concurrently treated with radiotherapy and temozolomide [26].

The prothrombotic effect of antiangiogenic agents is probably linked to an effect on the endothelium (decrease of antithrombotic activities and stimulation of a prothrombotic state), and appears as potentiating the prothrombotic conditions of the disease (myeloma, cancer) and the prothombotic effects of the associated treatments (chemotherapy, high-dose corticosteroids, erythropoietin).

Other agents

Cisplatin is a well-recognized risk factor for coagulation disorders and thrombosis, and at least two patients with cerebral dural sinus thrombosis following cisplatin therapy have been described [27]. One child developed dural sinus thrombosis one week after the first chemotherapy treatment with cisplatin, etopoxide, and bleomycin for a partially resected dysgerminoma [28].

A case of cyclosporine-induced dural sinus thrombosis has been published [29]. There are also several reports of CVT in patients undergoing allogeneic bone marrow transplantation treated with cyclosporine [30].

Mahadeo *et al.* described a 12-year-old male with ALL who developed subacute methotrexate-induced neurotoxicity and cerebral venous thrombosis after receiving intrathecal methotrexate. This case highlights the need for the differential diagnosis between different causes of neurological complications in patients with ALL, both those associated with the disease as well as those related to potential iatrogenic complications [31].

A massive thrombosis of the cerebral sinuses and veins was described in a woman with acute promyelocytic leukemia in complete morphological and molecular remission after treatment with all-trans retinoic acid and idarubicin [32].

A phase Ib/II trial was conducted in 16 patients to determine the response rate of renal cell carcinoma patients with pulmonary metastases treated with continuous infusion of interleukin-2 (IL-2) combined with granulocyte-macrophage-colony stimulating factor (GM-CSF). No significant antitumor activity was observed but autopsy in a patient who died revealed acute multifocal cerebral venous thrombosis as well as acute subdural and subarachnoid hemorrhage [33].

Hormonal therapies in the treatment of prostate cancer are known to be responsible for an increased vascular risk. The progestin chlormadinone and prostate cancer were proposed to be the cause of dural sinus thrombosis in one patient [34].

Hemostatic treatments

Isolated case reports of cerebral venous thrombosis as a potential hazard of different hemostatic treatments include: (1) prolonged epsilon-aminocaproic acid therapy, in a woman with menorrhagia [35], (2) tranexamic acid [36], (3) factor VII concentrate, in a baby with severe factor VII deficiency with postnatal intracranial haemorrhage [37].

Heparin-induced thrombocytopenia

Several cases of CVT were described in association with heparin-induced thrombocytopenia. Some were related with heparin [38,39], others with the synthetic heparinoid pentosan sulfate [40,41], and one with enoxaparin [42]. In a recent report, Fesler reviewed ten cases in the literature suggesting that heparin-induced thrombocytopenia-related CVT is often a fatal condition, particularly when diagnosed in comatose patients [42].

IV immunoglobulin therapy

A few cases of dural sinuses thrombosis have been published in patients to whom intravenous immunoglobulin (IVIG) was administered in different settings such as: (1) a 54-year-old woman with a diagnosis of IgG1 deficiency, starting symptoms from the lateral transverse and sagittal sinuses the day after an infusion of IVIG replacement treatment [43]; (2) an 11-year-old boy with humoral immunodeficiency on monthly IVIG infusions [44]; (3) a pediatric patient treated with high-dose IVIG for acute immune thrombocytopenic purpura in the absence of any hypercoagulable state [45].

Miscellaneous

A rare case of CVT was reported in a patient receiving peritoneal dialysis and epoetin alfa therapy. Epoetin alfa therapy, which had been initiated three months earlier, was associated with a problematic increase in hematocrit values, which could have been the precipitant of the venous thrombosis [46]. Also, there is a report of an amateur cyclist who suffered a CVT after using erythropoietin doping [47].

Antipsychotic drugs are associated with a risk of venous thromboembolism. We detected one case in the literature of CVT after treatment with clozapine [48].

A patient receiving IV dihydroergotamine (DHE) for relief of headache developed five hours later a severe diffuse headache and nausea, and a sagittal sinus thrombosis was confirmed. Dihydroergotamine has potent venoconstrictive effects and although there may be several explanations, the authors suggested that DHE helped precipitate neurologic deterioration in this patient who ultimately died [49].

Some so-called "natural products," believed to be harmless were associated with CVT in anecdotal reports. One case occurred after ingestion of a herbal tonic [50] and the other was associated with a large intake of phytoestrogens [51].

Interventions

Several medical and surgical procedures are listed among the transient risk factors for cerebral vein and dural sinus thrombosis [52–54]. The majority of the publications on this topic are single case reports or small case series. The evidence for the association between the procedure and CVT relies mostly on the temporal association, when the CVT closely follows after the procedure and no other plausible cause for CVT is found. In some cases, other potential causes for CVT are also present such as genetic or acquired prothrombotic conditions, infections (mostly CNS infections), malignancies, or drugs with a prothrombotic effect. In general the procedures that have been associated with CVT either produce a mechanical injury or a change of pressure on the dural sinus, cerebral veins, or meninges, or induce a transient prothrombotic state.

In the following paragraphs we review the literature reporting CVT patients associated with medical and surgical procedures (Table 23.2).

Lumbar puncture and related procedures

It is now well recognized that CVT is a possible, albeit rare, complication of diagnostic lumbar puncture. Lumbar puncture causes a cranio-spinal negative pressure gradient, a downward displacement of the brain, which eventually may cause traction on the sinus and bridging veins. A transcranial Doppler study performed before and after lumbar puncture demonstrated that lumbar puncture induces a decrease of 47% of the mean venous blood flow velocities in the straight sinus. This decrease in venous flow velocity is significant immediately at the end and also more than six hours after lumbar puncture [55].

Several of the first reports of CVT following diagnostic lumbar puncture were in patients with multiple

Table 23.2 Medical and surgical procedures associated with cerebral vein and dural sinus thrombosis.

Lumbar puncture and related procedures
Diagnostic lumbar puncture
Therapeutic lumbar puncture
Myelography
Spinal–epidural anesthesia
Lumbar drain

Procedures on the sinus and veins
Inferior petrosal sinus sampling
Jugular stenting
Jugular vein catheter
Brachial, subclavian, or superior vena cava catheter
Transvenous pacemaker catheter

Neurosurgery
Postoperative CVT after suboccipital, transpetrosal, and transcallosal approaches
Parasagittal meningiomas
Cervical disc arthroplasty
Ventriculoperitoneal surgery
Flowable topical hemostatic matrix
Treatment of vascular malformations

Transplantation
Allogenic bone-marrow transplantation
Renal transplant
Liver transplantation

Neck surgery
Radical neck dissection
Glomus jugulare tumor surgery
Hypoglossal nerve schwannoma surgery

Ear, nose, and throat surgical procedures
Acoustic neuroma surgery
Jugular bulb decompression
Nasal septum submucosal resection
Tracheostomy

Other surgeries
Thoracoscopic surgery
Coronary bypass surgery
Cardiopulmonary bypass

sclerosis who underwent a lumbar puncture as part of the initial diagnostic work-up and also received IV corticosteroid treatment in close temporal relationship with the lumbar puncture [56]. Aidi *et al.* in 1999 [57] stressed the changing pattern of headache after lumbar puncture, when a typical postdural puncture headache loses its postural component, becoming constant. In this circumstance, neuroimaging should be performed to rule out CVT.

Similarly, CVT has been reported after therapeutic lumbar puncture. Examples are intrathecal administration of methotrexate [58], or intrathecal [59] or epidural (with accidental dural puncture) corticosteroid infiltration for lumbar radiculalgia [60]. Cerebral venous thrombosis has also been described after myelography with iopamidol [61] and after placement of a lumbar drain after spinal surgery [62].

Cerebral venous thrombosis has also been reported after spinal–dural anesthesia for delivery, cesarean section or lower limb orthopedic surgery. In most cases the headache was initially a typical postlumbar puncture low CSF pressure headache [63], which was even treated in some patients with a epidural blood patch [64]. The headache then changed its characteristics, becoming constant and severe and not improving with horizontal position. In some patients, drowsiness, seizures, or focal signs developed. In one report the CVT manifested as a subarachnoid hemorrhage [65]. Epidural anesthesia was not the only risk factor for CVT in most cases. Many women were pregnant or in the puerperium or were taking oral contraceptives [66], all these conditions being well known risk factors for CVT. In some other patients, factor V Leiden mutation was identified [64,66].

Procedures on the sinus and veins

Interventions for the placement of diagnostic or therapeutic catheters in the dural sinuses or in the jugular or neighboring veins are other sources of iatrogenic CVT. Thrombosis begins at the tip of the cannula or at the local site of insertion and propagates through the vein. The first cases were reported in the 1980s following the insertion of long-term cannulas or catheters for administration of fluids, parenteral nutrition, and medications [52]. Two reports described dural sinus thrombosis following transvenous pacemaker implantation [67].

The majority of these cases occurred after placement of a catheter in the jugular vein, but CVT has

also been reported after implanted venous catheters in the brachial and subclavian veins [68] or the superior vena cava. Some of the cases were reported in neonates [69] and children. One child had leukemia and a prothrombin G20210A mutation [70]. Other patients were receiving chemotherapy [71] or parenteral nutrition [72] through the catheter.

Inferior petrosal sinus sampling is a useful diagnostic technique in ACTH-dependent hypercortisolism with normal or equivocal MR imaging. This procedure is believed to be safe but one case of brain stem venous infarction was reported among 44 patients who underwent this diagnostic procedure [73].

Jugular stenting is a controversial procedure to prevent progression in multiple sclerosis based on the assumption that "chronic cerebrospinal venous insufficiency" is a cause of progression in multiple sclerosis. The efficacy of this intervention is unproved. Internal jugular and dural sinus thrombosis is one of the potential complications of jugular stenting [74,75].

Neurosurgery

Neurosurgeons are well aware of the possibility of postoperative CVT after suboccipital, transpetrosal [76], and transcallosal approaches [77]. Nakase *et al.* [78] found an incidence of 0.3% (eight cases) of symptomatic CVT in patients who underwent neurosurgical interventions. Neurosurgery was performed for meningioma, acoustic neuroma (two cases each), metastasis, cavernoma, dural fistula, and trigeminal neuralgia (one case each). Postoperative CVT can be divided into acute and chronic [79]. The acute form manifests during surgery and is in general quite severe, causing brain edema and venous infarcts. It is caused mainly by damage or ligation of the petrosal vein. The chronic form is milder, manifests one or a few days after surgery as headache, seizure, or focal deficits, and it is due to damage or sacrifice of the bridging cortical veins. Some patients may have previous thrombotic venous events and acquired (e.g., antiphospholipid syndrome) or genetic thrombophilia [80].

Surgery of meningiomas has a 2 to 3% risk of CVT. The risk is higher (7%) in parasagittal meningiomas invading the superior sagittal sinus. Besides location (parasagittal, convexity, falx), other risk factors for CVT are tumor size and perilesional edema. To prevent venous infarction it is essential to maintain the intervening arachnoid plane as much as possible. The risk of CVT is reduced if an extended bifrontal surgical approach is used. Parasagittal meningiomas can initially be resected as extensively as possible, in the meantime avoiding manipulation of the vascular structures [81].

A case of CVT was reported during placement of a ventriculoperitoneal shunt [82] due to bipolar coagulation of a large paramedian cortical vein.

Flowable topical hemostatic matrix is applied via syringe injection in many neurosurgical procedures, to permit more rapid achievement of hemostasis. Iatrogenic cerebral venous occlusion induced by flowable topical hemostatic matrix occurred in 5 out of 651 infratentorial surgeries (0.8%), but in none of 3,318 supratentorial cases [83].

Finally, CVT can occur as a complication of the treatment of arteriovenous vascular malformations, either by endovascular or direct surgical procedures or by radiosurgery. The CVT can be asymptomatic, cause headache, seizures, or focal signs, or a massive sometimes fatal brain hemorrhage. It can also be a cause of delayed neurological deterioration following treatment of arteriovenous malformations of the brain.

Neck surgery

Surgeons have been aware for a long time of the possibility of "benign intracranial hypertension" following ligation of the external jugular vein during neck surgery for tuberculous glands or tumors. This was more frequent if the right jugular was ligated, because it usually drains the superior sagittal sinus when the left transverse sinus is hypoplasic [52]. Similarly, there are reports of transverse sinus thrombosis with cerebral venous infarction following radical neck dissection [84] and of a fatal cortical vein thrombosis with multiple hemorrhagic infarcts after ligation of the internal jugular vein during excision of a hypoglossal nerve schwannoma [85]. Glomus jugulare tumors invade the jugular bulb and the sigmoid sinus, making it difficult to resect the tumor without sacrificing the involved sinus [86], which may result in transverse sinus thrombosis [87]. However, with current treatment approaches (radiosurgery with or without surgical resection) CVT was not encountered in a systematic review of treatment-related morbidity of glomus jugulare tumors [88].

Ear, nose, and throat surgical procedures

The ear, mastoid, and nasal sinuses have close anatomical relationships with the jugular vein and the transverse sinus. Therefore damage to these venous structures with subsequent thrombosis is a possible, but fortunately infrequent, complication of ear, nose, and throat (ENT) interventions. Cerebral venous thrombosis was reported after jugular bulb decompression to correct for a dehiscent jugular bulb associated with hearing loss [89]. One case of venous infarction of the cerebellar vermis secondary to accidental sinus thrombosis was identified in a single center series of 432 cases of acoustic tumors [90]. Cavernous sinus thrombosis is a rare complication of submucous resection of the nasal septum [91]. A case of fatal intracranial hypertension following tracheostomy was reported in a patient with thrombosis of the left internal jugular vein after cannulation and a hypoplastic right-sided vein [92].

Transplantation

Cerebral venous thrombosis is listed among the possible neurologic complications of patients submitted to transplantation.

The majority of CVT cases reported after transplantation are related to allogenic bone-marrow transplantation. In 1998, Bertz *et al.* reported three patients with seizures after allogenic bone-marrow transplantation, due to sinus venous thrombosis [93]. Three other cases were described by Harvey *et al.* in 2000 [30]. Recently Motohashi *et al.* [94] described a case of extensive CVT presenting as severe headache in patients who received allogenic stem-cell transplantation for leukemia.

There are isolated case reports after renal transplantation [95], but the incidence of CVT after renal transplantation is very low: two cases of CVT in 132 adult recipients in the series of Yardimci *et al.* [96]. There is also a single case report of thrombosis of a developmental venous anomaly after liver transplantation [97].

In transplant recipients CVT has to be differentiated from other neurological complications, including infections, subdural hematoma, ischemic stroke, vasoconstriction syndrome, and subcortical encephalopathy. The appearance of severe headache, seizure, or focal deficits should prompt the ordering of MR with MR venography.

The pathogenesis of CVT after transplantation remains unclear but is probably multifactorial, with contributions from the underlying disease (e.g., leukemia, nephrotic syndrome), the transient prothrombotic state associated with the transplant procedure itself, and the immunosuppressive medication (e.g., corticosteroids, cyclosporine).

Other surgeries

Isolated case reports described CVT after types of surgery other than those described above include: (1) cardiopulmonary bypass for correction of a ventricular septal defect in a child with antiphospholipid syndrome [98]; (2) coronary artery bypass surgery [99]; (3) thoracoscopic microdiscectomy, complicated by cerebrospinal fluid leak, intracranial hypotension, and fatal CVT with cerebral and cerebellar hemorrhagic infarctions [100]; (4) thoracoscopic surgery for a benign pulmonary mass, with simultaneous pulmonary embolism [101]; and (5) cervical disc arthroplasty [102].

Iatrogenic CVT in the International Study in Cerebral Vein and Dural Sinus Thrombosis

In the ISCVT [53] there were 71 cases out of 624 patients (11.4%) for whom the cause, or if there were multiple causes, one of the causes of CVT was classified as "iatrogenic." The list of medical and surgical intervention included under this heading is listed in Table 23.3.

Not surprisingly, "iatrogenic CVTs" were more frequent among patients recruited in developed than in developing countries. Also, as comorbidities and frequency of medical encounters increase with age, patients with "iatrogenic CVTs" were on average 5.8 years older than the remaining CVT patients (44.2 vs. 38.5 years, P = 0.03). Presentation as a syndrome of isolated intracranial hypertension (12.7 vs. 24.2%, P = 0.29), papilledema (14.3 vs. 30.1%, P = 0.006), headache (81.7 vs. 89.7%, P = 0.045), diplopia/oculomotor palsies (5.6 vs. 14.5%, P = 0.40) were less frequent in the "iatrogenic" group. There were no other demographic, clinical, or neuroimaging differences between the two groups. Delays in admission and diagnosis were also similar in the two groups.

As is often typical of CVT, there was usually more than one contributing cause in 54 (76.1%) of the "iatrogenic CVTs" in the ISCVT. Other concomitant permanent or transient risk factors are shown in Table 23.4, and included 24 (33.8%) patients who had two or more additional risk factors. However, some of these risk factors were less prevalent in the "iatrogenic" subgroup. This was the case of "oral

Table 23.3 Medical and surgical interventions associated with CVT in the International Study of Cerebral Vein and Dural Sinus Thrombosis [53].

Intervention	Number of patients	%
Medications with prothrombotic action	47	66.2
Hormone replacement therapy	27	47.4[a]
Corticosteroids	9	12.7
Anabolic steroids	2	2.8
L-asparaginase	2	2.8
Other chemotherapeutic agents	4	5.6
Tamoxifen	1	1.4
Isotretinoin	1	1.4
Ergotamine	1	1.4
Recent surgery[b]	17	23.9
Neurosurgery	4	5.6
Other surgery	13	18.3
Recent lumbar puncture[b]	12	16.9
Epidural anesthesia	2	2.8
Jugular, subclavian, or other central venous catheter	7	9.9

Some patients had more than one iatrogenic cause.
CVT: cerebral venous thrombosis.
[a] Percent among 57 females
[b] performed <1 month before CVT onset.

contraceptives" (P <0.001), "pregnancy/puerperium" (P = 0.039), and "genetic prothrombotic conditions" (P = 0.036). On the other hand "malignancies" were more frequent among "iatrogenic CVT" patients (P <0.001). This association may be real, due to the prothrombotic state associated with cancer in general and with high white cell or platelet counts. However, it may be in part biased by confounding by indication, as patients with cancer are prescribed medications (e.g., L-asparaginase) and suffer interventions (e.g., lumbar puncture, central venous catheters, neurosurgery) which may also promote CVT.

The outcome of "iatrogenic CVT" was similar as for the remaining ISCVT cohort. Four patients died

Table 23.4 Concomitant risk factors for CVT in patients classified as iatrogenic CVT in the International Study of Cerebral Vein and Dural Sinus Thrombosis [53].

Risk factor	Number of patients	%
Oral contraceptives	8	14.0[a]
Pregnancy/puerperium	4	7.0[a]
Prothrombotic conditions		
Genetic	9	12.7
Acquired	14	19.7
Infections		
Ear, nose, throat	5	7.0
Other (non-CNS)	4	5.6
Malignancies		
CNS	4	5.6
Hematological	7	9.9
Other	6	8.5
Polycythemia/ thrombocythemia	6	8.5
Thyroid disease	2	2.8
Arteriovenous malformation	1	1.4
Beçhet's disease	1	1.4
Dehydration	1	1.4

CVT: cerebral venous thrombosis; CNS: central nervous system.
[a] Percentage among 57 females.

(5.6%) within 30 days from onset. At the last follow-up, 51 (71.8%) had completely recovered (modified Rankin Scale 0 or 1) and only 14 (19.7%) had died or were dependent (modified Rankin Scale 3 to 6). There was, however, a trend (P = 0.06) towards a 6.8% excess on the total number of deaths among the "iatrogenic CVT" subgroup: 10/71 (14.4%) vs. 42/553 (7.6%).

Conclusion

We reviewed the available evidence reporting the association between CVT and several drugs as well as numerous medical and surgical procedures. These "iatrogenic" cases represented 11% of all CVT in the ISCVT cohort. Most reports in the literature are single cases or small series without controls. The causality link is in general weak, except for the

temporal relationship between the intake of the drug or the intervention and CVT. Most patients had complex medical situations, notably cancer or other diseases associated with a prothrombotic state. Some were simultaneously treated with a mechanical intervention and a pharmacological treatment, which could cause venous thrombosis. In such patients, CVT must be considered among the differential diagnoses of neurological deterioration manifested as headache, seizures, decreased vigilance, and focal or multifocal signs.

References

1. de Bruijn S F, Stam J, Koopman M M, Vandenbroucke J P, Cerebral Venous Sinus Thrombosis Study Group. Case-control study of risk of cerebral sinus thrombosis in oral contraceptive users and in [correction of who are] carriers of hereditary prothrombotic conditions. *BMJ.* 1998; **316**:589–92.

2. Martinelli I, Sacchi E, Landi G, *et al.* High risk of cerebral-vein thrombosis in carriers of a prothrombin-gene mutation and in users of oral contraceptives. *N Engl J Med.* 1998; **338**:1793–7.

3. Jick S S, Jick H. Cerebral venous sinus thrombosis in users of four hormonal contraceptives: Levonorgestrel-containing oral contraceptives, norgestimate-containing oral contraceptives, desogestrel-containing oral contraceptives and the contraceptive patch. *Contraception.* 2006; **74**:290–2.

4. Kolacki C, Rocco V. The combined vaginal contraceptive ring, nuvaring, and cerebral venous sinus thrombosis: A case report and review of the literature. *J Emerg Med.* 2012; **42**:413–16.

5. Ou Y C, Kao Y L, Lai S L, *et al.* Thromboembolism after ovarian stimulation: Successful management of a woman with superior sagittal sinus thrombosis after IVF and embryo transfer: Case report. *Hum Reprod.* 2003; **18**:2375–81.

6. Oster J M, Shastri P, Geyer C. Cerebral venous sinus thrombosis after gender reassignment surgery. *Gend Med.* 2010; **7**:270–5.

7. Rajput R, Dhuan J, Agarwal S, Gahlaut P S. Central venous sinus thrombosis in a young woman taking norethindrone acetate for dysfunctional uterine bleeding: Case report and review of literature. *J Obstet Gynaecol Can.* 2008; **30**:680–3.

8. Aidi S, Chaunu M P, Biousse V, Bousser M G. Changing pattern of headache pointing to cerebral venous thrombosis after lumbar puncture and intravenous high-dose corticosteroids. *Headache.* 1999; **39**:559–64.

9. Ohta H, Kinoshita Y, Hashimoto M, *et al.* Superior sagittal sinus thrombosis presenting with subarachnoid

hemorrhage in a patient with aplastic anemia. *No To Shinkei.* 1998; **50**:739–43.

10. Kaito K, Kobayashi M, Otsubo H, *et al.* Superior sagittal sinus thrombosis in a patient with aplastic anemia treated with anabolic steroids. *Int J Hematol.* 1998; **68**:227–9.

11. Chu K, Kang D W, Kim D E, Roh J K. Cerebral venous thrombosis associated with tentorial subdural hematoma during oxymetholone therapy. *J Neurol Sci.* 2001; **185**:27–30.

12. Hamed L M, Glaser J S, Schatz N J, Perez T H. Pseudotumor cerebri induced by danazol. *Am J Ophthalmol.* 1989; **107**:105–10.

13. Satake R, Arakawa S, Hashimoto M, Minamide H, Takamori M. Successful direct thrombolysis in a patient with extensive dural sinus thrombosis induced by danazol. *Rinsho Shinkeigaku.* 1997; **37**:309–13.

14. Hassan K M, Varadarajulu R, Sharma S K, *et al.* Cerebral venous thrombosis in a patient of paroxysmal nocturnal haemoglobinuria following aplastic anaemia. *J Assoc Physicians India.* 2001; **49**:753–5.

15. Jaillard A S, Hommel M, Mallaret M. Venous sinus thrombosis associated with androgens in a healthy young man. *Stroke.* 1994; **25**:212–13.

16. Sahraian M A, Mottamedi M, Azimi A R, Moghimi B. Androgen-induced cerebral venous sinus thrombosis in a young body builder: Case report. *BMC Neurol.* 2004; **4**:22.

17. Grace R F, Dahlberg S E, Neuberg D, *et al.* The frequency and management of asparaginase-related thrombosis in paediatric and adult patients with acute lymphoblastic leukaemia treated on Dana-Farber Cancer Institute consortium protocols. *Br J Haematol.* 2011; **152**:452–9.

18. Levine M N, Gent M, Hirsh J, *et al.* The thrombogenic effect of anticancer drug therapy in women with stage II breast cancer. *N Engl J Med.* 1988; **318**:404–7.

19. Cuzick J, Powles T, Veronesi U, *et al.* Overview of the main outcomes in breast-cancer prevention trials. *Lancet.* 2003; **361**:296–300.

20. Deitcher S R, Gomes M P V. The risk of venous thromboembolic disease associated with adjuvant hormone therapy for breast carcinoma. *Cancer.* 2004; **101**:439–49.

21. Finelli P F, Schauer P K. Cerebral sinus thrombosis with tamoxifen. *Neurology.* 2001; **56**:1113–14.

22. Hitosugi M, Kitamura O, Takatsu A, Watanabe K, Kan S. A case of dural sinus thrombosis during the medication of medroxyprogesterone acetate. *Nihon Hoigaku Zasshi.* 1997; **51**:452–6.

23. Lenz R A, Saver J. Venous sinus thrombosis in a patient taking thalidomide. *Cerebrovasc Dis.* 2004; **18**:175–7.

24. Eudo C, Petit A, Mondon K, *et al.* Cerebral venous thrombosis in an individual with multiple myeloma treated with lenalidomide. *J Am Geriatr Soc.* 2011; **59**:2371–2.

25. Ozen A, Cicin I, Sezer A, *et al.* Dural sinus vein thrombosis in a patient with colon cancer treated with FOLFIRI/bevacizumab. *J Cancer Res Ther.* 2009; **5**:130–2.

26. Vargo J A, Snelling B M, Ghareeb E R, *et al.* Dural venous sinus thrombosis in anaplastic astrocytoma following concurrent temozolomide and focal brain radiotherapy plus bevacizumab. *J Neurooncol.* 2011; **104**:595–8.

27. Karam C, Koussa S. Cerebral dural sinus thrombosis following cisplatin chemotherapy. *J Clin Neurosci.* 2008; **15**:1274–5.

28. Latorre González G, López de Silanes de Miguel C, Escribano Gascón A B. Cerebral venous thrombosis in a chemotherapy patient with dysgerminoma. *An Pediatr.* 2008; **69**:485–6.

29. Al-Shekhlee A, Oghlakian G, Katirji B. A case of cyclosporine-induced dural sinus thrombosis. *J Thromb Haemost.* 2005; **3**:1327–8.

30. Harvey C J, Peniket A J, Miszkiel K, *et al.* MR angiographic diagnosis of cerebral venous sinus thrombosis following allogeneic bone marrow transplantation. *Bone Marrow Transplant.* 2000; **25**:791–5.

31. Mahadeo K M, Dhall G, Panigrahy A, Lastra C, Ettinger L J. Subacute methotrexate neurotoxicity and cerebral venous sinus thrombosis in a 12-year-old with acute lymphoblastic leukemia and methylenetetrahydrofolate reductase (MTHFR) C677T polymorphism: Homocysteine-mediated methotrexate neurotoxicity via direct endothelial injury. *Pediatr Hematol Oncol.* 2010; **27**:46–52.

32. Ciccone M, Rigolin G M, Viglione G M, *et al.* Thrombosis of the cerebral veins and sinuses in acute promyelocytic leukemia after all-trans retinoic acid treatment: A case report. *Blood Coagul Fibrinolysis.* 2008; **19**:721–3.

33. Hotton K M, Khorsand M, Hank J A, *et al.* A phase Ib/II trial of granulocyte-macrophage-colony stimulating factor and interleukin-2 for renal cell carcinoma patients with pulmonary metastases: a case of fatal central nervous system thrombosis. *Cancer.* 2000; **88**:1892–901.

34. Sakurai N, Koike Y, Hashizume Y, Takahashi A. Dural arteriovenous malformation and sinus thromboses in a patient with prostate cancer: an autopsy case. *Intern Med.* 1992; **31**:1032–7.

35. Achiron A, Gornish M, Melamed E. Cerebral sinus thrombosis as a potential hazard of antifibrinolytic treatment in menorrhagia. *Stroke.* 1990; **21**:817–19.

36. Humbert P, Gutknecht J, Mallet H, Dupond J L, Leconte des Floris R. Tranexamic acid and thrombosis of the superior longitudinal sinus. *Therapie*. 1987; **42**:65–6.

37. Worth L L, Hoots W K. Development of a subdural vein thrombosis following aggressive factor VII replacement for postnatal intracranial haemorrhage in a homozygous factor VII-deficient infant. *Haemophilia*. 1998; **4**:757–61.

38. Meýer-Lindenberg A, Quenzel E M, Bierhoff E, *et al.* Fatal cerebral venous sinus thrombosis in heparin-induced thrombotic thrombocytopenia. *Eur Neurol*. 1997; **37**:191–2.

39. Kyritsis A P, Williams E C, Schutta H S. Cerebral venous thrombosis due to heparin-induced thrombocytopenia. *Stroke*. 1990; **21**:1503–5.

40. Jacquin V, Salama J, Le Roux G, Delaporte P. Venous thrombosis in the brain and upper limbs associated with thrombopenia induced by pentosan polysulfate. *Ann Med Interne*. 1988; **139**:194–7.

41. Rice L, Kennedy D, Veach A. Pentosan induced cerebral sagittal sinus thrombosis: a variant of heparin induced thrombocytopenia. *J Urol*. 1998; **160**:2148.

42. Fesler M J, Creer M H, Richart J M, *et al.* Heparin-induced thrombocytopenia and cerebral venous sinus thrombosis: Case report and literature review. *Neurocrit Care*. 2011; **15**:161–5.

43. Evangelou N, Littlewood T, Anslow P, Chapel H. Transverse sinus thrombosis and IV Ig treatment: A case report and discussion of risk-benefit assessment for immunoglobulin treatment. *J Clin Pathol*. 2003; **56**:308–9.

44. Barada W, Muwakkit S, Hourani R, Bitar M, Mikati M. Cerebral sinus thrombosis in a patient with humoral immunodeficiency on intravenous immunoglobulin therapy: A case report. *Neuropediatrics*. 2008; **39**:131–3.

45. Al-Riyami A Z, Lee J, Connolly M, Shereck E. Cerebral sinus thrombosis following IV immunoglobulin therapy of immune thrombocytopenia purpura. *Pediatr Blood Cancer*. 2011; **57**:157–9.

46. Finelli P F, Carley M D. Cerebral venous thrombosis associated with epoetin alfa therapy. *Arch Neurol*. 2000; **57**:260–2.

47. Lage J M, Panizo C, Masdeu J, Rocha E. Cyclist's doping associated with cerebral sinus thrombosis. *Neurology*. 2002; **58**:665.

48. Werring D, Hacking D, Losseff N, *et al.* Cerebral venous sinus thrombosis may be associated with clozapine. *J Neuropsychiatry Clin Neurosci*. 2009; **21**:343–5.

49. Evans M S, Naritoku D K, Couch J R, Ghobrial M W. Onset of neurologic deficits after treatment with dihydroergotamine in a patient with sagittal sinus thrombosis. *Clin Neuropharmacol*. 1996; **19**:177–84.

50. Thorat J D, Ng I. Acute dural sinus thrombosis following ingestion of an herbal tonic: case report. *J Stroke Cerebrovasc Dis*. 2007; **16**:232–5.

51. Guimarães J, Azevedo E. Phytoestrogens as a risk factor for cerebral sinus thrombosis. *Cerebrovasc Dis*. 2005; **20**:137–8.

52. Bousser M G, Russell R R. Cerebral venous thrombosis. In Warlow C P, Van Gijn J, eds. *Major Problems in Neurology*. London, UK: WB Saunders; 1997; 27–9.

53. Ferro J M, Canhão P, Stam J, Bousser M G, Barinagarrementeria F, ISCVT Investigators. Prognosis of cerebral vein and dural sinus thrombosis: Results of the International Study on Cerebral Vein and Dural Sinus Thrombosis (ISCVT). *Stroke*. 2004; **35**:664–70.

54. Saadatnia M, Fatehi F, Basiri K, Mousavi S A, Mehr G K. Cerebral venous sinus thrombosis risk factors. *Int J Stroke*. 2009; **4**:111–23.

55. Canhão P, Batista P, Falcão F. Lumbar puncture and dural sinus thrombosis: A causal or casual association? *Cerebrovasc Dis*. 2005; **19**:53–6.

56. Albucher J F, Vuillemin-Azaïs C, Manelfe C, *et al.* Cerebral thrombophlebitis in three patients with probable multiple sclerosis. Role of lumbar puncture or intravenous corticosteroid treatment. *Cerebrovasc Dis*. 1999; **9**:298–303.

57. Aidi S, Chaunu M P, Biousse V, Bousser M G. Changing pattern of headache pointing to cerebral venous thrombosis after lumbar puncture and intravenous high-dose corticosteroids. *Headache*. 1999; **39**:559–64.

58. Bienfait H P, Gijtenbeek J M, van den Bent M J, *et al.* Cerebral venous and sinus thrombosis with cerebrospinal fluid circulation block after the first methotrexate administration by lumbar puncture. *Neuroradiology*. 2002; **44**:929–32.

59. Ergan M, Hansen von Bünau F, Courthéoux P, *et al.* Cerebral vein thrombosis after an intrathecal glucocorticoid injection. *Rev Rhum Engl Ed*. 1997; **64**:513–16.

60. Milhaud D, Heroum C, Charif M, *et al.* Dural puncture and corticotherapy as risks factors for cerebral venous sinus thrombosis. *Eur J Neurol*. 2000; **7**:123–4.

61. Brugeilles H, Pénisson-Besnier I, Pasco A, *et al.* Cerebral venous thrombosis after myelography with iopamidol. *Neuroradiology*. 1996; **38**:534–6.

62. Miglis M G, Levine D N. Intracranial venous thrombosis after placement of a lumbar drain. *Neurocrit Care*. 2010; **12**:83–7.

63. Ravindran R S, Zandstra G C. Cerebral venous thrombosis versus postlumbar puncture headache. *Anesthesiology*. 1989; **71**:478–9.

64. Kueper M, Goericke S L, Kastrup O. Cerebral venous thrombosis after epidural blood patch: coincidence or

causal relation? A case report and review of the literature. *Cephalalgia*. 2008; 287:769–73.

65. Oz O, Akgun H, Yücel M, Battal B, *et al*. Cerebral venous thrombosis presenting with subarachnoid hemorrhage after spinal anesthesia. *Acta Neurol Belg*. 2011; 111:237–40.

66. Wilder-Smith E, Kothbauer-Margreiter I, Lämmle B, *et al*. Dural puncture and activated protein C resistance: risk factors for cerebral venous sinus thrombosis. *J Neurol Neurosurg Psychiatry*. 1997; **63**:351–6.

67. Floyd W L, Mahaley M S. Cerebral dural venous sinus thrombosis following cardiac pacemaker implantation. *Arch Intern Med*. 1969; **124**:368–72.

68. Birdwell B G, Yeager R, Whitsett T L. Pseudotumor cerebri. A complication of catheter-induced subclavian vein thrombosis. *Arch Intern Med*. 1994; **154**:808–11.

69. Hurst R W, Kerns S R, McIlhenny J, Park T S, Cail W S. Neonatal dural venous sinus thrombosis associated with central venous catheterization: CT and MR studies. *J Comput Assist Tomogr*. 1989; **13**:504–7.

70. Mazzoleni S, Putti M C, Simioni P, *et al*. Early cerebral sinovenous thrombosis in a child with acute lymphoblastic leukemia carrying the prothrombin G20210A variant: A case report and review of the literature. *Blood Coagul Fibrinolysis*. 2005; **16**:43–9.

71. Holmes F A, Obbens E A, Griffin E, Lee Y Y. Cerebral venous sinus thrombosis in a patient receiving adjuvant chemotherapy for stage II breast cancer through an implanted central venous catheter. *Am J Clin Oncol*. 1987; **10**:362–6.

72. Souter R G, Mitchell A. Spreading cortical venous thrombosis due to infusion of hyperosmolar solution into the internal jugular vein. *Br Med J*. 1982; **285**:935–6.

73. Gandhi C D, Meyer S A, Patel A B, Johnson D M, Post K D. Neurologic complications of inferior petrosal sinus sampling. *Am J Neuroradiol*. 2008; **29**:760–5.

74. Burton J M, Alikhani K, Goyal M, *et al*. Complications in MS patients after CCSVI procedures abroad (Calgary, AB). *Can J Neurol Sci*. 2011; **38**:741–6.

75. Imperial College CCSVI Investigation Group, Thapar A, Lane T R, Pandey V, *et al*. Internal jugular thrombosis post venoplasty for chronic cerebrospinal venous insufficiency. *Phlebology*. 2011; **26**:254–6.

76. Keiper G L Jr, Sherman J D, Tomsick T A, Tew J M Jr. Dural sinus thrombosis and pseudotumor cerebri: Unexpected complications of suboccipital craniotomy and translabyrinthine craniectomy. *J Neurosurg*. 1999; **91**:192–7.

77. Garrido E, Fahs G R. Cerebral venous and sagittal sinus thrombosis after transcallosal removal of a colloid cyst of the third ventricle: case report. *Neurosurgery*. 1990; **26**:540–2.

78. Nakase H, Shin Y, Nakagawa I, Kimura R, Sakaki T. Clinical features of postoperative cerebral venous infarction. *Acta Neurochir*. 2005; **147**:621–6.

79. Roberson J B Jr, Brackmann D E, Fayad J N. Complications of venous insufficiency after neurotologic-skull base surgery. *Am J Otol*. 2000; **21**:701–5.

80. Lega B C, Yoshor D. Postoperative dural sinus thrombosis in a patient in a hypercoagulable state. Case report. *J Neurosurg*. 2006; **105**:772–4.

81. Jang W Y, Jung S, Jung T Y, Moon K S, Kim I Y. Predictive factors related to symptomatic venous infarction after meningioma surgery. *Br J Neurosurg*. 2012; **26**(5):705–9.

82. Son W S, Park J. Cerebral venous thrombosis complicated by hemorrhagic infarction secondary to ventriculoperitoneal shunting. *J Korean Neurosurg Soc*. 2010; **48**:357–9.

83. Singleton R H, Jankowitz B T, Wecht D A, Gardner P A. Iatrogenic cerebral venous sinus occlusion with flowable topical hemostatic matrix. *J Neurosurg*. 2011; **115**:576–83.

84. Mahasin Z Z, Saleem M, Gangopadhyay K. Transverse sinus thrombosis and venous infarction of the brain following unilateral radical neck dissection. *J Laryngol Otol*. 1998; **112**:88–91.

85. Garg N, Sampath S. Fatal delayed post-operative cerebral venous thrombosis after excision of hypoglossal nerve schwannoma. *Acta Neurochir*. 2008; **150**:605–9.

86. Sekhar L N, Tzortzidis F N, Bejjani G K, Schessel D A. Saphenous vein graft bypass of the sigmoid sinus and jugular bulb during the removal of glomus jugulare tumors. Report of two cases. *J Neurosurg*. 1997; **86**:1036–41.

87. Izadi S, Karkos P D, Krishnan R, Hsuan J, Lesser T H. Papilloedema secondary to venous sinus thrombosis following glomus jugulare tumour surgery. *J Laryngol Otol*. 2009; **123**:1393–5.

88. Ivan M E, Sughrue M E, Clark A J, *et al*. A meta-analysis of tumor control rates and treatment-related morbidity for patients with glomus jugulare tumors. *J Neurosurg*. 2011; **114**:1299–305.

89. Shah V A, Yang G S, Randhawa S, Hansen M R, Lee A G. Cerebral venous sinus thrombosis following jugular bulb decompression. *Semin Ophthalmol*. 2006; **21**:41–4.

90. Kania R, Lot G, Herman P, Tran Ba Huy P. Vascular complications after acoustic neurinoma surgery. *Ann Otolaryngol Chir Cervicofac*. 2003; **120**:94–102.

91. Haddad F S, Hubballa J, Zaytoun G, Haddad G F. Intracranial complications of submucous

resection of the nasal septum. *Am J Otolaryngol.* 1985; **6**:443–7.

92. Schummer W, Schummer C, Niesen W D. Unrecognized internal jugular vein obstruction: cause of fatal intracranial hypertension after tracheostomy? *J Neurosurg Anesthesiol.* 2002; **14**:313–15.

93. Bertz H, Laubenberger J, Steinfurth G, Finke J. Sinus venous thrombosis: an unusual cause for neurologic symptoms after bone marrow transplantation under immunosuppression. *Transplantation.* 1998; **66**:241–4.

94. Motohashi K, Hagihara M, Ito S, *et al.* Cerebral venous sinus thrombosis after allogeneic stem cell transplantation. *Int J Hematol.* 2010; **91**:154–6.

95. Nayak S G, Satish R, Gokulnath G. Extensive cerebral venous thrombosis in a renal allograft recipient. *Saudi J Kidney Dis Transpl.* 2008; **19**:90–3.

96. Yardimci N, Colak T, Sevmis S, *et al.* Neurologic complications after renal transplant. *Exp Clin Transplant.* 2008; **6**:224–8.

97. Ballarin R, Di Benedetto F, De Ruvo N, *et al.* Thrombosis of developmental venous anomalies of the brain after liver transplantation. *Transplantation.* 2009; **87**:615–16.

98. Emir M, Ozisik K, Cagli K, *et al.* Dural sinus thrombosis after cardiopulmonary bypass. *Perfusion.* 2004; **19**:133–5.

99. Zervakis D, Angelidakis P, Dedeilias P, Koutsoukou A. Cerebral vein thrombosis after coronary artery bypass surgery. *Interact Cardiovasc Thorac Surg.* 2007; **6**:514–16.

100. Cornips E M, Staals J, Stavast A, Rijkers K, van Oostenbrugge R J. Fatal cerebral and cerebellar hemorrhagic infarction after thoracoscopic microdiscectomy. Case report. *J Neurosurg Spine.* 2007; **6**:276–9.

101. Sakai T, Ogura Y, Kimura D, *et al.* Pulmonary embolism and cerebral venous thrombosis after thoracoscopic surgery for benign pulmonary disease. *Gen Thorac Cardiovasc Surg.* 2008; **56**:570–4.

102. Altaf F, Derbyshire N, Marshall R W. Cerebral venous sinus thrombosis following cervical disc arthroplasty. *J Bone Joint Surg Br.* 2010; **92**:576–8.

Chapter

24

Treatment of oral anticoagulant related intracranial hemorrhages

Mushtaq H. Qureshi, J. Alfredo Caceres and Adnan I. Qureshi

Introduction

Oral anticoagulants (OAC) are widely prescribed for the prevention of thromboembolic events in patients with atrial fibrillation, venous thrombosis, and artificial heart valves. Despite a reduction in thromboembolic events, there is a risk of intracranial hemorrhage (ICH) associated with OACs. In this chapter, we describe the treatment of OAC-related ICH and those related to other forms of anticoagulation.

Epidemiology

The global incidence of spontaneous ICH is 24.6 per 100,000 person-years with approximately 40,000 to 67,000 cases per year in the United States [1]. Anticoagulant-associated intracerebral hemorrhage (AAICH) is estimated to be responsible for approximately 20% of all primary ICH cases [2,3]. The incidence of AAICH has increased over the past years in the United States, but has apparently decreased in northern Europe. Independently of this disagreement, it is clear that the use of warfarin has quadrupled in the last two decades and that ICH comprise 70% of all intracranial hemorrhages that are related to the use of anticoagulants, with the remainder being mostly subdural hemorrhages [4]. The risk is associated with the use of anticoagulants and not consistently with the intensity of anticoagulation such as the international normalized ratio (INR) value; the incidence is high even in patients with normal INR values. Only 6% of AAICH had values above 3.0 according to one large study [5].

Mechanism of ICH related to OACs

Use of anticoagulants appears to be an added risk factor in the setting of an underlying vasculopathy, rather than the only cause of the ICH. The anatomic location of the ICH does not differ from those ICH events in patients not on anticoagulants, although those deep (non-lobar) ICHs tend to be significantly larger in volume compared to those in patients using OAC and could imply a higher susceptibility to the effects of anticoagulation from those deep perforating arteries [6].

Oral anticoagulants belong to the group of vitamin K antagonists (VKAs) and are represented by warfarin, acenocoumarol, and phenprocoumon, which differ in regards to plasma half-life. Although new anticoagulants have been recently approved by the US Food and Drug Administration (FDA) agency, warfarin remains the most widely available and utilized oral anticoagulant. Current approved indications include the acute treatment of venous thromboembolism (VTE), antiphospholipid syndrome (APS), prevention of cardioembolic stroke in atrial fibrillation (AF), in patients undergoing elective cardioversion, valvular heart disease and prosthetic valves, peripheral vascular disease, myocardial infarction and cardiomyopathy (although the use for this indication is now less common), pulmonary embolism (PE) and deep vein thrombosis (DVT), including cancer-associated DVT [7]. Warfarin interferes with the hepatic carboxylation of vitamin K-dependent coagulation factors II, VII, IX, and X via inhibition of vitamin K epoxide reductase complex 1 (VKORC1). Intracranial hemorrhage occurs as a consequence of bleeding diasthesis induced by warfarin [8].

The new agents can be divided accordingly in two groups: (1) direct thrombin inhibitor, represented by dabigatran, and (2) factor Xa inhibitors, represented by rivaroxaban, apixaban, and edoxaban.

As a direct thrombin inhibitor (DTI), dabigatran results in ICH by directly binding to thrombin, inhibiting its interaction with other coagulation factors and the activation of the coagulation cascade.

Treatment-Related Stroke, ed. Alexander Tsiskaridze, Arne Lindgren and Adnan Qureshi. Published by Cambridge University Press. © Cambridge University Press 2016.

Unlike heparin, dabigatran acts independently of antithrombin, inhibiting not only free and soluble thrombin but also the activated fibrin-bound thrombin. Subsequently, dabigatran also decreases the thrombin-mediated activation of platelets and reduces the rate of pulmonary embolism and death in patients with deep venous thrombosis [9–11]. Rivaroxaban and apixaban are oral agents that directly inhibit coagulation factor Xa and the subsequent activation of thrombin, resulting in bleeding diasthesis. Similar to DTIs, factor Xa inhibitors act on soluble and fibrin-bound thrombin. These agents have renal excretion, which may result in accumulation in patients with renal insufficiency [12].

Laboratory measurement of intensity of anticoagulation by OACs

At the time of occurrence of OAC-related ICH, serial measurements of concentration of anticoagulation are important to determine the risk of hematoma expansion and efficacy of reversal.

A brief explanation of various coagulation assays is provided below:

Prothrombin time (PT)

Warfarin is monitored in the lab with prothrombin time and INR. Prothrombin time is the time required in seconds for plasma to coagulate after the addition of calcium and thromboplastin to citrated plasma [13]. Most often warfarin levels are measured using this assay because it inhibits factors II, VII, IX, and X. Inhibition or absence of these factors causes prolongation of PT. Varying sensitivities of the available thromboplastin agents to the reduction in coagulation factors is one of the disadvantages of the PT assay [14].

International normalized ratio (INR)

To correct the varying sensitivity of thromboplastin, PT is converted to normalized ratio using a mathematical calculation that accounts for the manufacturer's international sensitivity index. Once calculated, the INR can be evaluated without regard to the thromboplastin reagent used in the PT assay [14].

Dilute prothrombin time (dPT)

Although it has been used to screen lupus anticoagulant, its use may be helpful in monitoring the intensity of anticoagulation with newer anticoagulants. It differs from the prothrombin time in terms of using a diluted thromboplastin reagent [15].

Thrombin time (TT)

This test measures the activity of thrombin in plasma and can measure the activity of various anticoagulants. It carries a very high sensitivity in measuring the activity of newer anticoagulants (e.g., dabigatran), which work by directly inhibiting the activity of thrombin [16].

Ecarin clotting time

Ecarin – an enzyme derived from snake venom – is the primary reagent in the Ecarin clotting time test. It functions by activating prothrombin, which in turn stimulates meizothrombin, a precursor to thrombin [17].

Activated partial thromboplastin time (aPTT)

This assay is commonly used to monitor heparin in an inpatient setting, and is reflective of the activity and presence of factors II, V, VIII–XII, and fibrinogen. Therefore anticoagulants that inhibit these factors will cause an increase in aPTT [18].

Heptest

This test is indicated for the quantification of intensity of anticoagulation with heparin, low molecular weight heparin (LMWH) and heparinoids, and possibly new anticoagulants [19]. The Heptest is based on the ability of heparin to catalyze the inactivation of factor Xa; however, it is not specific for factor Xa and can be influenced by other agents that inhibit factor IIa [20].

Prothrombinase-induced clotting time (PiCT)

The prothrombinase-induced clotting time assay measures the coagulation time after the combination of factor Xa, phospholipids, and an enzyme that activates factor V, is activated when patient plasma is added. Currently the test is only approved for measuring the effects of unfractionated heparin (UFH) and LMWHs but it is also being evaluated to measure the effect of newer anticoagulants [21].

Chromogenic assays

In these assays, the ability of the factor to cleave a chromogenic-linked substrate is assessed (Table 24.1).

Table 24.1 Utility of various assays for the newer anticoagulants.

Assay	Dabigatran	Rivaroxaban	Apixaban
PT	Not ideal; widely available	Widespread availability makes PT useful	Widespread availability makes PT useful
dPT	Not widely available; lacks FDA approval	Not widely available; lacks FDA approval	Not widely available; lacks FDA approval
Thrombin time	Sensitivity limits utility in quantifying anticoagulation	Not useful	Not useful
Ecarin clotting time	Limited availability; lacks FDA approval	Not useful	Not useful
aPTT	Availability and sensitivity support use	Not ideal; widely available	Not ideal; widely available
Heptest	Not likely to be useful	Not widely available; lacks FDA approval	Not widely available; lacks FDA approval
PiCT	Not likely to be useful	Not widely available; lacks FDA approval	Not widely available; lacks FDA approval
Chromogenic antifactor IIa	Minimal data and not currently available	Most promising assay	Most promising assay

PT: prothrombin time; dPT: dilute prothrombin time; FDA: Food and Drug Administration; aPTT: activated partial thromboplastin time; PiCT: prothrombinase-induced clotting time.

Treatment

Following the diagnosis, current guidelines indicate that reversal of the anticoagulation should be promptly initiated.

The initial approach to a patient with an AAICH is similar to other medical emergencies. The first consideration is given to protecting the airway. Endotracheal intubation may be required in patients with a Glasgow Coma Scale score below 8, impairment in reflexes that protect the airway, or patients with brain stem dysfunction [22]. Rapid sequence intubation is typically the preferred approach in the acute setting. Depending on the general medical and neurological condition, admission to an intensive care unit (ICU) should be considered, frequently for intracranial pressure (ICP) monitoring and treatment. Blood pressure should be under close control, hyperglycemia and fever should be prevented, and seizure prophylaxis be considered. A rapid neurosurgical evaluation should also be requested [23].

The overall concept of anticoagulation reversal is aimed at correcting and normalizing the INR with a target goal of ≤1.4 to ≤1.2 [24]. Early treatment is critical as it is known that hematoma expansion

occurs in the acute stage (27% during the first 3 hours from the onset of symptoms and reported up to 17 hours). Early reversal is recommended to reduce the chance of further hematoma expansion and allow urgent surgical evacuations in neurologically deteriorating patients with anticoagulation-related ICH [25]. Agents available for the reversal of anticoagulation are vitamin K, fresh frozen plasma (FFP), prothrombin complex concentrates (PCC), and recombinant factor VIIa (FVIIa). Newer anticoagulants, for example dabigatran, lack antidotes and their reversal requires supportive treatment [9]. The preferential use of the reversal agents differs in different parts of the world according to local availability and scientific societies guidelines (Table 24.2).

Vitamin K

Vitamin K is the first-line agent in the acute treatment of AAICH. Intravenous administration is the preferred route due to unpredictable absorption rate by the intramuscular and subcutaneous route. Vitamin K should be started promptly at a dose of 5 to 10 mg and given slowly over 30 minutes due to the potential for anaphylaxis, which is rare and is estimated to occur

Table 24.2 Recommendations for the treatment of AAICH according to scientific societies.

Scientific society (year)	Preferred choice	Secondary choice	Use of vitamin K (route of administration)
ASTH (2004)	FFP + PCC	–	Yes (IV)
AHA/ASA (2010)	FFP	PCC	Yes (IV)
ACCP (2012)	PCC	FFP	Yes (IV)
BSH (2011)	PCC	FFP	Yes (IV)
EUSI (2006)	FFP or PCC	–	Yes (IV)

FFP: fresh frozen plasma; PCC: prothrombin complex concentrates; IV: intravenous.

in 3 per 10,000 doses and infrequently fatal [27]. A second or third dose of 5 to 10 mg may be administered every 12 hours, not exceeding a total dose of 25 mg. Vitamin K has a slow onset of action requiring on average time ranging from 6 to 24 hours to normalize the INR [28].

Fresh frozen plasma

Fresh frozen plasma (FFP) is obtained from the separation of cellular components in whole blood collections and stored at −18°C within 6 to 8 hours of phlebotomy. It contains all coagulation factors and is prepared in bags of 200 to 250 ml for infusion [29].

The main advantages of FFP are its widespread availability and relative low cost; however, one of the major disadvantages is the delay in correction of the INR and the anticoagulation status within the first 24 hours. For every 30 minutes of delay in the first dose of FFP, there is an associated 20% decrease in the odds of INR reversal within 24 hours [30]. To utilize FFP therapy, the blood type from the donor has to match the recipient's blood type, which could incur a delay of up to 60 minutes for determination of the blood type after the frozen units are thawed (may take 30 to 45 minutes). Due to the high sodium content, units have to be infused slowly at a rate of at least 30 minutes per unit to avoid circulatory overload [31].

The use of FFP is also associated with the risk of developing adverse events that include (1) transfusion-related acute lung injury (TRALI), with a reported mortality rate of 5 to 25% [32]; (2) volume overload, the initial dose is 10 to 15 mL/kg, which could imply up to 2 liters of extra volume; (3) allergic reactions, which are usually mild and self-limited and have an incidence of about 1:591 to 1:2,184 per unit of plasma transfused; and (4) transmission of infectious agents, which is less frequently reported [33].

Prothrombin complex concentrate

Prothrombin complex concentrate (PCC) is a highly concentrated combination of coagulation factors extracted from plasma. There are currently two commercially available forms of PCC that primarily differ in the content of factor VII. The three-factor PCC contains factors II, IX, and X and was the only form available in the United States for many years. This product is commercialized as Bebulin (Baxter Healthcare Corporation, Westlake Village, CA, USA) and Profilnine (Grifols Biologicals, Inc., Los Angeles, CA, USA). The four-factor PCC contains factors II, VII, IX, and X and is available in many regions of the world including Canada, Europe, and Australia. In the United States, the only four-factor PCC was approved by the FDA in April of 2013 "for the urgent reversal of anticoagulation in adults with major bleeding". It is currently marketed under the name of Kcentra (CSL Behring, King of Prussia, PA, USA).

Treatment with PCC reverses anticoagulation more rapidly than FFP [34]. Prothrombin complex concentrate administration was associated with a reduced incidence and extent of hematoma growth compared with FFP and VKA in one study, presumably due to more rapid INR reversal. However, the rates of hematoma growth and death or disability showed no difference between the patients who were treated with either PCC or FFP, if the INR was completely reversed within two hours of admission [35,36].

Recombinant factor VIIa

Recombinant factor VIIa (rFVIIa) has been approved to treat the bleeding episodes in type A and B hemophiliacs with inhibitors to factors VIII or IX, patients with congenital factor VII deficiency, and acquired hemophiliacs. In the European Union it is also approved for the treatment of Glanzmann thrombasthenia [26]. In the management of AAICH there have been many case reports that explain the successful use of rFVIIa in normalizing the INR, but there are concerns that the effect on patient outcomes may be limited [37]. rFVIIa has been shown to be effective in reversing therapeutic INRs to normal at varying doses (10 μg/kg to a maximum of 400 μg/kg) in healthy volunteers and in reversing supratherapeutic INRs and/or bleeding in patients on warfarin. Dager *et al.* [38] found that a dose of approximately 16 μg/kg was adequate for rapid reversal. The significance of rFVIIa in spontaneous ICH patients who were not on warfarin anticoagulation reduces growth of the hematoma if administered within four hours of onset [39], although survival or functional outcome were not improved [40]. Another trial compared increasing doses of rFVIIa with placebo in patients with traumatic ICH who were not on VKAs [41], and in those patients there was no significant difference in mortality or adverse events among treatment groups, although asymptomatic deep vein thrombosis was more frequent in patients who received any dose of rFVIIa. Higher rFVIIa dose was associated with lower hemorrhage volume and less hematoma progression, although the association was not statistically significant. A meta-analysis of various randomized controlled trials concluded that rFVIIa could reduce hemorrhage progression in ICH, but there was no significant improvement in mortality or function status and it was associated with increased risk of thromboembolic events [42]. Although guidelines have been published that describe the off-label use of rFVIIa in AAICH (Table 24.3), the most recent ones proscribe against use of rFVIIa for treating AAICH [43,44].

Current guidelines

Early diagnosis and initiating treatment is of utmost importance. The sudden eruption of an ICH displaces brain tissue and can result in an increase in ICP [48]. Neurological status should be assessed at frequent intervals using standard stroke scales such as the National Institutes of Health Stroke Scale (NIHSS) [49] and coma scales such as the Glasgow Coma Scale (GCS) [50]. Systemic arterial pressure should be monitored in patients whose neurological status is deteriorating and who require continuous IV

Table 24.3 Recommendations regarding use of recombinant factor VIIA.

Society (year)	Recommendations
SABM/UHC (2005) [45]	Appropriate for spontaneous or traumatic intracranial bleeding in patients on warfarin
EU societies (2006) [46]	Patients on warfarin anticoagulation not addressed
Northern Ireland (2007) [13]	If ongoing significant hemorrhage after correction of clotting factor deficiencies
ASH (2008) [47]	Not indicated

SABM: Society for Advancement of Blood Management; UHC: University Hospitals Consortium; EU: European Union; ASH: American Society of Hematology.

administration of antihypertensive medications. Pulse oximetry and respiratory status can be used to assess airway and oxygenation. There is evidence that admission of ICH patients to a neuroscience intensive care unit may result in a reduced mortality rate [51]. Metabolic and hemodynamic variables assessment by multimodal monitoring can provide crucial information at the cellular level. Continuous or frequent assessment of these variables in terms of brain tissue oxygenation, CBF, and intracerebral microdialysis provide critical physiological information about brain function in acute brain injury patients, but their efficacy in ICH patients has not been tested in randomized clinical trials.

The growth of the hematoma is promoted by the anticoagulant in the first 3 to 6 hours and reaches plateau by 24 hours after the onset, so it is important to rapidly reverse the anticoagulant action to mitigate poor outcome and mortality. Higher INR (>3) is associated with a larger hematoma volume and growth, which in turn is a predictor of poor outcome and mortality [52]. According to a study performed by Davis *et al.* [52] for each cubic centimeter increase in baseline ICH volume, the hazard ratio of death increases by 1%, and the patient is 6% more likely to have a one-point worsening of the modified Rankin scale for survivors. The combined use of IV vitamin K, PCC, or FFP and rFVIIa is usually recommended even though one regimen is not superior to the other [53]. According to the AHA/ASA Stroke Council the PCC, factor IX concentrate, and rFVIIa normalize the laboratory elevation of the INR with lower volumes of fluids as compared to FFP and rapidly, however, with a greater thromboembolic potential [54]. Fresh frozen plasma is an alternative, but with much longer infusion times and greater fluid volume requirement (Class IIb, LOE B). Patients with ICH related to anticoagulants should receive treatment with IV vitamin K to counteract the effects of warfarin, and replacement of clotting factors (Class IIb, LOE B). The reversal of warfarin-induced ICH can be achieved promptly by PCC or rFVIIa; however, due to the short half-lives of these agents there may be an increase in the INR in the ensuing hours and hence the patient requires monitoring [25].

Taking into account the heterogeneity in the guidelines by professional societies in the management of AAICH, the following management strategy is recommended:

- Patient's ABO/Rh blood type should be determined.
- Vitamin K (5 to 10 mg) should be started by slow intravenous infusion over 30 minutes and again in 12 hour period.
- Prothrombin complex concentrate and fresh frozen plasma (see below for calculation of dose and volume requirements).
- rFVIIa – there is not any fixed recommendation on the dose; however, fixed-vial dosing of 2 mg would provide 20 to 40 u/kg for patients between 50 kg and 100 kg of body weight.

Calculating the dose of PCC or the volume of FFP

- Decide on the "goal" INR.
- Convert INR to percent (%) functional prothrombin complex, using table below.

INR range	Functional prothrombin complex (%)
>5	5
4.0–4.9	10
2.6–3.2	15
2.2–2.5	20
1.9–2.1	25
1.7–1.8	30
1.4–1.6	40
1.0	100

How to calculate dose: (target in % PC – current level in % PC) × body weight (kg) = ml of FFP or IU of PCC needed.

For example: a patient arrives with an INR of 4.5, target INR is 1.5, body weight is 80 kg. Therefore (40 – 10) × 80 = 2,400. So the required dose calculated is 2,400 mL of FFP or 2,400 IU of PCC [55].

Reversal of INR as part of quality metrics for intensity of care in patients with ICH

Reversal of the INR has been included as one of the evidence-based dataset of elements as part of the quality metrics for intensity of care in patients with ICH [25]. Two measures were selected among a total of 26 quality indicators related to 18 facets of care with thresholds for quality response that were identified.

The two indices associated with the reversal of INR were (1) rapid reversal, and (2) use of multiple agents for reversal.

Various studies have shown the significance of and have validated the rapid reversal of INR. Huttner et al. [35] in one of the studies showed a trend for reduced extent of hematoma among patients with early INR reversal compared with those without reversal (38% vs. 54%). According to one study by Goldstein et al. [30] every 30-minute delay in FFP and vitamin K administration was independently associated with a 20% decrease in the probability of successful INR reversal in 24 hours. On the other hand, at least two agents within two hours of first INR >1.4 were recommended. The agents were not specified, but a combination of IV vitamin K, PCC, or FFP and rfVIIa is usually recommended without clear evidence of superiority of one regimen over another [53].

Validation of the ICH-specific intensity of care quality metrics has been provided by Qureshi et al. in a study that supports their broader use for improving and standardizing medical care among patients with ICH [56]. The intensity of care quality metric score ranged from 17 to 26 points. The mean score was higher in those who survived compared with those who died (23 ± 3 vs. 21 ± 2; P = 0.02). The receiver operating characteristic curve demonstrated a high discriminating ability of intensity of care quality metrics for in-hospital mortality (0.730, 95% CI 0.591 to 0.869) and a C-statistic of 0.91 (95% CI 0.90–0.92). The correlation of the new ICH-specific intensity of care quality metric with in-hospital mortality supports the therapeutic value of early and effective reversal of INR when used in combination with other medical interventions.

Reversal of new oral anticoagulants

For dabigatran, since there is no antidote, supportive treatment is needed initially and dabigatran should be stopped immediately [11]. Further management should be individualized based on the severity of bleeding. Since dabigatran is primarily excreted in the urine adequate diuresis is required. In cases of thrombocytopenia and use of antiplatelet drugs, transfusion with FFP, platelets and red cell concentrates may be needed. Various diagnostic tests such as TT, aPTT, and ECT may be helpful in guiding therapy [9]. Although we lack published data to support their

use [57], specific reversal agents such as recombinant activated factor VII (rFVIIa) [58] and PCCs [59] may be considered. Both rFVIIa and PCCs have been reported to have thrombogenic potential; therefore, as in all emergency situations, a risk–benefit evaluation regarding the use of this treatment is mandated. Surgical consideration is an option in life-threatening conditions. Finally, if all the above measures fail, hemodialysis can remove about 60% of the drug in 2 to 4 hours [60].

When do we restart the patient on anticoagulants?

The indication for restarting oral anticoagulation should be carefully balanced with the risk of a new warfarin-associated ICH. There are currently no

Table 24.4 Studies that reported data on restarting oral anticoagulation in patients with AAICH[a].

Studies (years)	Number of patients	Restarting anticoagulation and outcomes
Punthakee et al. (2002) [62]	7	Warfarin therapy was started at a mean of 14 days (9–15 days in 4 patients); thrombotic events or ICH enlargement not noted.
Bertram et al. (2000) [66]	13	Full dose of IV heparin was administered on days 1 and 2, in 7 patients. Hematoma enlargement was noted in 2 of 6 patients given low-dose heparin, 3 had ischemic strokes on the 2nd, 4th and 5th day. (All previously treated with prothrombin complex concentrates.)
Butler & Tait (1998) [67]	4	Heparin administered on day 3 (range, 1–6) and warfarin was given on day 7 (range, 3–19) in 10 patients with ICHs (n = 4) or subdural hematomas (n = 6); no ICH enlargement or thrombotic events.
Phan et al. (2000) [63]	87	Anticoagulation withheld for a mean of 10 days, acute treatment to reverse anticoagulation was not reported, and 1 ischemic stroke; the 30-day thromboembolism rate was estimated to be 3% for those patients who had prosthetic cardiac valves.
Leker & Abramsky (1998) [65]	4	4 patients were administered intravenous heparin 24–36 hours as soon as INR was <1.5 after vitamin K and plasma infusion; no worsening was noted.
Kawamata et al. (1995) [68]	13	6 patients underwent surgery; of 20 patients with intracranial hemorrhages and prosthetic valves, 1 thromboembolism was noticed in the setting of early postoperative heparin.
Babikian et al. (1988) [69]	3	Of 6 patients with prosthetic cardiac valves (3 with ICH and 3 with subdural), warfarin therapy was interrupted for a mean of 19 days without any incidence of thromboembolism.
Gomez et al. (1988) [70]	1	Heparin was administered on day 10 without hemorrhagic worsening in 1 patient.

[a] Reports and/or cases with surgical evacuation are excluded.

ICH: intracerebral hemorrhage; INR: international normalized ratio.

studies that provide us with an accurate approximation of the risk of recurrent ICH in patients who have survived AAICH and who are subsequently undergoing anticoagulation [28]. There is a wide range of data that mentions about withholding warfarin from four to six weeks [61] to one to two weeks [62–64], and to the use of intravenous heparin [65,66] immediately after the INR is normalized. Overall the data (8 studies involving 132 patients) suggest a low risk of thromboembolic complications between 7 and 14 days after anticoagulation reversal in patients with warfarin-associated ICH (Table 24.4).

Conclusion

Successful management of AAICH includes a wide range of treatments in the absence of adequate data. Limitations to successful management include unfamiliarity with the need for IV administration of vitamin K by clinicians and hospital pharmacies and the challenging inventory management strategies for providing emergency plasma therapy. In addition, approval status and availability of four-factor PCCs is limited, whereas three-factor PCCs are not approved for replacing the vitamin K-dependent clotting factors except for factor IX. Close collaboration between emergency department personnel and treating physicians, transfusion medicine, hematology, and neurology and/or neurosurgery services, as well as pharmacy, is of supreme importance to achieve timely normalization of the INR and to control bleeding.

References

1. van Asch C J, Luitse M J, Rinkel G J, *et al.* Incidence, case fatality, and functional outcome of intracerebral haemorrhage over time, according to age, sex, and ethnic origin: A systematic review and meta-analysis. *Lancet Neurology.* 2010; **9**:167–76.

2. Flaherty M L, Kissela B, Woo D, *et al.* The increasing incidence of anticoagulant-associated intracerebral hemorrhage. *Neurology.* 2007; **68**:116–21.

3. Huhtakangas J, Tetri S, Juvela S, *et al.* Effect of increased warfarin use on warfarin-related cerebral hemorrhage: A longitudinal population-based study. *Stroke.* 2011; 42:2431–5.

4. Hart R G, Boop B S, Anderson D C. Oral anticoagulants and intracranial hemorrhage. Facts and hypotheses. *Stroke.* 1995; **26**:1471–7.

5. Jeffree R L, Gordon D H, Sivasubramaniam R, Chapman A. Warfarin related intracranial haemorrhage: A case-controlled study of

6. Dequatre-Ponchelle N, Henon H, Pasquini M, *et al.* Vitamin K antagonists-associated cerebral hemorrhages: What are their characteristics? *Stroke.* 2013; **44**:350–5.

7. Keeling D, Baglin T, Tait C, *et al.* Guidelines on oral anticoagulation with warfarin – fourth edition. *British Journal of Haematology.* 2011; **154**:311–24.

8. Limdi N A, Veenstra D L. Warfarin pharmacogenetics. *Pharmacotherapy.* 2008; **28**:1084–97.

9. Watanabe M, Siddiqui F M, Qureshi A I. Incidence and management of ischemic stroke and intracerebral hemorrhage in patients on dabigatran etexilate treatment. *Neurocritical Care.* 2012; **16**:203–9.

10. Di Nisio M, Middeldorp S, Buller H R. Direct thrombin inhibitors. *New England Journal of Medicine.* 2005; **353**:1028–40.

11. van Ryn J, Stangier J, Haertter S, *et al.* Dabigatran etexilate – a novel, reversible, oral direct thrombin inhibitor: Interpretation of coagulation assays and reversal of anticoagulant activity. *Thrombosis and Haemostasis.* 2010; **103**:1116–27.

12. Yeh C H, Fredenburgh J C, Weitz J I. Oral direct factor Xa inhibitors. *Circulation Research.* 2012; **111**:1069–78.

13. Kamal A H, Tefferi A, Pruthi R K. How to interpret and pursue an abnormal prothrombin time, activated partial thromboplastin time, and bleeding time in adults. *Mayo Clinic Proceedings.* 2007; **82**:864–73.

14. Miyares M A, Davis K. Newer oral anticoagulants: A review of laboratory monitoring options and reversal agents in the hemorrhagic patient. *American Journal of Health-System Pharmacy.* 2012; **69**:1473–84.

15. Samama M M, Martinoli J L, LeFlem L, *et al.* Assessment of laboratory assays to measure rivaroxaban – an oral, direct factor Xa inhibitor. *Thrombosis and Haemostasis.* 2010; **103**:815–25.

16. Samama M M, Guinet C. Laboratory assessment of new anticoagulants. *Clinical Chemistry and Laboratory Medicine.* 2011; **49**:761–72.

17. Stangier J, Rathgen K, Stahle H, Gansser D, Roth W. The pharmacokinetics, pharmacodynamics and tolerability of dabigatran etexilate, a new oral direct thrombin inhibitor, in healthy male subjects. *British Journal of Clinical Pharmacology.* 2007; **64**:292–303.

18. Lippi G, Favaloro E J. Activated partial thromboplastin time: New tricks for an old dogma. *Seminars in Thrombosis and Hemostasis.* 2008; **34**:604–11.

19. Wong P C, Crain E J, Xin B, *et al.* Apixaban, an oral, direct and highly selective factor Xa inhibitor: In vitro,

antithrombotic and antihemostatic studies. *Journal of Thrombosis and Haemostasis*. 2008; **6**:820–9.

20. Bara L, Mardiguian J, Samama M. In vitro effect on Heptest of low molecular weight heparin fractions and preparations with various anti-IIa and anti-Xa activities. *Thrombosis Research*. 1990; **57**:585–92.

21. Harder S, Parisius J, Picard-Willems B. Monitoring direct FXa-inhibitors and fondaparinux by prothrombinase-induced clotting time (PiCT): Relation to FXa-activity and influence of assay modifications. *Thrombosis Research*. 2008; **123**:396–403.

22. Qureshi A I, Tuhrim S, Broderick J P, *et al.* Spontaneous intracerebral hemorrhage. *New England Journal of Medicine*. 2001; **344**:1450–60.

23. Goldstein J N, Gilson A J. Critical care management of acute intracerebral hemorrhage. *Current Treatment Options in Neurology*. 2011; **13**:204–16.

24. Masotti L, Di Napoli M, Godoy D A, *et al.* The practical management of intracerebral hemorrhage associated with oral anticoagulant therapy. *International Journal of Stroke*. 2011; **6**:228–40.

25. Qureshi A I. Intracerebral hemorrhage specific intensity of care quality metrics. *Neurocritical Care*. 2011; **14**:291–317.

26. Goodnough L T, Shander A. How I treat warfarin-associated coagulopathy in patients with intracerebral hemorrhage. *Blood*. 2011; **117**:6091–9.

27. Riegert-Johnson D L, Volcheck G W. The incidence of anaphylaxis following intravenous phytonadione (vitamin K1): A 5-year retrospective review. *Annals of Allergy, Asthma & Immunology*. 2002; **89**:400–6.

28. Aguilar M I, Hart R G, Kase C S, *et al.* Treatment of warfarin-associated intracerebral hemorrhage: Literature review and expert opinion. *Mayo Clinic Proceedings*. 2007; **82**:82–92.

29. Benjamin R J, McLaughlin L S. Plasma components: Properties, differences, and uses. *Transfusion*. 2012; **52**(Suppl 1):9S-19S.

30. Goldstein J N, Thomas S H, Frontiero V, *et al.* Timing of fresh frozen plasma administration and rapid correction of coagulopathy in warfarin-related intracerebral hemorrhage. *Stroke*. 2006; **37**:151–5.

31. Goodnough L T. A reappraisal of plasma, prothrombin complex concentrates, and recombinant factor VIIa in patient blood management. *Critical Care Clinics*. 2012; **28**:413–26.

32. Silliman C C, McLaughlin N J. Transfusion-related acute lung injury. *Blood Reviews*. 2006; **20**:139–59.

33. Pandey S, Vyas G N. Adverse effects of plasma transfusion. *Transfusion*. 2012; **52**(Suppl 1):65S-79S.

34. Fredriksson K, Norrving B, Stromblad L G. Emergency reversal of anticoagulation after intracerebral hemorrhage. *Stroke*. 1992; **23**:972–7.

35. Huttner H B, Schellinger P D, Hartmann M, *et al.* Hematoma growth and outcome in treated neurocritical care patients with intracerebral hemorrhage related to oral anticoagulant therapy: Comparison of acute treatment strategies using vitamin K, fresh frozen plasma, and prothrombin complex concentrates. *Stroke*. 2006; **37**:1465–70.

36. Switzer J A, Rocker J, Mohorn P, *et al.* Clinical experience with three-factor prothrombin complex concentrate to reverse warfarin anticoagulation in intracranial hemorrhage. *Stroke*. 2012; **43**:2500–2.

37. Wiedermann C J, Stockner I. Warfarin-induced bleeding complications: clinical presentation and therapeutic options. *Thrombosis Research*. 2008; **122**(Suppl 2):S13–18.

38. Dager W E, King J H, Regalia R C, *et al.* Reversal of elevated international normalized ratios and bleeding with low-dose recombinant activated factor VII in patients receiving warfarin. *Pharmacotherapy*. 2006; **26**:1091–8.

39. Mayer S A, Brun N C, Begtrup K, *et al.* Recombinant activated factor VII for acute intracerebral hemorrhage. *New England Journal of Medicine*. 2005; **352**:777–85.

40. Mayer S A, Brun N C, Begtrup K, *et al.* Efficacy and safety of recombinant activated factor VII for acute intracerebral hemorrhage. *New England Journal of Medicine*. 2008; **358**:2127–37.

41. Narayan R K, Maas A I, Marshall L F, *et al.* Recombinant factor VIIa in traumatic intracerebral hemorrhage: Results of a dose-escalation clinical trial. *Neurosurgery*. 2008; **62**:776–86.

42. Yuan Z H, Jiang J K, Huang W D, *et al.* A meta-analysis of the efficacy and safety of recombinant activated factor VII for patients with acute intracerebral hemorrhage without hemophilia. *Journal of Clinical Neuroscience*. 2010; **17**:685–93.

43. Morgenstern L B, Hemphill J C, 3rd, Anderson C, *et al.* Guidelines for the management of spontaneous intracerebral hemorrhage: A guideline for healthcare professionals from the American Heart Association/ American Stroke Association. *Stroke*. 2010; **41**:2108–29.

44. Pernod G, Godier A, Gozalo C, *et al.* French National Authority for H. French clinical practice guidelines on the management of patients on vitamin K antagonists in at-risk situations (overdose, risk of bleeding, and active bleeding). *Thrombosis Research*. 2010; **126**:e167–74.

45. Shander A G L, Ratko T, *et al.* Consensus recommendations for the off-label use of recombinant human factor VIIa (novoseven) therapy. *Pharmacol Ther*. 2005; 644.

46. Vincent J L, Rossaint R, Riou B, *et al.* Recommendations on the use of recombinant activated factor VII as an

adjunctive treatment for massive bleeding: A European perspective. *Critical Care.* 2006; **10**:R120.

47. Rosovsky R P, Crowther M A. What is the evidence for the off-label use of recombinant factor VIIa (rFVIIa) in the acute reversal of warfarin? ASH evidence-based review 2008. *Hematology.* 2008;36–8.

48. Fernandes H M, Siddique S, Banister K, *et al.* Continuous monitoring of ICP and CPP following ICH and its relationship to clinical, radiological and surgical parameters. *Acta Neurochirurgica. Supplement.* 2000; **76**:463–6.

49. Brott T, Adams H P, Jr., Olinger C P, *et al.* Measurements of acute cerebral infarction: A clinical examination scale. *Stroke.* 1989; **20**:864–70.

50. Teasdale G, Jennett B. Assessment of coma and impaired consciousness. A practical scale. *Lancet.* 1974; **2**:81–4.

51. Diringer M N, Edwards D F. Admission to a neurologic/neurosurgical intensive care unit is associated with reduced mortality rate after intracerebral hemorrhage. *Critical Care Medicine.* 2001; **29**:635–40.

52. Flaherty M L, Tao H, Haverbusch M, *et al.* Warfarin use leads to larger intracerebral hematomas. *Neurology.* 2008; **71**:1084–9.

53. Steiner T, Rosand J, Diringer M. Intracerebral hemorrhage associated with oral anticoagulant therapy: Current practices and unresolved questions. *Stroke.* 2006; **37**:256–62.

54. Webb H D, Griffin C A. Cytogenetic study of acoustic neuroma. *Cancer Genetics and Cytogenetics.* 1991; **56**:83–4.

55. Schulman S. Clinical practice. Care of patients receiving long-term anticoagulant therapy. *New England Journal of Medicine.* 2003; **349**:675–83.

56. Qureshi A I, Majidi S, Chaudhry S A, Qureshi M H, Suri M F. Validation of intracerebral hemorrhage-specific intensity of care quality metrics. *Journal of Stroke and Cerebrovascular Diseases.* 2013; **22**:661–7.

57. Fernlof G, Sjostrom B M, Lindell K M, Wall U E. Management of major bleedings during anticoagulant treatment with the oral direct thrombin inhibitor ximelagatran or warfarin. *Blood coagulation & Fibrinolysis.* 2009; **20**:667–74.

58. Monroe D M, Hoffman M, Oliver J A, Roberts H R. Platelet activity of high-dose factor VIIa is independent of tissue factor. *British Journal of Haematology.* 1997; **99**:542–7.

59. Leissinger C A, Blatt P M, Hoots W K, Ewenstein B. Role of prothrombin complex concentrates in reversing warfarin anticoagulation: A review of the literature. *American Journal of Hematology.* 2008; **83**:137–43.

60. Stangier J, Rathgen K, Stahle H, Mazur D. Influence of renal impairment on the pharmacokinetics and pharmacodynamics of oral dabigatran etexilate: An open-label, parallel-group, single-centre study. *Clinical Pharmacokinetics.* 2010; **49**:259–68.

61. Crawley F, Bevan D, Wren D. Management of intracranial bleeding associated with anticoagulation: Balancing the risk of further bleeding against thromboembolism from prosthetic heart valves. *Journal of Neurology, Neurosurgery, and Psychiatry.* 2000; **69**:396–8.

62. Punthakee X, Doobay J, Anand S S. Oral-anticoagulant-related intracerebral hemorrhage. *Thrombosis Research.* 2002; **108**:31–6.

63. Phan T G, Koh M, Wijdicks E F. Safety of discontinuation of anticoagulation in patients with intracranial hemorrhage at high thromboembolic risk. *Archives of Neurology.* 2000; **57**:1710–13.

64. Wijdicks E F, Schievink W I, Brown R D, Mullany C J. The dilemma of discontinuation of anticoagulation therapy for patients with intracranial hemorrhage and mechanical heart valves. *Neurosurgery.* 1998; **42**:769–73.

65. Leker R R, Abramsky O. Early anticoagulation in patients with prosthetic heart valves and intracerebral hematoma. *Neurology.* 1998; **50**:1489–91.

66. Bertram M, Bonsanto M, Hacke W, Schwab S. Managing the therapeutic dilemma: Patients with spontaneous intracerebral hemorrhage and urgent need for anticoagulation. *Journal of Neurology.* 2000; **247**:209–14.

67. Butler A C, Tait R C. Restarting anticoagulation in prosthetic heart valve patients after intracranial haemorrhage: A 2-year follow-up. *British Journal of Haematology.* 1998; **103**:1064–6.

68. Kawamata T, Takeshita M, Kubo O, *et al.* Management of intracranial hemorrhage associated with anticoagulant therapy. *Surgical Neurology.* 1995; **44**:438–42.

69. Babikian V L, Kase C S, Pessin M S, Caplan L R, Gorelick P B. Resumption of anticoagulation after intracranial bleeding in patients with prosthetic heart valves. *Stroke.* 1988; **19**:407–8.

70. Gomez C R, Sandhu J, Mehta P. Resumption of anticoagulation during hypertensive cerebral hemorrhage with prosthetic heart valve. *Stroke.* 1988; **19**:407.

Index

Locators in *italic* refer to figures.
Locators in **bold** refer to tables.